Armageddon Medicine

How to Be Your Own Doctor in 2012 and Beyond

An Instruction Manual

Seldom does one read a book that is truly "definitive." But Dr. Cynthia Koelker has indeed written one. . . *Armageddon Medicine* will save countless lives in coming disasters, but only if its collected wisdom and knowledge are put into action.

James Wesley, Rawles
Editor, SurvivalBlog.com
August, 2011

Infection – the bane of mankind since the dawn of civilization. And when civilization comes to an end, that fact won't change. Unless you're prepared to treat pneumonia, sepsis, MRSA, *C. diff,* and a host of other infections on your own, what you don't know may kill you. In down-to-earth language, *Armageddon Medicine* tells you how to care for yourself and loved ones without a doctor, should society fall apart.

Stephen A. Farkas, MD, FACP
Associate Professor of Medicine
Northeast Ohio Medical University
October, 2011

Armageddon Medicine

How to Be Your Own Doctor in 2012 and Beyond

An Instruction Manual

Cynthia J. Koelker, MD

MD BOOKS USA

Published by
MD Books USA
213 Massillon Road
Akron, OH 44312

First MD Books USA printing, January, 2012
10 9 8 7 6 5 4 3 2 1

Library of Congress Cataloging-in-Publication Data in Progress

Koelker, Cynthia J.
Armageddon medicine: how to be your own doctor in 2012 and beyond, an instruction manual /
Cynthia J. Koelker.
p. cm.
Includes index
ISBN 978-0-9825081-2-1
1. Medicine, Popular. 2. Survival skills. 3. Survivalism. 4. Preparedness I. Title II. Title: Armageddon medicine: how to be your own doctor in 2012 and beyond, an instruction manual.

Printed in the United States of America

Publisher's Note

All product names, brand names, and services used in this book are trade names, trademarks, or registered trademarks. Neither the publisher nor the author is associated with any company or vendor of any pharmaceutical or nutraceutical product or medical device.

While the author and publisher have been conscientious in the preparation of this manual, it is not meant to offer professional medical advice. The use of this book does not establish a doctor-patient relationship with either the author or publisher. The reader must seek the services of a qualified professional for such advice. Neither the author nor publisher makes any warranty with respect to the completeness or accuracy of the contents of this manual. The publisher and author disclaim any and all responsibility for any liability, loss, or risk, personal or otherwise, which is incurred as a consequence of the use of this information.

At the time of publication the author and publisher have made every effort to provide accurate Internet addresses. However, neither the publisher nor the author assumes any responsibility for errors, or changes that occur after publication. The author and publisher have no control over and assume no responsibility for cited Web sites or their content.

Dedication

This book is dedicated to my children and grandchildren, with the hope that they never need to use it.

Acknowledgments

Though this manual has been a full year in the making, I could spend many more teaching readers of *Armageddon Medicine* how to care for themselves when there's no other choice. As always when I write, I thank my family for forbearance and encouragement, when the task seems to overshadow all else.

I am especially grateful to my longtime friend and colleague, Dr. Stephen Farkas, for lending his expertise to the portions of the manuscript relating to infectious disease. As a respected specialist in the field, Dr. Farkas has spent decades not only healing patients of every sort of infection, from TB to tetanus, but also teaching the next generation of physicians how to do the same. Thank you, Steve, for helping all of us.

It has been an honor to serve as Medical Editor for SurvivalBlog and to work with blog-editor Jim Rawles. Jim has done our country and the world-at-large a great service in bringing together a wealth of information relating to self-reliance and preparedness. I appreciate so much your willingness to contribute the Foreword for this work, Jim, and your encouragement in its creation.

Few authors are fortunate enough to have an agent who is also a friend. In seeking works that "advocate and elevate," Terrie Wolf and AKA Literary do the same for their clients. Thank you, Terrie and Neil, for all your help on this project.

I am also grateful to the readers and contributors to my own blog, ArmageddonMedicine.net. It has truly become a community of concerned individuals willing to share their knowledge and experience with others. The collective wisdom is truly amazing.

As I write this, I wonder about Armageddon. Will God permit such a disaster to occur in my lifetime or that of my children? I'm hoping not, yet often fear that the writing is on the wall. I thank Him for the prolonged prosperity he has lent our country and for the love He continues to shower upon us. I pray this volume offers hope and healing to many.

Table of Contents

Foreword

by James Wesley, Rawles

Editor, SurvivalBlog.com

Seldom does one read a book that is truly "definitive." But Dr. Cynthia Koelker has indeed written one, in *Armageddon Medicine*. Her book does an excellent job of detailing the key topics and skills that families need to master to be well-prepared for the medical aspects of disaster situations.

Life is full of imponderables, and recent events in the modern era have taught us that the future is truly unpredictable. The 9-11 terrorist attacks of 2001, Hurricane Katrina in 2005, and the earthquake, tsunami, and subsequent nuclear meltdowns in Japan in 2011 together introduced us to a cold, hard, new reality: we simply can no longer blithely expect tomorrow to be a repeat of today. Nor can we expect government agencies to be capable of providing for our needs in the event of disasters. Time and time again, governments have proven that they simply don't have the manpower, the transport, or the logistics to make that happen in a timely manner. In the next disaster it will be what I call YOYO time — which stands for "You're On Your Own." YOYO time may last for many months. Are you ready for it?

There are many looming threats to our health and safety, ranging from floods, fires, earthquakes, hurricanes and tornadoes, to pandemics and nuclear terrorism. The future is uncertain, and at times this realization can seem overwhelming. But with the grounding knowledge of human physiology, some training, and some fairly modest supplies, we can at least be prepared to guard our physical health, regardless of what the future brings. Cynthia Koelker brings this all together, in *Armageddon Medicine*.

In the chapters ahead, you will learn the essentials to keep you and your loved ones sane, healthy, and avoid having them "assume room temperature." Her chapters detail mental health, acute infections, skin conditions, pain management, acute injuries, health issues for women, nuclear warfare, bioterrorism, and much more.

Quite importantly, Dr. Koelker discusses some topics not found in mainstream texts. For example, she describes in detail how to obtain alternative antibiotics during situations where access to pharmacies is limited or non-existent. She also dares to walk the path that the AMA establishment fears to tread, in discussing herbal medicine and other natural remedies.

To supplement the main text of the book, Dr. Koelker includes three very valuable appendices. The first one outlines key resources both in print and on the Web that you should gather as reference material. The others include outstanding detailed lists of medical supplies that you should assemble for your family.

Don't just read this book and put it on the shelf. Consider it a challenge and a call to action. Start assembling your medical supplies *now*. Get enrolled in advanced first aid and CPR training immediately. Practice what you've learned, and keep learning. Be ready to adapt and overcome times of adversity.

You need this book. In fact you'll need *two* copies, so that you will have one available to lend to friends, relatives, co-workers, and fellow church congregants.

Armageddon Medicine will save countless lives in coming disasters, but only if its collected wisdom and knowledge is put into action. Don't dawdle and don't hesitate. **When the time to perform is at hand, the time to prepare has passed.**

James Wesley, Rawles

Editor, SurvivalBlog.com

August, 2011

Introduction

What if the unthinkable happens? World War III? Global economic collapse? Worldwide plague? An asteroid collision? Biblical Armageddon?

Assuming you're fortunate enough to live through the initial event, will you be able to care for yourself in an era of no doctors, no hospitals, no pharmacies? No doubt a smattering of physicians will survive, but where are they? Can the few remaining assume care for the devastated population?

2012. It's upon us. Is the threat real or imagined? What about our less-than-friendly nuclear neighbors? Or a pandemic eclipsing the *Andromeda Strain*? Or perhaps an economic meltdown extinguishing our currency as well as the national power grid?

I am not an alarmist. My lifetime has been one of unrivaled American prosperity. But I often wonder, how long can it last? In recent years I have come to doubt the continued stability of our nation, our society.

Although I don't claim to be an expert on end-of-world survival, I do possess decades of practical experience as a family physician. If such an unthinkable event occurs, how will people care for themselves? The young and healthy have little know-how when it comes to injuries, infections, childbirth, and nutrition. Millions of middle-aged souls suffer from diabetes, depression, heart disease, asthma, arthritis, back pain, and ulcers. What about the elderly with poor eyesight, poor digestion, poor mobility, and a poor prognosis? Who will care for them?

If the power grid is destroyed there will be no water, no food, no social services – at least not with the abundance and availability to which we're all accustomed. What will you do if you contract pneumonia? How long can your diabetic mother survive? Might your infant son die of scarlet fever?

These are just a few of the questions I've asked myself. Though the situation sounds grim, there is hope.

Although Rawles[1] and others have written excellent books regarding surviving the end of the world as we know it, the medical information contained therein is limited. If society is to continue, those who remain must know how to care for themselves. Today's common maladies will continue to plague mankind. No doubt new and unforeseen threats will emerge.

This book is written to aid the survivors – and those who hope to survive. How should you prepare if you have young children? What will you do if you're diabetic? Is there any hope for your parents with heart disease and arthritis?

You'll find chapters on preparedness, acute injuries, infections, women's health, chronic disease, mental illness, and nutrition. Checklists will help you know what to do before the big event and how to prepare for life afterward. Detailed instructions on common illnesses will tell you what a physician would do and how you can treat yourself effectively. Practical advice on managing chronic disease will assure those with serious problems of continued survival.

[1] *How to Survive the End of the World as We Know It: Tactics, Techniques, and Technologies for Uncertain Times*, James Wesley, Rawles

Even if nothing happens (and let's hope it doesn't), this manual is chockfull of practical advice for every patient. Catastrophe or not, the same principles apply. Either way, medical knowledge will remain a powerful tool in assuring your loved ones' survival.

Cynthia J. Koelker, MD

November 2011

Preface

The Four Phases of Medical Armageddon

Floundering, Fading, Forgotten, Future

Medical Armageddon: *the end of modern medicine as we know it.*

As terrible as recent disasters have been, they don't hold a candle to a true national or global catastrophe. Although 9/11 and hurricane Katrina were truly horrific, could America recover if the carnage were magnified ten-fold, a hundred-fold, a thousand-fold? True, fallen nations have been revived, but only with the aid of willing outsiders or long periods of convalescence. What if there's no one left to help?

The 2009 H1N1 influenza pandemic taught us how unprepared we are to prevent widespread affliction. Vaccine supplies were unavailable in many areas until *after* the flu had passed, leaving thousands dead in its wake. When the vaccine was finally shipped, many medical offices still received not a single dose, and endless lines at community centers dissuaded uncounted patients from being immunized at all.

Fortunately, H1N1 wasn't the killer flu it might have been. Consider these statistics: in 2009, approximately 57 million Americans contracted H1N1 influenza. Of these, about 11,690 died.[2] Compare this to 1918–1919 when 850,000 of 20 million infected patients met their death of influenza or pneumonia – 650,000 died in four months alone![3] Had this same flu epidemic hit America in 2009, over a million deaths might have occurred. One might suppose that the reason for fewer deaths was the miracle of modern medicine, but this is not the case. The 2009 H1N1 was simply not as lethal. Had it been a true "killer flu" in the same unimmunized population, deaths may have multiplied a thousand-fold, even with antiviral medication. And an epidemic can still happen. Authorities say we're overdue.

No matter what nationwide disaster someday hits America, the health care system *will* be overwhelmed. Perhaps we should hope for something as minor as a flu epidemic. Only a few per cent of the population would likely succumb, and life would eventually return to normal. A protracted power outage, or severe fuel shortage, or (heaven forbid) war on American soil would soon result in chaos. In a global Armageddon scenario, with two-thirds of the population annihilated, the health care system would **flounder**, perhaps never to return to its former state.

As communication, transportation, and production grind to a halt, hospitals would soon exhaust available supplies. Health care workers will need to safeguard their own families, leaving suffering patients to fend for themselves. Within days, or weeks, or months, medical scavenging and self-treatment may become the norm.

---

[2] Updated CDC Estimates of 2009 H1N1 Influenza Cases, Hospitalizations and Deaths in the United States, April 2009–April 2010, at www.cdc.gov/h1n1flu/estimates_2009_h1n1.htm

[3] The Pandemic of Influenza in 1918–1919, at www.history.navy.mil/library/online/influenza%20pan.htm

Yet the memory of modern medicine will not disappear overnight. Many Americans possesses a fair degree of sophisticated knowledge, enough to read a textbook and figure out how to help their loved ones. Diabetics realize they need insulin, and have been taught to check their blood sugar and how to inject themselves. Asthmatics understand that inhalers relieve their obstructed breathing. It's no secret that nitroglycerin and morphine help a heart attack. Who doesn't know that antibiotics are the treatment for pneumonia or a kidney infection? As long as supplies can be found, people can treat themselves for many conditions, perhaps for years to come. But as these supplies dwindle, if production, transportation, and communication are not revived, modern medicine will eventually **fade**.

As with ancient societies, ours, too, will someday pass away. CAT scanners will become relics of a **forgotten** past. Handy gadgets such as home blood glucose monitors will no longer function, as batteries die and testing strips disappear.

And then what?

If mankind continues to populate the planet, eventually technology will re-emerge, perhaps in new and exciting directions. The **future** may hold cures we've never imagined, answers for the aging, help for today's hopeless.

Though I cannot see this future, I fear the pathway spirals downward before it ascends to new heights. I trust some along the journey may find answers in this humble book. Today's medical care is marvelous, and I pray it never flounders. I wonder, though, what my great-great-grandchildren will think if, a hundred years hence, they come upon my writing.

I'm hoping they never need my advice.

SECTION ONE

The Basics

Chapter 1

Preparedness

What you can do now to help yourself then

Today . . . the sun is shining. The kids are in school, grocery stores are full to overflowing, the house is warm, and gasoline hasn't reached $5 a gallon. American Idol is in its eleventh season. All is well.

Tomorrow . . . who knows? Will it be $10-a-gallon gasoline? Food shortages? Unaffordable heating? Bioterrorism? Do you have what it takes to survive?

Human beings – what amazing creatures! – at least when we're not busy killing each other. We can learn, laugh, love, adapt, grow, and most importantly, plan. You, not the government, are your own most valuable resource. Although animals may have the instincts to store food, migrate to a warmer climate, and flee from danger, as a human being, *you* can do much more. You can plan ahead.

Much of our life *is* planned, but in a fairly haphazard way. We sometimes get immunizations (if we feel like it, or happen to be at the doctor's office). We buy enough groceries for a day or a week, whatever happens to be on sale, or is appealing for the moment. We pay our bills, mostly on time, and trust that our heat, water, and electricity will be there tomorrow. If we need more food, we can drive to the store and buy it.

And this works – at least for now. But *what if* you believed that three months hence, they'd all be gone? You'd start preparing, of course. And if, like Y2K, nothing happened, you'd be none the worse for your provisions.

In the realm of medicine, preparations fall into both general and specific categories. General recommendations apply to the population as a whole, whereas specific advice is dependent on age, state of health, location, mobility, and other factors.

If you have medical problems, no doubt you're quite worried. Diabetes, asthma, and heart disease won't disappear just because no doctor's around. If you're well, what about your loved ones? Can your parents, or grandparents, or children thrive without a physician's care?

Fortunately, there is much you can do. Reading this book – *and acting on it* – is a good place to start. A single volume cannot cover every aspect of medical care, but it can get you started in the direction of securing your own health and that of your family.

The first thing that comes to mind is **vaccine-preventable disease**. Americans think very little about this because we haven't seen diphtheria, or tetanus, or typhus first-hand, and scarcely believe these diseases kill people. But I remember having mourned babies who died of meningitis in the 1980s, before the HIB (*Haemophilus influenzae* B) vaccine, and doctors older than I can't forget the devastating effects of diphtheria and polio. Nowadays people worry about their babies developing autism or attention deficit disorder from vaccines (unfounded concerns from my point of view), rather than being grateful that their children haven't succumbed to terrifying childhood infections. For parents who have chosen not to immunize your children, please realize that the reason your children haven't been exposed to one of these deadly diseases is because the other children *have* been immunized. When this "herd immunity" becomes diluted through lack of universal vaccination, your children *will* be susceptible as these infections re-emerge in the population.

Vaccine-preventable disease is a concern that will only escalate in the future, if and when vaccines become unavailable. And does this next thought worry you? Most American doctors have never even seen a case of diphtheria, or tetanus, or rabies. Younger physicians have never treated measles, mumps, rubella, polio, pertussis, or *Haemophilus influenzae* meningitis. Do you want your child to be their first case? The generation of health care workers (as well as grandmothers) familiar with many of these diseases is dying off, and all that remains is book knowledge.

Hepatitis (A and B), chicken pox, shingles, and meningococcal meningitis still occur sporadically in the American population, despite vaccine availability, and influenza and pneumonia remain quite common. Some overseas travelers may have received vaccines to diseases not currently seen in the U.S., such as yellow fever, cholera, or typhus. Could these diseases reach American shores? Infectious disease has not been conquered, merely held at bay for the time being.

If national supply chains are disrupted, within mere weeks immunizations to common diseases will become unavailable. With a major catastrophe, it would take years to decades to re-establish the production of safe and effective vaccines.

Therefore, it is vitally important not only to receive currently available vaccines *now*, but also to learn something about each illness. Though you will be prepared and (hopefully) immunized, others may not be. If you encounter an ill person, how will you determine what infection they have and whether you're protected against a contagious disease they may harbor?

Which diseases may re-emerge? These are primarily those to which infants and children are routinely immunized. In the United States, this includes hepatitis A and B, rotavirus, diphtheria, tetanus, pertussis (whooping cough), *Haemophilus influenzae* B, pneumococcal pneumonia, polio, influenza, measles, mumps, rubella, and varicella (chicken pox).

Why are immunizations so important? Largely because no medication works. The majority of these illnesses are caused by viruses. Antibiotics do not kill viruses. The few antiviral drugs we have are generally ineffective against these microbes. Although antibiotics are often effective against bacteria which cause pneumonia, meningitis, or pertussis, without additional supportive care (such as I.V. fluids, oxygen, tube-feeding, or breathing treatments) antibiotics alone may not resolve life-threatening infections, and babies with insufficiently developed immune systems are susceptible to overwhelming infection.

Older children may also be immunized against meningococcal meningitis and human papilloma virus (venereal warts and cervical cancer). Older adults add varicella zoster (shingles) to this list. (Many older adults have not been vaccinated against certain childhood diseases, but catch-up doses are not generally advocated.)

Childhood vaccines are quite expensive, running into hundreds of dollars.[4] Fortunately, most are covered by insurance plans. For those without insurance, check with your local health department or hospital clinic, where prices may be considerably less than at a private office.

---

[4] CDC Vaccine Price List, updated May, 2011 at http://www.cdc.gov/vaccines/programs/vfc/cdc-vac-price-list.htm

Americans who travel overseas are currently encouraged to receive various other vaccines, depending on destination. These may include cholera, Japanese encephalitis, rabies, tick-borne encephalitis, tuberculosis, typhoid fever, and yellow fever. Depending on your personal situation, you, too, may want to consider these vaccinations. Your family physician will not have any of these available, so you should consult with your local or state health department or travel clinic.

At a bare minimum, all adults should update their tetanus shot, which now includes a booster for diphtheria and pertussis (Tdap) for everyone through age 64 (Td alone for older adults).

Next, what is the depth of your medical knowledge? Is someone in your family a doctor, nurse, physician's assistant, or midwife? If so, perhaps you can rely on them, but educating yourself may become a matter of life or death.

Before people survived long enough to die of heart attacks and cancer, they died prematurely of injuries, infection, dehydration, and malnutrition. These are the primary focus of this book. Many injuries are preventable, as will be stressed in a later chapter. Major injuries (gunshot wounds, head injuries, cervical spine fractures) may well be fatal without intensive (and likely unavailable) medical intervention. Less severe injuries should be treatable and survivable (as long as infection is avoided), though the outcome may be less than ideal compared to current standards. A broken hip can heal without pinning, though chronic pain and permanent disability may result.

Depending on your own health and that of your family, you may want to arm yourself with specific disease-oriented knowledge. Or, if you're expecting a child, you will want to learn all you can about labor, delivery, and newborn care. If your mother is diabetic, you may want to educate yourself about injecting insulin. Can a needle be re-used? How should she treat her blood sugar if testing is unavailable? Many of these issues will be addressed in later chapters, but thinking about specific health problems now and projecting into the future will bring questions to light that should be discussed with your personal physician.

Appendix A lists helpful books and resources for medical care in situations where doctors and other health care resources are unavailable. Again, depending on your situation in life, you may want to invest in some or all of these.

Appendix B lists supplies and medications to consider for your medical kit, with recommendations for family, community, and professional care.

Appendix C offers a list of over-the-counter medications you may want to stockpile for use by your family or survival group. Later chapters cover questions about using expired medications, alternate therapies, and prescription drugs, with special attention to antibiotic use.

Lastly, what is your level of fitness? Can you walk a mile carrying two gallons of water? When transportation and supplies are not readily available, people will no longer exercise because they should, but because they must. Perhaps planting and caring for your own garden would be a good place to start developing stronger muscles. You'll want to be at your best in case you must rely on your body as much as your mind. Are you overweight? Approaching your ideal weight is a good idea, though a few extra pounds may see you through lean times.

Identifying health concerns and goals is a first step toward preparing for the worst. But before moving on to specific medical concerns, we'll address items even more vital to life itself: water, food, and shelter.

Food for Thought

If I had lived a hundred years ago I'd be dead already.

That is to say, the average lifespan has increased 30 years over the past century.

Why is this? According to the CDC, 25 of the 30 added years were due to public health measures, not fancy medical interventions. Most of these are within your control.

Here is the CDC's list of

America's Ten Great Public Health Achievements, 1900–1999:

- Vaccination
- Motor-vehicle safety
- Safer workplaces
- Control of infectious diseases
- Decline in deaths from coronary heart disease and stroke
- Safer and healthier foods
- Healthier mothers and babies
- Family planning
- Fluoridation of drinking water
- Recognition of tobacco use as a health hazard

See: http://www.cdc.gov/mmwr/preview/mmwrhtml/00056796.htm

Chapter 1 – Checklist

- ☐ All adults, update your tetanus shot by receiving a Tdap booster (or Td, for those older than 64 years.)

- ☐ All children, update all vaccines according to age.

  All vaccine recommendation schedules are available at: http://www.cdc.gov/vaccines/recs/schedules/default.htm

- ☐ Consider special vaccines for travelers and special situations.

- ☐ Educate yourself about once common childhood illnesses. The *Diseases and Conditions* link at the Mayo Clinic Web site is a good place to start.

  http://www.mayoclinic.com/health/DiseasesIndex/DiseasesIndex

- ☐ Obtain both a new and 40-year-old version of *Baby and Child Care* by Dr. Benjamin Spock.

- ☐ Identify disease-specific questions and needs for the future.

- ☐ Maximize your own health and fitness: exercise, lose weight, stop smoking, and avoid excess alcohol intake.

Chapter 2

The Essentials: Water, Food, Clothing, Shelter

Water, Electrolytes, Calories, Protein, Vitamins, Minerals, Clothing, and Shelter

The Garden of Eden – I picture it like Hawaii, but without the rain. Abundant food, ripe for the picking. No mosquitoes nor malaria. No scavenging wolves or stinging insects. No rusty nails to pierce your foot. Plenty of sun, but plenty of shade. Will you be in the Garden of Eden or more likely Detroit when the crisis hits? If you're lucky enough to have a productive garden, will you reap the rewards? Will packs of dogs threaten your children? Do you have enough shoes to last the rest of your life? Or enough water to last even a week?

A diabetic will die quicker without water than without insulin. Hypothermia is more rapidly fatal than pneumonia. Starvation will kill you faster than cancer.

Water

What good is all the medication in the world without clean drinking water? Can your body fight infection if your immune system is weak from malnutrition? Assuring a dependable supply of potable water is THE single most important thing you can do to safeguard your health. Don't count on the government doing this for you. If the public water supply runs dry (which will happen if the grid goes down and pumps are offline), it'll be up to you to solve your own dilemma. Other sources (see **Appendix A**) describe how to procure safe drinking water in adverse conditions. I'm only reiterating that as far as your health goes, you must think of water first.

The body is about 60% water by weight, but where is all this water? Not in the blood stream. Only about 1/12 of your total body water is coursing through your veins. Most of the water, about two thirds, resides inside the cells of your body, the so-called intracellular fluid. When a person becomes dehydrated, they not only lose water from their bloodstream, but from the inside of the cells. This is the difference between a grape and raisin. You don't want to become a human raisin.

So how much water does a person require? Is it really true that you need eight 8-ounce glasses of water a day? And what does that even mean, that a person *needs* so much water? What actually happens when the body is deprived of water?

Generally speaking, human beings and other adult animals maintain a fairly stable body weight. Since most of the body consists of water, this implies the amount of water in your body should remain fairly constant. No doubt you realize that you lose water whenever you urinate, or sweat, or spit, or bleed, or have diarrhea, or even a menstrual period. You're probably unaware of the amount of water lost just by breathing, or by evaporation from your skin (aside from sweating). These are called insensible fluid losses.

Emergency Disinfection of Drinking Water

1. Allow murky water to settle and then siphon off clearer water toward the top. Filter settled water through a clean cloth, coffee filter, or water filter.

2. **Boiling** water is the best method of disinfection, and will kill microorganisms such as *Giardia lamblia* and *Cryptosporidium*, which are often found in lakes or rivers.

   Allow water to come to a rolling boil, then boil vigorously for 1 minute at sea level (or 3 minutes at altitudes above 1 mile).

   Let cool; avoid pouring into contaminated containers. Improve taste by adding a pinch of salt to each quart (or liter).

3. If boiling is impractical, the second best choice is **chemical disinfection** with chlorine (preferable) or iodine (good).

   Chlorine: use *unscented, unthickened* household bleach with 4–6% available chlorine. Add 2 drops per quart or liter (8 drops/gallon) and allow water to sit for 30 minutes before drinking.

   (If water is cloudy or very cold, double the amount of chlorine.)

   Iodine: add 5 drops of 2% household iodine per quart or liter. Allow water to sit 30 minutes before drinking.

   (For cloudy water, use 10 drops of iodine per quart or liter.)

To stay the same weight, the amount of water lost daily must be replaced by an equal volume. One simple way to determine the amount required is to weigh yourself daily on an accurate scale and simply drink enough water (or other non-diuretic fluids) to maintain the same body weight. If you happen to drink more water than you need, your body will simply flush it out in the form of urine. Doctors frequently weigh patients who are taking diuretics (water pills) or receiving I.V. fluids (or both) in order to determine their water balance.

Unfortunately, things are not always this simple. If you are able to stay at home where your handy (non-electronic) scale is readily available, weighing yourself daily is a great way to determine proper fluid replacement. But in an Armageddon scenario, this may well be unrealistic.

So back to the question, how much water do you really need? The short and simple answer for the impatient reader is, ideally, 2 to 3 liters (or quarts) of fluids a day. If there is no cause to suspect greater water loss than usual, even one quart a day may suffice. This gets to the heart of the matter, the real reasons for urination. Obviously, the first reason is to rid your body of excessive water. But the second is equally important, that is, to cleanse your body of toxic waste. If your kidneys do not cleanse your blood of urea and other waste products, they will build up and eventually kill you. Your own body will become a toxic waste dump.

Although 1 quart of water a day may suffice under conditions of minimal loss, a multitude of situations accelerate fluid depletion, and therefore increase the need for additional water intake. Conditions that are will increase a person's need for water include:

- fever
- hyperventilation (from work, illness, or fever)
- high ambient temperature
- low humidity
- sweating (from work, illness, or environment)
- diarrhea (especially secretory diarrhea)
- certain medications (most notably diuretics, including caffeine)
- excessive urinary loss (from medication or illness)
- bleeding (internal, menstrual, or other)
- nursing an infant
- internal fluid sequestration due to injury or illness
- injury or illness that increases the amount of waste produced

Under any of these conditions it becomes extremely difficult to measure the amount of water a person requires. Does a fever double insensible fluid losses? Can intractable diarrhea triple the amount of water needed? The answer to both is yes.

Under stressful circumstances healthy kidneys will do their best to compensate for fluid loss by concentrating the urine as much as possible. The least amount of urine necessary to rid the body of its daily waste production is about half a liter, or 2 cups of water. Obviously, you cannot urinate solid waste, and the colon can only eliminate unabsorbed food, not waste products of cellular metabolism that enter the bloodstream.

The best way to assess the proper amount of fluid intake is to weigh sick patients daily. Even with no caloric intake, few patients lose as much as a pound a day of their own fat or muscle tissue (though we may wish we could).

Anything beyond a weight loss of several ounces is actually fluid loss, which must be replaced.

What if the patient's weight increases? It is nearly impossible for a person with functioning kidneys and a good heart to get too much water by oral intake alone. However, it is very easy to administer too much fluid intravenously, especially in a sick or elderly patient. I've seen patients gain ten pounds overnight when excess fluids are administered in hopes of stabilizing blood pressure. This often throws the patient into congestive heart failure, and sometimes cause the legs to balloon out to the extent the skin begins weeping. Patients like this are very difficult to handle: the fluids are keeping them alive yet killing them at the same time.

When a patient cannot be weighed, the next best thing is to measure their daily urine output. Hospitalized patients with any sort of fluid balance concern (fever, diarrhea, vomiting, inability to eat, heart failure, kidney disease, swelling, or diuretic use) should have both done, that is, be both weighed and have their urine output monitored. Urine output below 30 cc per hour indicates an acute need for additional fluids.

In children the water requirement is proportionately much larger. The calculations for fluid replacement become more complex. It is safe to assume that even an infant will need as much water as an adult. If you have young children, purchase an appropriately-sized balance scale or spring scale (electronic scales should be avoided due to the need for batteries or electricity). Whereas it may be difficult to weigh a bedbound adult, it's a simple matter to place a small child on a scale. As a parent you should monitor a sick child's fluid intake closely and increase it accordingly if necessary to maintain a stable weight. A child who has lost 5% of his or her body weight and cannot drink enough to make up the difference is in danger of serious dehydration. Without I.V. fluids, such dehydration may prove fatal. Although in a catastrophic scenario professional medical care may be difficult to come by, this information will at least alert you as to when to attempt to seek it.

Another population at increased risk is the elderly. The thirst mechanism is much less reliable in individuals in their 70s and beyond. Complicating this are both medical problems and their treatments. Diuretics place a person at significant risk for dehydration, especially when accompanied by loss of appetite, fever, confusion, or even swelling. The older generation is at additional risk because they often do not understand their multiple health problems thoroughly or simply forget what the doctor has told them. Conversely, some are so concerned about following doctor's orders that they continue their medication even when they should not. Taking a water pill when you are dehydrated is as dangerous as injecting insulin when you cannot eat.

If you are concerned about losing your parents or grandparents in the face of a crisis, now is the time to educate yourself about their medical conditions. As a physician I always appreciate it when a child or grandchild accompanies their elderly relative to the doctor. Two heads are better than one, and a younger person may have less trouble remembering, or may bring additional issues to light, or pose additional questions relevant to their relative's condition or environment.

One final note: it seems unlikely that anyone would consider concocting their own intravenous fluids, but just in case, a word of warning: DO NOT use plain water. It can cause serious electrolyte imbalance and even death. Doctors always use solutions containing either dextrose (usually 5%) and/or saline.

Electrolytes

With the advent of Gatorade everyone's heard of electrolytes. But what are they? What do they actually do?

Electrolytes are basically salts dissolved in water, most importantly sodium, chloride, and potassium. They are involved in metabolic processes as diverse as regulation of heart rate, kidney function, cognition, and the circulation. The flow of water to and from cells is dependent on the concentration of electrolytes both inside and outside cells.

Plain drinking water does not contain electrolytes, but this is not a problem in a person who is eating. Food contains electrolytes in liquid or crystallized form. As water and food mix together in the stomach and intestines, the fluids and electrolytes are absorbed in proper concentrations to maintain a healthy body . . . unless something goes wrong.

In a healthy person on a normal diet, it is unusual to see an electrolyte imbalance. However, in a dehydrated person, or one with vomiting or diarrhea, or someone on multiple medications, electrolyte disturbances are common.

Serum potassium levels may drop with diarrhea or vomiting, or secondary to certain diuretics. Low potassium levels may cause weakness, impaired thinking, heart rhythm problems, or even paralysis. A patient's potassium level may rise when the kidneys are not functioning adequately, or secondary to ACE inhibitors or potassium-sparing diuretics, or due to tissue breakdown. High potassium levels may also cause weakness, paralysis, and cardiac arrhythmias. High sodium levels are often a marker for dehydration, although dehydration with low sodium levels is common among patients taking diuretics. Clearly the situation can be confusing, even for doctors, especially without access to blood testing.

The take-home lesson here is that if a person is not able to eat regular food, electrolytes must be added to oral or I.V. fluids, in amounts similar to those normally found in the blood stream. This way, if electrolyte levels are low, they'll be replenished; if too high, they'll be diluted.

One of the most significant lessons of the 20th century is that fluids are absorbed more efficiently in the presence of sugar and electrolytes. Grandma had it right when she said a little chicken soup and ginger ale would be good for you. Sports drinks such as Gatorade include the proper amount of salts and sugar for optimal absorption. You can make your own oral rehydration fluid by adding a little table salt and sugar (or fruit juice) to water.

To make your own oral rehydration fluid, combine:

- 1 liter (about 5 cups) clean drinking water
- 6 teaspoons sugar
- ½ teaspoon salt
- ½ cup orange juice (optional, adds potassium)

One of the most important supplies to stockpile is iodized table salt. The body needs about 1 teaspoon of sodium chloride (table salt) daily to replace that which is lost in sweat and feces. Eating today's American diet it is difficult to become sodium depleted (unless you're taking a diuretic). However, if all your food must be grown, the diet may become deficient in sodium. Certainly your food will taste better if you have a little salt to add. A teaspoon may sound like a lot, but a single bowl of canned soup often contains this amount. Our table salt is iodized to prevent goiter and thyroid dysfunction. Unless you live near a steady supply of seafood (the best natural source of iodine) make sure it is the iodized salt that you purchase.

Potassium is found in plants, and therefore is not crucial to stockpile separately. High potassium foods include citrus fruits, tomatoes, bananas, melons, prunes, raisins, beans, spinach, squash, beets, carrots, potatoes, milk, molasses, nuts, seeds, and to a lesser degree, most fruits, vegetables, and legumes.

Calories

Beyond water, beyond electrolytes, the next most basic need is calories. Many patients can go months without their thyroid medication or diabetic pills. Few asthmatics will suffocate over the next season without access to their inhalers. But nearly everyone will die in a month or two without food. Calories provide the energy our bodies require to stay warm, to think, to breathe, and to move.

Gone are the days when we'll worry about too many calories. In times of scarcity, too few calories will be our major concern.

In a crisis situation your caloric requirement is likely to increase as you are forced to walk more. Under current conditions a sedentary adult can maintain his or her body weight on about 1800 to 2400 kcal per day. (Note: "kilocalories," or kcal, is actually the correct term, but this is abbreviated to "calories" for popular use.) This amount may double when physical activity increases dramatically.

When stockpiling food for a crisis situation, calorie-dense foods become critical. Although fruits and vegetables provide needed vitamins and minerals (see below), they are generally low in calories. Carbohydrates and proteins have about equal calories based on dry weight, with fats being the ultimate energy-dense form of nutrition.

Aim for at least 2,000 cal per day of stockpiled food per individual. One 8-ounce jar of peanut butter contains about 2,800 calories. If you ate only that you'd need a good 200 jars per person to sustain you through a single year. Of course, a well-balanced diet is preferable to peanut butter alone, but starvation is directly related to inadequate caloric intake. Vitamin deficiency diseases will take months to years to develop, whereas a child can starve to death in a matter of weeks.

It also makes little sense to stockpile food your family won't eat. My kids would have to be truly starving before they'd willingly choke down tofu. Peanut butter is a great option not only because it is nutrient-dense, but because most everyone likes it, even young children. It is also easy to store and quite inexpensive. After the 2010 Haiti earthquake, peanut butter was one of the prime foods distributed among disaster survivors. Due to dental concerns among the indigent, the smooth variety was preferred over chunky. Chocolate hazelnut cream (such as Nutella) makes a tasty alternative.

I am not advocating peanut butter as the sole source of nutrition, but rather stress it for its ease. Dried fruits, canned beans, energy bars, tuna canned in oil, beef jerky, nuts, shelled sunflower seeds, fruit canned in heavy syrup, condensed milk, and dry cereal are all calorie-dense alternatives that require no preparation and have a long shelf life. Remember that food needing preparation may also require a source of heat and/or water.

The Church of Jesus Christ of Latter-day Saints encourages their members to have sufficient food and supplies on hand to be self-sufficient for three months to a year. The Web site About.com features a calculator based on their recommendations to help you estimate amounts needed per year according to family size.[5]

Food for a year, per LDS recommendations.		
	Over age 7 years	**Child 0–6 years**
Grains (wheat, flour, corn meal, oats, rice, pasta)	**300 lb.**	**148 lb.**
Fats and Oils (shortening, cooking oil, salad dressing, mayonnaise, peanut butter)	**13 lb.**	**7 lb.**
Legumes (dried peas, beans, lentils)	**60 lb.**	**24 lb.**
Sugars (honey, sugar, brown sugar, syrup, jams, etc.)	**60 lb.**	**29 lb.**
Milk (dry and evaporated, cheese, other)	**75 lb.**	**37 lb.**
Don't forget baking soda, baking powder, vinegar, yeast, salt, and seasonings.		

[5] Food Storage Calculator at: http://lds.about.com/library/bl/faq/blcalculator.htm

Carbohydrates

Carb-conscious Americans seek to limit their intake of bread, potatoes, pasta, rice, cereal, flour, and sugar. While this may slim the waistline, the message gets lost that some carbohydrate is necessary for proper metabolism and to prevent ketosis. About 100–150 grams per day (400–600 kcal) are needed to prevent cannibalizing your own muscles. When times are lean, you'll be happy to snarf down a baked potato or a bowl of pasta (not that you aren't now).

Dried carbs are easy to stockpile in the form of enriched rice, dehydrated potatoes, egg-free noodles, dried or canned pasta, fortified cereals, sugar, and flour. Although the whole-grain forms are preferable with their higher vitamin, mineral, and fiber content, they may not remain fresh as long as the refined products, and may cost a little more. A diet high in vitamin- and mineral-containing plant foods would be ideal, but fortified cereals (think Total) may bridge the gap until you can plant, gather, or harvest your own.

Meal worms or their eggs are sometimes found in corn meal and other grains, so it may be prudent to package grain products in smaller lots so your entire store does not become infested.

Protein

Have you ever gone a year without a steak dinner? Better get used to the idea.

Our bodies are made of meat, which will be self-cannibalized for calories if our diets are deficient in energy-yielding foods. Unless you want to catabolize your own muscles, you will need sufficient calories to maintain your lean body weight. Calories in the form of carbohydrates are generally easier to acquire, store, and afford than protein calories (see above). Although meat and cheese are the traditional sources of protein in our culture, eggs, beans, nuts, and legumes are additional options. Storing canned products (tuna or salmon in oil, canned chicken, stew, bacon, beef chunks or ravioli) is safer than frozen products unless you have a reliable source of refrigeration.

The most important reason to include protein in your diet is because the body cannot manufacture 8 of the 22 amino acids necessary for protein synthesis. Muscle is the largest reservoir of protein in the body, but proteins also circulate in the blood and are essential for metabolic function. A minimum of 0.8 gm/kg body weight is required daily (about 50 grams, or two ounces) for the average man. This really isn't that much – about as much meat as in a small McDonald's hamburger. A double Whopper is overkill.

Animal proteins are considered complete proteins, containing all the necessary amino acids. Plant foods are relatively lacking in certain amino acids, however including a variety of both grains *and* legumes in your diet (not necessarily at the same meal) will supply sufficient essential amino acids. Notice that the LDS chart above does not include animal protein beyond milk. Meat-lovers will want to include canned meats in their stores.

Remember those pictures of starving children with hugely swollen bellies? **Kwashiorkor** is a special type of childhood starvation, rare in the U.S., but common in developing countries. Previously thought to be due to calorie and protein starvation alone, it is now understood to involve additional factors (such as the ingestion of moldy food). Other signs of kwashiorkor include loss of teeth, irritability, loss of appetite, enlarged liver, and thinning hair. Though such children are protein-malnourished, they can die of liver failure if given too much protein too quickly. Fortunately, your child will not develop kwashiorkor unless first deprived of sufficient calories and protein.

Vitamins and minerals

Would you recognize scurvy if you saw it? Would your doctor? How about pellagra or rickets? Are vomiting and difficulty walking obvious signs of beriberi?

Vitamin-crazed Americans have never seen true vitamin-deficiency diseases. We know vitamins are good for us, and figure that more must be better. Most people don't understand that vitamins were discovered by analyzing serious illness. Consumers believe vitamin C will ward off a cold, and thus consume quantities unheard of in prior generations. But vitamins and minerals are trace nutrients, needed in very small amounts. If we all ate enough fresh fruits and vegetables, vitamin deficiencies would be quite rare. In one sense we might be healthier in a future where we are forced to grow our own food. But few Americans are farmers possessing the knowledge and ability to grow sufficient food to live on.

Therefore, it would be wise to stockpile inexpensive multivitamins to supplement your diet, especially for the children within your group. Look for something that supplies 100% of both water-soluble (B_1 (thiamine), B_6 (pyridoxine), B_{12}, C, niacin, riboflavin, folic acid) and fat-soluble vitamins (A, D, E, K), as well as zinc, copper, cobalt, iodine, manganese, iron, and chromium, and possibly nickel, molybdenum, silicon, selenium, and fluorine.

Essential fat

You may believe you need to eat no fat at all, but this is untrue. Linoleic acid and arachidonic acid are essential nutrients. Linoleic acid must be supplied in the diet, or signs of essential fatty acid (EFA) deficiency may develop, including hair loss, growth retardation, dermatitis, and low platelets.

Common sources for linoleic acid include nuts, eggs, cereals, cashews, and most cooking oils (corn, safflower, sunflower, vegetable). Only a small amount is needed daily, on the order of a few nuts, or one egg.

Vitamin Deficiency Diseases at a Glance

Lack of . . .	Leads to . . .	Symptoms . . .
Folate	Megaloblastic anemia Neural tube defects	Fatigue Birth defects (when mothers deficient)
Niacin	Pellagra	The 3 D's: diarrhea, dermatitis, dementia
Riboflavin	Riboflavin deficiency Anemia	Sore throat, lips, mouth, or tongue Seborrheic dermatitis Fatigue
Thiamin	Beriberi	Polyneuropathy, high-output heart failure, Wernicke-Korsakoff syndrome
Vitamin A	Vitamin A deficiency	Night blindness, poor immunity, rashes
Vitamin B6	Pellagra-like illness	Dermatitis, depression, confusion, seizures
Vitamin B12	Megaloblastic anemia White matter lesions	Fatigue Dementia, numbness of hands or feet
Vitamin C	Scurvy	Fatigue, depression, rash, petechiae, internal bleeding, impaired healing
Vitamin D	Rickets in children Osteoporosis in adults	Weak or curved bones, compression fractures, muscle weakness, bone pain
Vitamin E	Anemia Neurologic deficits	Fatigue Various brain and nerve problems
Vitamin K	Bleeding disorders	Easy bleeding, bruising, hemorrhagic disease of the newborn

Dietary fiber

Did you ever experience the pleasure of being manually disimpacted? Having hard, stale poop dug out of your rectum is no barrel of laughs. Likewise, serious constipation can hurt every bit as bad as labor pains or kidney stones, and unless you've experienced a blockade of rock-like feces, you may not appreciate the value of dietary fiber.

A diet limited to protein, simple carbohydrates, and fats *will* cause constipation even in the best of us. Count on it. If you don't plan for enough fiber, better lay in a supply of medical gloves for future disimpaction.

Americans already eat only about half the 25 gm of fiber recommended daily. As you plan your food stores, make sure to include more high fiber foods than you are currently including in your diet.

Soluble fiber (the type that draws moisture into our bowel movements and keeps them the proper consistency) is found primarily in plant sources. If you'll be growing your own produce, include broccoli, carrots, root tubers, root vegetables, onions, grapes, apples, and plums. For stockpiling, include oats, rye, barley, prunes, raisins, other dried or canned fruit, beans, peas, and peanuts. As a general rule, anything that comes from a plant will be higher in fiber than an animal product.

If none of your favorites are here, check out www.metamucil.com which features lists of foods and their associated fiber content. And if you just can't stand the thought of any of these, purchase a powdered supplement such as Metamucil or Citrucel, which may be mixed with fluids or sprinkled on your food for additional fiber. If you do use these supplements, you *must* also ingest sufficient fluid for the powder to absorb (otherwise: sawdust in, rocks out). Dried fruits, vegetables, beans, or any other dried food must absorb water as well to help keep the stools soft. Fresh fruits and vegetables already possess sufficiently high water content without adding extra.

Clothing

Blisters, bug bites, burns, bleeding. These are just a few of the problems you'll avoid by having proper clothing for a disaster-related scenario.

In northern climes, winter promises frostbite and hypothermia for those unprepared. Children and the elderly are especially susceptible to the effects of cold. If the streets aren't plowed, how will you get around? Do you and your family have well-fitting boots, coats, hats, and gloves to gather enough firewood when it's 20 below zero, or enough warm clothes to sleep and live in sub-freezing temperatures? Medical preparedness is irrelevant if you freeze to death.

In southern climates excess heat may lead to sunburn, dehydration, and heatstroke. Light-weight, light-color, body-covering clothing is essential to preventing many heat-related illnesses. Electric air-conditioning will be for the privileged few. Shade and evaporative cooling may be insufficient to allow adequate regulation of body temperature, especially for those who cannot supply and fulfill their own hydration needs, particularly the young and the old.

Foot injury leads to amputation in diabetics. Walking a mile in poorly-fitting shoes may lead to blisters that never heal. Proper, protective shoes are as important as insulin in a medical Armageddon and should be considered a vital part of everyone's preparations.

Mosquitoes may increase exponentially when chemical spraying ceases. Long sleeves and long pants help prevent the bite of mosquitoes, ticks, and other critters that may spread malaria, West Nile virus, encephalitis, Lyme disease, Rocky Mountain spotted fever, and other viral infections.

Shelter

Lastly, shelter is as vital as food, often more so, depending on the weather. The best protective clothing cannot withstand a hurricane, tornado, blizzard, flood, sandstorm, or lightning strike. A roof over your head trumps antibiotics when it comes to winter pneumonia.

And don't forget a warm spot for Lassie and Mr. Ed.

Chapter 2 – Checklist

- ☐ Obtain a good spring or balance scale (without batteries or electricity)
- ☐ Begin a medical chart for each member of your family or group, including their height and weight as a baseline
- ☐ Educate yourself about your loved ones' illnesses, risks, medications, and alternative treatments
- ☐ Assure an adequate and renewable supply of potable water (minimum 2 liters of water per person day); also household bleach and iodine for water disinfection
- ☐ Stock iodized salt and food sources of potassium
- ☐ Stock sufficient food to provide 1800–2400 calories per person per day
- ☐ Stock sufficient protein-rich foods to provide 50 grams per person per day
- ☐ Stock multi-vitamins with minerals for every family member
- ☐ Stock calcium supplements for women (and maybe everyone)
- ☐ Stock sources of essential oils and soluble fiber
- ☐ Procure appropriate clothing for expected (and unexpected) environments
- ☐ Assure adequate shelter, with appropriate heating and cooling (and the same for your pets)

SECTION TWO

Mental Illness

Chapter 3

Reacting to Stress and Devastation

Separating the normal from the abnormal

Your job is no more. You're in danger of losing your home. Your parents have lost their pension and moved in with you. You cringe at the thought of watching your children go hungry. Can you defend your family against marauders? Things look hopeless as society crashes around you. What will happen if you can't provide for your loved ones? Can you endure the stress? Should you fear a mental breakdown?

Stress – probably the number one complaint family doctors encounter, even in good times – life stress, not colds, not diabetes, not hypertension. People can tolerate pain or ignore a terrible rash. But stress makes a person feel they've lost control – often because they indeed have. Wounds that damage the inner person cause psychic pain, and often require psychic (emotional or spiritual), not medical, answers.

For the purpose of this chapter stress reactions will be addressed separately from other mental illness. True mental illness is a deviation from the norm, a problem that causes a disturbance of thinking or emotion serious enough to interfere with everyday function, judgment, or relationships, sometimes resulting in self-destructive behavior. Stress reactions may fulfill this definition, except perhaps for being a deviation from the norm in times of overwhelming disaster. Of course, in modern American society, all sorts of problems have been labeled mental illness that may well be variants of normal. Is Internet addiction a true mental illness? What about attention-deficit disorder? The same behavior that is now condemned in U.S. culture may be met with approval at other times or in other places.

The point is not to debate the definition of mental illness, but to say that stress reactions can and do occur in everyday people. Severe stress reactions can afflict anyone – including “normal” people caught up in abnormal situations. You (or I) may be one of them. How will we react? Will we succumb?

If we cannot control our surroundings, do we at least have a choice whether or not we cross the invisible line separating us from mental illness? I contend that we do.

Devastating life stress will be the norm for survivors of Armageddon. The abnormal will become the normal. Though I hope to never confront the traumatic death of a loved one, I am doing what I can to prepare.

And what is that?

As a physician I learned long ago that I’m not in control. Sure, I have some input into the outcome of certain life and death situations. But I cannot save everyone – that’s a given in this imperfect world. Doctors cannot function if we are crippled by every failure. Although accepting guilt or responsibility is a sign of mature adulthood, feeling guilty is deadening. It sucks the life right out of a person.

Guilt – the slayer of happiness, hope, and health – and often the reason a severe stress reaction devolves into true mental illness. However, there is a huge difference between acknowledging guilt and feeling guilty. That difference lies in the art of self-forgiveness.

Have you ever said, "I could never forgive myself if . . ." or "Life wouldn't be worth living if . . ." or "I'd kill myself if . . .?" Thinking this way is setting yourself up for a downward spiral, possibly into mental illness. These potential "unforgiveable" tragedies must be considered before they occur, and thought through to a positive solution. You *can* forgive yourself and life *is* worth living regardless of circumstances.

An interesting thing about guilt is the question of to whom one feels accountable. Is it the government? Your family? Your inner spirit? God? If society collapses, no one will be chasing you down to pay a speeding ticket or collect child support. As for moral responsibility, if you cannot prevent your own children's death, consider: will others forgive you, perhaps other hurting parents shouldering the same burden? Surely if you (and God) can forgive another's shortcomings, you can forgive your own.

The best way to become stronger at forgiving yourself is to practice it now. Most of us have some fault we wish were otherwise, or a past action that torments our spirits. If God can forgive you (and He can), it is only right that you forgive yourself. Perhaps you need to ask forgiveness of another, but whether or not that is granted, you are permitted to forgive yourself. Then after forgiving yourself, appreciate what you do have and move on. You are not responsible for that which you cannot control.

A second trait that paralyzes people in times of trouble is **worry**. Often I have patients who say that they're just worriers, as if they have no control over the trait. But people do have the option of worrying or not. As Mark Twain put it, "I have known a great many troubles, but most of them never happened."

Or, as Wallace D. Wattles advised, "You can never become a great man or woman until you have overcome anxiety, worry, and fear. It is impossible for an anxious person, a worried one, or a fearful one to perceive truth; all things are distorted and thrown out of their proper relations by such mental states, and those who are in them cannot read the thoughts of God."

> Or, as Jesus put it, "*Do not worry about your life, what you will eat or drink; or about your body, what you will wear. Is not life more than food, and the body more than clothes? Look at the birds of the air; they do not sow or reap or store away in barns, and yet your heavenly Father feeds them. Are you not much more valuable than they? Can any one of you by worrying add a single hour to your life? . . . So do not worry, saying, 'What shall we eat?' or 'What shall we drink?' or 'What shall we wear?' For the pagans run after all these things, and your heavenly Father knows that you need them. But seek first his kingdom and his righteousness, and all these things will be given to you as well. Therefore do not worry about tomorrow, for tomorrow will worry about itself. Each day has enough trouble of its own.*"
>
> (Excerpted from Matthew 6, New International Version, © 2011)

Apparently worry is a choice, and a harmful one at that. Perhaps we should aim to be like Esther of Old Testament renown, who, in doing good in a potentially dangerous situation said, "and if I perish, I perish."

The audio teaching entitled "Christian First-Aid Kit" from Andrew Wommack Ministries (www.awmi.net) offers a whole series of free downloads relating to "let not your heart be troubled" in times of crisis, or how to control your emotions when your first instinct is despair.

Lastly, what about **grieving**? Isn't this a normal reaction? Yes, it is, and grief must be worked through or it begins to stifle the spontaneity and joy that characterize a healthy life. But even when we grieve, we have a choice as to when. Sometimes a crisis necessitates that grieving be postponed until a danger has passed. When the adrenaline has worn off, the work of grieving can occur.

Grief is not only a response to personal loss, but a reaction to all that's wrong with the world (and there's plenty of material there). The wish for peace and happiness is a universal one, and the lack of it disturbs our innermost being. But opposing grief stands hope for a better tomorrow and a new existence where goodness reigns. Holding on to this hope is essential for maintaining mental health when everything around you appears hopeless.

I begin with stress because this is the one health problem that will affect all survivors of an Armageddon event. Optimizing your reaction begins with preparation – emotional, spiritual, and physical. If you are able to function and carry on despite how you feel, I would classify your reaction as normal in terms of mental health. If your functioning becomes a liability to your family or your survival group, I would classify this as a mental illness, possibly requiring medical treatment (per the next chapter). When making plans to survive a national or global disaster, don't neglect preparing your spirit for the extreme challenges ahead.

Dealing with loss – the stages of grief

(adapted from Elisabeth Kubler-Ross)

1. **Shock** – initially after a loss, a person experiences a feeling of disbelief, numbness, or paralysis. This is similar to extreme physical trauma, where the patient may initially perceive no pain from a broken bone or amputated body part. This stage generally passes in hours to days.
2. **Denial** – when a loss is too painful to absorb, the mind often chooses to deny the event happened, especially when a person feels at fault, such as in a divorce or the death of a child. This stage is also usually short-lived.
3. **Anger** – once the loss is perceived, emotions come into play, particularly anger. *This is the first danger point.* Crying, screaming, or lashing out against others is common and usually normal. However, when people get stuck here, unresolved grief may lead to unhealthy bitterness, hostility, or aggression, tainting one's life long-term.
4. **Depression** – *this is where many of my patients experience difficulty.* It is normal to feel sad or unhappy for weeks or months, depending on the degree of loss. This stage may also be accompanied by excess guilt, physical symptoms, panic, or anxiety. Perhaps it is true that your life never will be the same. However, it is not normal or healthy to remain sad or depressed for months on end without improvement. Unhappiness can lead to changes in brain chemistry, sometimes requiring medication.
5. **Acceptance** – this is a gradual process, often beginning before the actual loss, as in the case of a chronically ill parent. Interest in normal activities revives as hope is renewed and the loss is accepted as part of life.

Chapter 3 – Checklist

- ☐ Learn the difference between acknowledging guilt and feeling guilty, and the consequences of each.
- ☐ Analyze in what way self-forgiveness needs to play a role in your preparedness training for unforeseen events.
- ☐ Analyze your tendency toward worry, fear, and hopelessness, and how you have reacted to stressful situations in the past, and how you might react in the future.
- ☐ Thoughtfully consider alternative action plans to replace unproductive patterns of reaction.
- ☐ Make spiritual and emotional vigor as high a priority as physical health.
- ☐ Download the "Christian First-Aid Kit" from Andrew Wommack Ministries at www.awmi.net.

Chapter 4

Mental Illness

Universal impact, individual preparedness

Universal Impact

How dare I proclaim that the problem of mental illness will impact everyone at TEOTWAWKI? Because it does so already.

Depression, anxiety, alcoholism, drug abuse, psychosis, bipolar disorder, Alzheimer's disease – is there a single reader unacquainted with the destructive forces of these diseases? And that's only to name a few. What about phobias, obsessive-compulsive disorder, eating disorders, anger disorders, autism, personality disorders, and attention deficit disorders? Will any of these improve if society collapses?

Every family doctor sees patients suffering from one or more of these problems on a daily basis. Perhaps you might argue that not all are diseases, but will the tendency toward alcoholism or uncontrolled anger improve when stress is multiplied a hundred-fold?

The National Institute of Mental Illness offers the following disturbing statistics:

- In any given year, about 1 in 4 adults suffers from a diagnosable mental disorder
- About 1 in 17 Americans suffers from a serious mental illness.
- Mental disorders are the leading cause of disability in the U.S. and Canada.

One could assume that these statistics won't improve at the end of the world as we know it. Of course, many of the elderly will not survive without on-going care, and so the prevalence of Alzheimer's and other dementias may decrease as the elderly population dies off. Attention deficit disorder may no longer be a problem when surviving children are not required to sit at a desk all day, and compulsive eating may be cured when there's no food available.

But, overall, in times of stress, people decompensate. Anxious people grow panicky, depressed patients become suicidal, psychotics hallucinate a different reality, alcoholics drink themselves into oblivion, Alzheimer's patients wander off, and anorexics starve themselves.

Death, divorce, disaster, disease – these are among the common triggers for acute mental illness, as well as exacerbations of chronic conditions. Any actual, perceived, or feared loss can knock a stable person out of equilibrium, or send a borderline patient into a tailspin.

Even if your family is prepared, of course others won't be. And people who believe they are prepared to face any contingency may find themselves horrified and debilitated by the suffering around them. Though your doctor may no longer be available to diagnose post-traumatic stress disorder, you or someone you know will suffer from it nevertheless.

So what's a person to do? Although this book cannot tackle the entire field of post-Armageddon psychiatry, here are some building blocks for your mental health arsenal.

For patients and loved ones who are medication-dependent, start stockpiling now. Ask your doctor under what circumstances he or she would consider dispensing a long-term supply. Building a trusting relationship is essential. If your doctor thinks you will not return for follow-up if you have a year's supply of medicine, convince him otherwise by your actions. (Note: controlled drugs cannot be dispensed in amounts greater than a six-month supply, and you will have to prove yourself very trustworthy to convince your doctor to write even that much.) Insurance will not pay for advance prescriptions beyond the coming one to three month period, so you will likely have to pay on your own, which may be a problem for the more expensive medications. If this is the case, ask your physician whether there might be an older (hence cheaper) drug that may work as well, or nearly so. For patients using as-needed medications, refill your prescriptions regularly, even if you have not used them up. Alternative treatments for common mental illnesses will be reviewed at the end of this chapter.

Medication is not now nor will it ever be the answer for all mental problems. Modern medicine does not have any therapy to improve brain function in people of diminished mental capacity, including those with Alzheimer's disease, but there are ways to help such a person function in daily life. If you have a parent with dementia, a sibling with Down syndrome, or a special needs child, the time is now to make plans for when community resources are unavailable. Also, along with diminished mental capacity often comes diminished physical capacity. Will your granny be able to make it to the bathroom at night? Does she need a hospital bed or bedside commode? Will accommodations be needed to assure safety?

Any person living in a nursing home, assisted living, or similar facility will face dire risk in the event of a global or national disaster. Paid caregivers may well abandon their position in favor of safeguarding their own families. If you can't care for your institutionalized loved ones now, how will you do so when the situation becomes critical? This is not to say you cannot do so. I have seen many families provide care superior to that of professionals. The American lifestyle is one of the primary reasons so many elderly and disabled are in extended care facilities, all the better not to interfere with our busy American lives. Investigate now what it will take to care for those who may have no choice but depend on you for survival.

Continuing in the vein of non-pharmaceutical aids, seven come to mind that I have seen work as well as any medicine:

- **love** (sense of community, companionship, essential for women)
- sense of **purpose** or usefulness (essential for men)
- taking time to **play** (good for all, essential for children)
- abundant physical **exercise**
- adequate **rest**
- abiding **faith**
- renewed **hope**

It is more blessed to give than to receive. – Jesus

The purpose of human life is to serve, and to show compassion and the will to help others.
– Albert Schweitzer

A merry heart doeth good like medicine. – King Solomon

And who doesn't feel better after a good night's sleep? – Doc Cindy

More important than being loved is having someone (or something) to love. As a mother, I get more out of loving my children (and messy goldendoodles) than I receive in return. Remember "Wilson" in *Castaway*?

Although the above may sound trite, it is true nevertheless – and also backed by science. We could discuss how sleep resets brain wave cycles, or how physical exercise stimulates the production of mood-stabilizing serotonin and norepinephrine, but mere common sense affirms that healthy living is more likely to produce a healthy mind than unhealthy living would. Over and over I've seen people make themselves sick by working too much, sleeping too little, spending too much time alone, and perceiving no purpose in life.

If life doesn't make sense to you now, will it suddenly seem purposeful when the population is decimated? Maybe you'll find faith and hope when nothing else is left to you, but would it not be better to ground yourself now in the God of the universe? Einstein said, "I do not believe that civilization will be wiped out in a war fought with the atomic bomb. Perhaps two-thirds of the people of the earth will be killed." How would you respond to such a disastrous scenario? If you survive, will the aftermath leave you dysfunctional or able to continue on with a positive attitude?

Depression and **anxiety** are the two most common forms of mental illness doctors encounter. Either may be pathological (chemical) or stress-induced. People responding to difficult life challenges do have a choice in the extent of their own response. Many a patient has said to me, "You know I'm just a worrier," but that implies, at least to some extent, that they have chosen this reaction, or that it is a conditioned response. Though making mental changes may seem more difficult than making physical changes, it is possible. For readers with a Judeo-Christian background, consider that the opposite of fear is not courage, but rather faith.

In the event of widespread catastrophe, fear and grief will be among the immediate problems (see **Chapter 3**). Some people will experience anger as well, and may risk growing violent. Consider the following thought experiment to help plan for the future: what do you fear the most? The loss of your children? Debilitating physical illness? Supporting yourself? Being alone? Whatever it is, face it now in your mind, and work through how you could cope with the situation. Would it kill you? Or only be difficult? Could you find a way to go on? Then after facing the feared consequences of a theoretical problem, analyze how you could make your current position more secure against future threats. Perhaps you need to learn a new skill, or acquire more friends, or assure a way of communicating with distant loved ones.

Both fear and grief may lead to acute anxiety and/or depression. However, in the acute situation, antidepressant medications are generally not helpful. Anti-anxiety medications (such as Ativan, Xanax, Klonopin, or Valium) do work quickly to settle a person's nerves. However, these are all controlled drugs, and it will be difficult to procure a supply of them for a future, unknown crisis. In olden days, and even now, people comfort themselves with alcohol (which is actually a depressant in the long run). If you are a person who is not prone to addiction or alcoholism, a small amount of alcohol may be helpful in coping with tragedy. For the addiction-prone, it is best avoided.

A better alternative might be to request a short-term supply of a mild nerve medication from your doctor. Most doctors would be willing to prescribe Vistaril (hydroxyzine pamoate, a non-addicting anxiety medication, usually dosed at 25 to 50 mg up to four times daily) for any acute, anxiety-producing situation, including stage fright, a death in the family, family stress, or other common difficulty. Sleep is a natural cure for overcoming short-term stress-induced anxiety, and therefore sleep-inducing medication may be helpful, such as prescription Ambien (zolpidem). Over-the-counter sleep aids are also effective and contain a sedating antihistamine such as diphenhydramine or doxylamine succinate.

Non-habit-forming treatments for chronic anxiety include the SSRIs (discussed below, for depression), as well as buspirone (5–15 mg up to three times daily). Over-the-counter drugs that may help combat acute anxiety include meclizine, diphenhydramine, and possibly cetirizine.

One problem with acute grief is that it sometimes evolves into true depression. Though difficult to explain, prolonged unhappiness seems capable of altering the neurochemistry of the brain. Knowing this, you may be able to ward off true depression by purposefully pursuing happiness and enjoyable experiences, even if you can't believe this would possibly help. To some degree, happy thoughts can help normalize brain chemistry.

However, this is not always possible. If you (or a loved one) are suffering from chronic feelings of unhappiness, medical treatment should be considered. Be aware, though, that depression is not merely a feeling. The problem with true depression is actually poor functioning: inability to work, a change in sleep patterns (insomnia or excess sleep), decreased (or increased) food intake, irritability or anger, and self-isolation. Other physical symptoms may include headaches, tight muscles, stomachache, diarrhea or constipation, fatigue, or even chest pain. Women seem more attuned to these changes than men do, and are more likely to seek professional care.

Stockpiling inexpensive antidepressant medication for future potential use among your family or group members should be considered, though this may be difficult to achieve. (I, myself, would not be willing to dispense such medication unless I knew the patient very well.) For the layman, the simplest and safest antidepressants to use are Paxil, Prozac, and Celexa.[6] The standard dose for any of these is 20 mg a day. The dose may be cut in half for small or elderly people, or for those who experience annoying side-effects, or doubled for larger people, or if no improvement is noted within about a month. Each of these medications comes in generic form for about $4 for 30 pills. Unlike tricyclic antidepressant drugs, accidental or intentional overdose of these three is unlikely to cause a serious heart arrhythmia or death. This group of medicines (SSRIs, or selective serotonin reuptake inhibitors) is also useful for chronic anxiety, menopausal symptoms, severe PMS, obsessive-compulsive disorder, and sometimes chronic pain, including headaches, back pain, and nerve pain. Wellbutrin and Effexor are two other commonly employed anti-depressants, but even generic versions remain fairly expensive.

Antidepressant medications take 2–4 weeks to begin to have an effect, often with physical symptoms starting to remit before feelings of unhappiness improve. Outside observers (family, friends) may notice these changes before the patient himself. It generally requires 3–4 months to achieve complete remission of symptoms. If no apparent benefit is perceived by a month or two, a higher dose or a different medication should be considered (as should the diagnosis itself – physical problems such as hypothyroidism sometimes mimic depression). In general, the antidepressant should be taken for a minimum of six months, though a full year is usually advisable to prevent relapse, at least if the

---

[6] Lexapro may also be dosed at 20 mg daily, but is expensive and no generic is currently available. Zoloft is also effective, but the dosage is different and may require additional adjustment.

medication is readily available. (Additional options include lithium or combination drug therapy, but these are beyond the scope of this book.)

What about **psychosis**? Anyone suffering hallucinations, mania, or delusions is likely to worsen when their support system collapses. Who will insist these patients continue their medications? Who will help them distinguish between the real and the imagined? Psychiatrists and community service groups will not be readily available to cope with a crisis, and any remaining hospitals will be overrun with people suffering from trauma or infection.

First, if you have a loved one taking antipsychotic medication, talk to his or her doctor about both long-term and alternative management options. (Note – physicians may be unwilling to share this information due to the HIPPA laws unless the patient signs a release or is present during the discussion.) Are they willing to prescribe a sufficient supply in case of serious emergency? If so, can you afford the medication? Some of the newer meds run hundreds of dollars monthly (Abilify, Geodon, Risperdal, Zyprexa), and insurance will not pay more than three months ahead. If cost is a concern, ask about older (hence cheaper) alternatives (haloperidol or thioridazine). The primary concern with older antipsychotic drugs is side-effects, particularly movement disorders including irreversible tardive dyskinesia. However, this occurs primarily with prolonged administration of the drug. For an older patient, this may be less of a concern. (In fact, for all of us, this may be a lesser concern.)

If you end up with a minimal supply of essential medication, and can foresee that you'll run out, realize that tapering a drug is better than stopping it cold turkey. Cutting the dose of most antipsychotic medicines by half every week or two should minimize withdrawal or discontinuation symptoms. For example, if a full dose is 100 mg daily, decrease to 50 mg daily for 1–2 weeks, then 25 mg for 1–2 weeks, then 12.5 for 1–2 weeks, then 12.5 every other day for a week, then stop altogether. Also, half the current dose may be better than none at all. Some patients cope just fine while still experiencing mild hallucinations or delusions. Rationing the medication may help a borderline person function in society for a longer period of time.

When medications run low, bizarre behavior may occur. Patients may wander off, or become "stuck" in certain behaviors, or lose interest in eating, or occasionally become violent. Physical restraints may become necessary, though in certain cases this only makes the problem worse. As with infants, restrain these patients as little as possible, but sufficient to avoid their hurting themselves or others. Encourage them, love them, feed them, care for them. But do not allow them to become dangerous if at all possible. Also, do not leave their care to one person alone, as this often becomes too great a burden. Don't assume that a nurse in your midst wants to spend all her time supervising a "crazy" patient – she not only does not, but cannot.

And what if you are unable to control the situation? What if your loved one simply cannot be managed, or what if a stranger – acting strangely – wanders into your group?

The answer must be to do only as much as you are able with limited resources. No one can handle every problem. You may be forced to decide if it's better to restrain a person physically (or chemically) or to send them from the group. This will not be an easy decision. However, the demands of a truly psychotic, strong and angry young man may threaten the survival of your entire group. A non-violent individual may be allowed to wander around acting peculiar, as long as he or she is not a threat. Please realize that the bizarre behavior is a response to what the person believes to be true, and so in a sense *is* rational. If *you* truly believed you were surrounded by hungry demons, would it not be reasonable to shriek and seek escape?

Finally, is there a role for herbal therapy? One good review article, entitled *Complementary Medicine for Psychiatric Disorders in Children and Adolescents* may be found online at: http://www.medscape.com/viewarticle/575412. The following is a summary of their findings:

1. Omega-3 Fatty Acids are possibly effective for adult and pediatric patients suffering from schizophrenia, mania, or depression. Side-effects of Omega-3s include stomach upset, headache, decreased appetite, sleep disturbance, and fishy breath.
2. St. John's wort has often been used to treat depression, and is probably effective in adults for mild to moderate symptoms of acute (short-term) depression. One study in adults showed that 900–1800 mg/day worked as well as 20–40 mg of paroxetine (generic Paxil) over the course of 6 weeks, and helped prevent relapse over the next 4 months. Few studies have been done in children, and overdose may cause seizures.
3. Gingko biloba has been shown to improve the thinking process slightly in older adults with Alzheimer's disease and other dementias, but did not improve the patient's mood otherwise. One concern about using ginkgo in older adults is that of drug interactions, particularly those on blood thinners and risperidone. This may be less of a concern after an Armageddon event when such medicines become unavailable.
4. Kava has shown a small positive effect in treating anxiety, but liver damage is a concern. Likewise, lemon balm and valerian may be helpful alone or in combination. However, the effect may be dose-

dependent, with a low dose lowering anxiety somewhat, but a higher dose worsening the condition. As with many medications, herbs known to benefit certain people sometimes have the opposite effect on others, just as alcohol is energizing to some, but sleep-inducing to many.

For patients with true schizophrenia, does the future appear grim without medication? In looking for an alternative, keep in mind that it is *much* easier to find a substance that worsens brain function than one that improves it. The National Center for Complementary and Alternative Medicine lists no other herbal product (besides Omega-3 fatty acids) as potentially beneficial for schizophrenia. Some have questioned whether cannabis (marijuana) use improves specific cognitive functions in a subset of schizophrenic patients, but until this is better understood, cannabis is best avoided, since it is also known to trigger the condition.

The prognosis for schizophrenics in developing countries might surprise you. According to a 1983 article in the journal *Psychiatry*,[7] the billions of dollars spent annually on the treatment of schizophrenia have not yielded better rates of recovery than in Third World countries. In fact, evidence supports a better outcome for schizophrenia in these less affluent societies, at least partly due to easier re-integration of the recovering patient into a community less driven by technology. A simpler life at a slower pace may allow many patients to function adequately without medication.

[7] Recovery from schizophrenia in the Third World, *Psychiatry*. 1983 Aug;46(3):197–212.

Chapter 4 – Checklist

- ☐ Analyze and prepare for the mental health needs of each potential member of your group, including medications, restraints, housing, special accommodations, and supervision.

- ☐ Develop a trusting relationship with your primary physician and discuss the possibility of obtaining medication for potential future use.

- ☐ Assess your own mental health and take steps to overcome current addictions or unhealthy behaviors using non-pharmacologic means.

- ☐ In your preparations, don't forget to include activities you find enjoyable. Include (non-electronic) games and hobby supplies in your stockpiles. A deck of cards, a chessboard, or book of parlor games may do more for your future mental health than medication.

- ☐ Make sure you have comfortable, warm sleeping quarters available. Nothing brings on fear, anxiety, worry, fatigue, and depression as quickly as inadequate rest and sleep deprivation.

- ☐ Stockpile the medications and herbal products mentioned above for potential future use.

- ☐ Download *Complementary Medicine for Psychiatric Disorders in Children and Adolescents* at: http://www.medscape.com/viewarticle/575412.

SECTION THREE

Acute Infection and Symptoms

Chapter 5

Introduction to Acute Infection

Understanding, prevention, and rational treatment

Understanding infection

Infections in human beings are caused by a frightening array of microorganisms. Bacteria, viruses, fungi, yeast, worms, amoeba, parasites, and prions invade the human body, spreading fear and misery throughout the world.

In a very real sense, every infection is caused by an interaction with our environment. You've all seen the "bubble boy" who cannot leave his plastic shell without fear of death. Interacting with the normal human environment would be fatal due to his inadequate immune system. Fortunately, most of us have excellent immune systems, but a good immune system is not the only barrier to infection.

To understand human infection you must understand the human environment, both external and internal. The world is a germy place, and it's amazing we're all as healthy as we are. The food we eat, the water we drink, the air we breathe, and everything we touch are all potential sources of infection. Even our own bodies may betray us. Our skin is a playground for mites and bacteria. Our mouths and intestines are a nursery for a whole civilization of microorganisms.

All infections result from tiny organisms penetrating barriers designed to protect us. They may enter our body through any opening: eyes, ears, nose, mouth, urethra, rectum, vagina – occasionally even our belly buttons. A tiny crack in the skin, a bug bite, or irritated hair follicle is all that's needed to afford a portal for entry. Once these unwelcome visitors get a foot in the door *(literally!)*, they may take over without our knowledge or permission.

Humans and animals share multiple barriers to infection. Skin, hair, fur, scales, hooves, and feathers all help keep microorganisms from invading. The naked ape adds shoes and clothing to this armamentarium, as well as bathing and other sanitary practices. Additionally, the germs that thrive on healthy individuals, our "normal human flora," protect their own territory from nasty invaders. Having good intestinal germs helps limit the harmful ones. The mucus that coats our airways and intestines helps trap undesirable microorganisms, and the action of cilia (tiny hairs) helps carry them away. Stomach acid tolls a death knell to most bacteria. Skin oil helps keep our protective dermis supple and healthy. Tears wash dust and germs from our eyes. Earwax not only helps keep the bugs out, but helps prevent infection. Our bodies are wonderfully designed to repair themselves and to prevent outside invasion.

Preventing infection

Obviously, prevention is the name of the game. Just as automobiles perform best with clean oil, proper tire pressure, and adequate gasoline, the human body performs best when well cared for. Prevention encompasses far more than avoiding sick people and rabid dogs.

The primary goal is to keep germs from invading the body by maintaining intact natural barriers. Preventing infection via a well-functioning immune system is actually a secondary goal, and does not activate until a microorganism has penetrated a first-line physical or chemical defense system.

The largest and most obvious barrier to infection is the skin. Hair and nails may be considered extensions of the skin. Healthy skin requires a healthy diet with sufficient calories, protein, essential fats, vitamins, minerals, and other nutrients, as discussed in **Chapter 2**. Unless you have a skin disease, adequate nutrition, gentle cleansing, and adequate lubrication are the keys to maintaining intact skin.

What is appropriate cleaning? In America, we bathe too much. Many problems are caused by the chemicals we use to clean, deodorize, perfume, shave, exfoliate, tan, bleach, and otherwise camouflage our skin. Just leave it alone! Bathing with clean water and *perhaps* a gentle soap is all you need, focusing on areas prone to natural accumulations of bacteria: armpits, groin, hands, and feet. Doing more dries the skin, allowing cracks to form and bacteria, fungi, and viruses to invade. We need skin oil to keep our leathery layer elastic and intact. Although using moisturizing cream certainly does help, it's not the same as allowing your self-made lubricant and sealer to do the job it was designed to do. Anyone with a history of cellulitis who is prone to dry skin *should* use a moisturizer twice daily in winter, and once daily otherwise.

Proper drying of the skin is also essential. Maceration (skin deterioration and rawness) occurs when skin folds remain moist for prolonged periods. Yeast and bacteria thrive in warm, wet areas, irritating the skin especially where it rubs together, which sometimes allows the microbes to invade deeper tissues. The skin may become red, raw, itchy, and oozing, leading to a cycle of more of the same. This problem is more common in overweight individuals, especially diabetics. Prevent intertrigo by allowing skin folds to air dry, or blot them gently. Rubbing irritated areas will only make the problem worse.

How NOT to Clean Your Hands

Do not try this at home.

Try cleaning your hands with carburetor cleaner. *(No, don't!)*

One day my hands were covered with a spray adhesive that ordinary cleansers wouldn't budge. Becoming desperate, I stupidly doused them with carburetor cleaner, which assuredly did remove the gummy goo. Not only that, it took *all* the natural oils from my skin, leaving them dry as parchment for a month. No amount of hand cream restored them until my skin was able to manufacture sufficient natural oil and the damaged epidermis was replaced with fresh skin cells.

Also, wearing appropriate clothing may lessen the need for frequent bathing, and serves as additional protection. Wear socks and good-fitting shoes, long pants, long sleeves, and head-covering whenever there is threat of contamination or physical harm. Injury to the skin and subsequent infection also occur from shaving, plucking, trimming, and cutting. In a post-apocalyptic world, who cares if you have hairy legs or armpits, or a clean-shaven face? Don't trim your nails too short, consider not shaving, don't pull a hang-nail, and don't pop a zit.

Even small injuries can lead to major infections. I've seen people require hospitalization when a sunburn or bug bite, a blister or simply dry skin became infected. Watch out for scratches, frostbite, lacerations, abrasions, chemical burns, friction, poison ivy, and insect stings. Any time the skin is damaged, the likelihood of infection skyrockets.

Hand sanitizer may be somewhat effective at preventing the spread of cold and flu viruses, but with its high alcohol content, it also results in drying of the skin or cracks, which may become portals of entry for infection.

Starting at the head and working down, here are several other ways to prevent infection:

1. **Don't use Q-tips.** Many patients suffer ear infections after removing the protective coating of earwax, or from scraping their ear canals in the process. Additionally, Q-tips often pack the wax in deeper, sometimes requiring professional removal. As with the skin, just leave your ears alone. The natural design of the ear allows gradual movement of earwax from the inner canal to the outer ear. Earwax also keeps the bugs out – reason enough to leave it alone.
2. **Don't rub or touch your eyes.** Bacteria and virus particles are often transmitted to the eyes via the hands, causing conjunctivitis (pink eye) and respiratory infections. (The eyes are connected to the nose via the tear drainage ducts.) As with the ears, leave your eyes alone. Rubbing the eyes may cause tiny abrasions, allowing infection to invade. If you must rinse your eye, use clean, warm water, or stand in a shower if available. This often helps to relieve itchy eyes as well.

3. **Don't pop your pimples.** It didn't help the last time and it won't help this time. Surely you know it only makes things worse. Although acne bacteria cause inflammation (not true infection), breaching the skin may allow staph and strep germs to invade, causing a true infection.
4. **Don't touch your mouth or nose.** Many microorganisms that cause colds, flu, bronchitis, and viral pneumonia are often transmitted to the nose via the hands – probably 90%. Avoiding contact with infected individuals is best, but it's not always possible to know, so clean your hands thoroughly before touching your face or eating.
5. **Avoid food and drink that leaves the mouth raw or inflamed**, including hot liquids, spicy food, tobacco, and (possibly) excess alcohol. Although such exposure is more likely to cause uncomfortable inflammation than true infection, viruses such as herpes are more likely to invade damaged skin and mucosal membranes.
6. **Avoid potentially contaminated food and drinks**, to decrease the possibility of food poisoning, giardia, worms, hepatitis A, and gastroenteritis.
7. **Cherish your stomach acid.** With the increased use of acid-lowering drugs in recent years, there has been growing concern that gastrointestinal infections may increase. Hydrochloric acid is a potent sterilizing agent, killing off most germs that we ingest along with our food and drink. When acid levels are decreased using the super-strong proton pump inhibitors (PPIs, including Prilosec, Prevacid, Nexium, Aciphex, Dexilant, Protonix), the potential exists for microorganisms to survive the passage through the stomach. In 2010 it was demonstrated that *Clostridium difficile* (popularly known as *C. diff*) colitis organisms are more difficult to eradicate in patients taking PPIs than in those not prescribed these medications. Although other ways to treat heartburn

exist, Americans have become lazy, preferring the easy answer PPIs afford. If you are taking a PPI, be sure to read the entries on heartburn and GERD.

8. **Avoid bubble baths or strong soaps in the genital areas**, especially in little girls and women. The minor irritation this causes often leads to urinary infections. Drinking plenty of liquids and urinating frequently also helps flush the urinary system of bacteria. Women should be sure to urinate shortly after sexual intercourse to decrease the likelihood of "honeymoon cystitis."
9. **Practice safe sex.** Monogamy with a trusted infection-free partner (or total abstinence) is the only way to be 100% safe. If this is impossible, stock up on condoms to protect yourself and society from spread of disease. If you're worried, get checked now for sexually transmitted diseases, and treat yourself and partner if needed. Tests for STDs will be hard to come by at TEOTWAWKI, as will cures.
10. **Check your feet regularly.** For diabetics, or people with poor circulation or numb feet, checking your feet daily should be part of your regular routine. For others, watch for blisters, bug bites, athlete's foot, warts, injuries, abrasions, and rashes. Feet are among the dirtiest parts of the body, and minor injuries may lead to infection that travels up the legs or into the bones, occasionally requiring amputation.
11. **Avoid antibiotics when possible.** For decades the use (and overuse) of antibiotics has resulted in iatrogenic (physician-caused) yeast infections and resistant bacterial strains. Now the problem is worsened with the widespread prevalence of both *Clostridium difficile* colitis (antibiotic-related colitis, or *C. diff.*) and *methicillin-resistant Staphylococcus aureus* (MRSA, pronounced "mersa") (see **Chapters 11** and **13**), both potentially lethal infections. Although antibiotics can be lifesaving, they can take a life as well.

Strengthening the immune system

Although many natural medicine practitioners advise *Echinacea* and other herbs to strengthen the immune system, I've found very little scientific corroboration. What is true is that a person on a healthy diet weighted toward fresh fruits, vegetables, and whole grains should have sufficient amino acids, vitamins, and other nutrients essential to maintain a well-functioning immune system.

Treating infection and rational rationing

Despite your best precautions, infections will inevitably occur. The pages that follow outline how to diagnose and treat common infections.

Before going on, however, a few words about antibiotics and rationing.

Nowadays – in times of plenty – most patients take antibiotics out of fear: fear of discomfort, fear of missing work, fear of being inconvenienced. Every day patients request antibiotics for minor problems or questionable indications, and every day doctors comply.

In times of scarcity, people will still take antibiotics out of fear, but the stakes will be higher. No more antibiotics for acne, for viruses, for minor infections. People will take antibiotics out of fear of death, disability, or deformity.

Who should be treated? Who should not? The question of health care rationing raised its ugly head during the health reform debates. But that was child's play compared to the rationing that will – that must – occur when Armageddon strikes.

Although I can tell you what medicine to use for a specific problem, I cannot tell you precisely who should receive treatment. In modern society, we think mostly of ourselves, and our own survival. In uncertain times the survival of the family, the clan, or humanity itself may be at risk. Is a child more important than a breadwinner? Is a physician more vital than a priest? Will you find yourself in a group that must decide?

Until manufacturing capabilities are reestablished, medical supplies will be limited. Rationing *will* occur, but will rationing be rational? Or will the greedy and powerful prevail? Is it fair for a person who has carefully prepared to be forced to share with those who have not?

The chapters on specific diseases suggest how to treat many problems with the least amount of medication likely to be effective, based on my experience seeing thousands of patients over multiple decades. These are only guidelines and specifics will vary according to each patient, but preserving medical supplies to aid the greatest number of people is the goal.

For myself, I've already realized that though my medical knowledge may be useful, compared to the younger, potentially child-bearing generation, I am genetically expendable. My children are grown, my generation is approaching retirement, our strength is waning. Although I would hope to contribute unselfishly to a society in chaos, acquired knowledge (and better yet, wisdom) may be the gift I am most able to share. I cannot run fast; I cannot protect my family from armed intruders; I am but an amateur farmer. Yet we all have something to offer, and the true test of Armageddon may be how we choose to care for one another. If you only have one bottle of penicillin, seek wisdom in your rationing.

Food for thought . . . from www.ArmageddonMedicine.net

Antibiotics - 5 Reasons to Avoid Them

Have a cold? Take an antibiotic?

Ear pain? Take an antibiotic.

Acne? Take an antibiotic.

That's what people think anyway. *But is this really the best course of action? Does the short-term gain outweigh the long-term consequences? And is there a short-term gain to begin with?* Antibiotics don't help colds caused by a virus. Most ear infections clear just as quickly without antibiotics. True, bad acne improves with oral antibiotics, but what about the millions of teens who take them for just a few zits?

Every day doctors see problems related to the use of antibiotics. Here are five reasons doctors try to limit their use and why you should think twice yourself before taking one.

1. Yeast infection. Often patients are unaware that our body is covered with germs, both inside and out. The skin, the mouth, the vagina, the intestine – all have their own population of bacteria. For the most part, these microbes stay where they belong and do what they're supposed to. One function of the normal flora (normal population of bacteria) is to keep the bad ones at bay. There are always a few harmful bacteria around, but usually they are crowded out by the good ones. However, taking an antibiotic often kills off the population of good bacteria and allows a different microbe to take over. Most commonly, yeast is the intruder. Once the bacteria get out of the way, the few yeast that linger on the skin, in the vagina, or in the colon claim the territory as their own. The overgrowth of yeast often leads to symptoms of vaginal yeast infection or a yeast skin infection, usually in warm areas such as the armpits, groin, or under the breast.

2. *Clostridium difficile* colitis. Just as the overgrowth of yeast can occur and produce infection when the normal bacteria are killed off, so may harmful bacteria. Frequently the normal flora of the intestine is susceptible to an antibiotic taken for an illness. However, *Clostridium difficile* (or *C. diff.*) is not killed by common antibiotics such as penicillin, sulfa drugs, or erythromycin. The few *C. diff.* bacteria that you may harbor in your intestine will not harm you as long as their numbers remain limited. But when overgrowth occurs, foul-smelling diarrhea occurs, sometimes accompanied by fever, dehydration, or the need for hospitalization. *C. diff.* colitis requires a different antibiotic to rid your body of this harmful organism, and may be fatal without treatment.

3. Resistance. As mentioned above, certain bacteria are already resistant to antibiotics. However, the potential exists for many bacteria to become resistant to useful antibiotics. What if penicillin became ineffective for strep throat? In some cases it already is. MRSA (*methicillin-resistant Staph aureus*) is a harmful bacteria that has emerged in recent years due to the overuse of antibiotics. If you remember your high school genetics, you may know that when bacteria (or people) multiply by the billions, a few mutations are inevitable. In the microbe population this often means that when billions of bacteria reproduce, a few of the daughter-bacteria inherit a mutation that makes them resistant to certain antibiotics. Usually these mutated bacteria, though stronger in the sense that they could live through an "attack" of penicillin, are actually weaker in other ways and die a natural but premature death. However, if the entire population of bacteria is subject to a round of antibiotics, the weaker but penicillin-resistant bacteria may live to repopulate the environment. Then the next time penicillin is used, it will not work. Doctors see antibiotic resistance everyday. It IS a real threat, and at least for now, we don't have new antibiotics on the horizon to use against these resistant bacteria.

4. Nausea, vomiting, and diarrhea. Even apart from killing off the normal flora of the body, antibiotics may cause nausea, vomiting, or diarrhea by themselves. These are chemicals after all, chemicals which the body may reject as foreign. The erythromycin class of antibiotics is especially notorious for causing gastrointestinal symptoms by stimulating the naturally occurring contractions of the gut.

5. Drug allergy. Any patient can be allergic to any medication, and antibiotics are no exception. Though often an antibiotic allergy may manifest as only a rash, true anaphylaxis may occur with the use of any antibiotic. Anaphylaxis is a total body allergic response which may include hives, nausea, light-headedness, itching, swelling, and trouble breathing, much like a bee-sting allergy. Any time you think you are having a reaction to a medication, call your doctor. If you are having trouble breathing or feel like you might faint, call 911. This is a medical emergency.

Just writing this reminds me to be careful when prescribing antibiotics to my patients. Next time your doctor orders you a round of penicillin or other antibiotic, ask how necessary the drug really is. Often they are prescribed for convenience more than necessity.

Chapter 5 – Checklist

- ☐ Learn how to care for your skin now to achieve optimum texture and integrity, in particular how to avoid dry skin, cracking, flaking, fissuring, callus and blister formation, especially on the hands and feet.

- ☐ Stockpile dye-free perfume-free skin cream or moisturizer appropriate for use by persons of all ages and genders.

- ☐ Include hand sanitizer in your supplies to be used only on rare occasions.

- ☐ Among your supplies include gentle shampoo and soap, appropriate for all family members. Watered-down baby shampoo may also be used as an eye rinse.

- ☐ Don't forget the toilet paper. Residual fecal matter at the anus can easily result in skin irritation and sometimes local yeast infection.

- ☐ Include terrycloth towels for thorough drying.

- ☐ Among your toiletries include: nail clippers and nail files for optimum nail care; a mirror not only to see your face, but to view difficult-to-access areas; a pumice stone to minimize callus formation; a nit comb in case of lice; and good razor blades and tweezers (which can double as surgical instruments)

- ☐ Consider stocking a lifetime supply of condoms for yourself, your teenagers, and others who won't remember to do so.

- ☐ Consider discussing potential future medical rationing among your family or survivalist group now, before the necessity arises, to develop a sensible plan.

- ☐ Decide where you fit in personally in the grand scheme of things and prepare accordingly. It may be more important to stockpile milk for your grandchildren than medication for yourself.

Chapter 6

Medical Quarantine and Isolation

Who, what, when, where, why

Plague. Yellow fever. Cholera. Diphtheria. TB. Smallpox. SARS. Hemorrhagic fever. Influenza. With which of these diseases would you feel comfortable sharing your home?

Protecting your family

Each of the above is on the current presidentially ordered "List of Quarantinable Communicable Diseases" per Executive Order 13295 April 4, 2003 and subsequent revisions. For over a century the federal government has been active in preventing individuals with certain contagious diseases from entering our country. As a practicing physician in the United States for a quarter of a century, to date of these I have encountered only tuberculosis (TB) and influenza – and I'd like to keep it that way.

Though less likely to cause a fatal illness, you might also be leery about sharing living quarters with a person suffering from hepatitis, strep throat, methicillin-resistant staph, *C. diff.*, pneumonia, vomiting, diarrhea, a cough, lice, fleas, a rash, fever, stiff neck, swollen glands – or any type of potentially contagious symptom or disease. If your immunizations – or those of your children – are not up to date, you should also be concerned about measles, mumps, rubella, chicken pox, *Haemophilus influenzae*, polio, and whooping cough (pertussis).

Hundreds of years ago, quarantines against ships carrying potential infection were imposed to reduce the risk of plague among port cities. *How will you respond if a sick person shows up at your doorstep? Or a family with a feverish child? Or even someone apparently well?*

Assuming contagious disease is the only reason for turning a person away (which is admittedly unlikely to be the case in an Armageddon scenario), how will you balance "loving your neighbor" versus protecting your own family?

Medical quarantine and/or isolation offer a possible solution.

According to the CDC, "the difference between quarantine and isolation can be summed up like this:

- ***Isolation*** applies to persons who are known to be ill with a contagious disease.
- ***Quarantine*** applies to those who have been exposed to a contagious disease but who may or may not become ill."

The term "quarantine" can also be applied to material items that may be implicated in the spread of disease, for example, food and animal products.

Imagine someone ill approaches, seeking shelter. *What should you do? Or what if someone in your own household succumbs to what may be a contagious illness?*

First, let's consider how our government would handle it. If you were a Haitian orphan entering the U.S. after the 2010 earthquake disaster, per the CDC you would be examined and screened for: bacterial and protozoal diarrhea, hepatitis A and E, typhoid fever, dengue fever, malaria, leptospirosis, tuberculosis, syphilis, intestinal parasites, *Giardia spp., Cryptosporidium*, rotavirus antigen (if symptomatic), and strongyloides (if your blood showed eosinophilia). Additionally, your immune status would be evaluated and updated for diphtheria, pertussis, tetanus, measles, rubella, polio, hepatitis A and B, *Haemophilus influenzae* B, meningococcus, pneumococcus, and varicella (chicken pox).

Lacking the means to do any of this, what constitutes a reasonable approach to strangers seeking help? Can you trust their claims of wellness? Is it likely that a stranded family (who hasn't read this book) will be carrying their immunization records?

With the modern understanding that transmissible microbes are accountable for the spread of much disease, common sense dictates that an obviously ill person should be isolated from apparently well individuals. Clues to contagious illness include such common symptoms as fever, chills, fatigue, nausea, vomiting, diarrhea, cough, runny nose, sore throat, swollen glands, and rash. Of course, there are non-contagious causes of each of the above symptoms, but if in doubt, better to be safe than sorry. Other symptoms occasionally associated with contagion include headache, ear pain, weight loss, muscle aches, joint pain, chest pain, mouth soreness, irritability, stiff neck, abdominal pain, change in mental status, and genital symptoms. Almost any physical or mental symptom has, at one time or another, been associated with a transmissible illness.

Unfortunately, certain illnesses such as chicken pox and influenza are often highly contagious even before infection is apparent. A child with a single blister, mistaken for a bug bite, may spread varicella to an entire class. Other times, a person can be a carrier of disease without showing signs of the infection personally. Remember Typhoid Mary, who spread typhoid fever a century ago without ever exhibiting signs of illness? In other cases, what causes a minimal illness in one person may cause long-term suffering in another. For example, a toddler infected with infectious mononucleosis may simply have a runny nose for a day or two, whereas the twenty-year-old parent may suffer debilitating fatigue for months.

This is the basis for quarantining apparently healthy individuals. If your own group is healthy, you must keep it that way by isolating newcomers from the established group until it is clear that the newcomers remain healthy over a period of time. Even then, this cannot assure that an asymptomatic carrier is not in your presence, but the risk decreases as evidence of prolonged health accumulates.

Quarantine and isolation measures depend on potential routes of transmission: airborne, droplet-borne, waterborne, direct contact, vector-borne (mosquitoes, fleas), fomite-borne (doorknobs, clothing, equipment, toys, or other inanimate object that may allow transmission of virus particles, bacteria, or possibly lice, scabies, bedbugs, or fleas), food-borne, and blood-borne.

First, to address the case of one of your own who falls ill: a family or group that has been isolated from others for less than three weeks is still susceptible to illnesses originating from the outside. There are, of course, certain illnesses that may take longer to manifest themselves, including infectious mononucleosis and hepatitis A, which have an incubation period of up to about six weeks. When infection is suspected, the individual should be isolated in a separate room if at all possible, preferably one vented to the outside. Keeping a window cracked can create a negative pressure environment, making it more likely that air from the uncontaminated portion of the house will be sucked into the sick-room, rather than having contaminated air rush into the rest of the house every time the door is opened. Keeping a rug or towel rolled along the bottom of the door may help as well. Don't forget about ductwork that may connect a sickroom with other parts of the house. Any room that can be effectively isolated from the remainder of the home may be used as a sickroom. The living room couch is a poor choice for a sick bed. Airborne infections include tuberculosis and the varicella (chicken pox) virus. For a true airborne disease, any person coming in contact with the infected patient should wear personal protective equipment, most importantly a mask.

Fortunately, most illnesses are not purely airborne. Both viral and bacterial infections are much more likely to be spread through droplets from secretions via contact with the hands, eating utensils, doorknobs, bathroom items, toys, or other fomites. The hand sanitizer folks have capitalized on this fact. Studies have shown equal benefit using either hand sanitizer or hand-washing with soap and water.

Whereas with an airborne infection you might become infected simply by entering a contaminated room, most common illnesses will not be transmitted unless you actually touch a contaminated surface, then touch your eyes, nose, or mouth before washing your hands. Keep in mind that anything else you touch may become contaminated as well: a thermometer, a stethoscope, a cup or plate, a toothbrush, the remote control, telephone, light switch, etc. Generally speaking, you are unlikely to become ill if you merely enter a sickroom, sit across the room when conversing, and avoid touching any objects. Even doctors who have close but brief contact with their patients rarely become ill when they adhere to strict hand-washing. I avoid inhaling when examing a patient's nose or mouth, and try to stand off to the side rather than directly in the line of fire of a cough or sneeze. I never touch my face until I've washed my hands between patients.

In an isolated group that has an established track record of good health, when symptoms occur suggesting an infectious organism, additional causes should be considered including allergies, food intolerances or poisoning, toxins or poisons, radiation, immune reactions, insect bites or bee stings. Isolating the individual until the question is clarified is a reasonable precaution.

If a sickroom is established, if possible limit the interaction with the sick individual to only one or two others, who themselves should be semi-isolated from the remainder of the group. Establish separate sleeping quarters for the caregivers if space allows, along with separate eating and bathroom arrangements until the situation is clarified or resolved.

The more difficult question is how to deal with outsiders. If a group or individual approaches you for shelter, it may not be apparent if they are sick. As discussed above, the incubation period for many contagious diseases is up to three weeks, though 10 days or less is more common. Avoiding contact with newcomers for at least a week is advisable, no matter how well they look. This will allow time to sort out diseases with a short incubation period, though there is no way to know if someone is an asymptomatic carrier (until they make someone else sick, a pattern that is difficult to identify).

What does avoiding contact mean? If you have the space to allow them use of an outbuilding such as a freestanding garage or barn, that would be ideal. Or, if you live in a neighborhood, are there other homes standing empty that could be used? If not, a basement or an inside room, preferably one vented to the outside, is a consideration. Plan to keep food utensils and waste disposal entirely separate. Do not feel you are being a bad host if you don't offer to wash their dishes. Use disposables, if you have them. (Large leaves may be used as disposable plates if needed.) To avoid cross-contamination from used dishes, serve food by dropping it onto plates or bowls from a height where splash-back onto your own dishware will not occur. Keep an extra 5-gallon bucket with attached toilet seat handy for use as a commode for guests (preferably with sturdy, disposable plastic bags as well). If you use an interior room for quarantine, have your guests fold their arms across their chests as they enter and approach the assigned room to avoid potential contamination of walls, doorknobs, and other surfaces.

If someone among your guests is ill and you are able to provide two areas, one for isolation and one for quarantine, this may decrease the spread of sickness within the new group. However, if you only have a single space to use, consider all the newcomers infected until sufficient time has passed to ascertain their health.

How long is long enough?

There is no definitive answer for every situation. This is where common sense, patient history, and physical examination come into play. Restricting a family of six to a single bedroom for three weeks would be very difficult (though not as difficult as watching your own family die of pandemic influenza). If hepatitis A, or typhoid fever, or Avian flu, or some new superbug is known to be circulating, the answer would be tailored to the specific infection. However, assuming today's microbial environment, ten days of quarantine would eliminate the likelihood of most transmissible infections. Among apparently well individuals, even five days would probably decrease the risk of contagion by close to 90%.

The evaluation does not end there, though. Interviewing should be an ongoing process. If your would-be guests on the doorstep look like death warmed over or disclose that they've all been infected with the Andromeda strain, it would be ill-advised to allow them to enter your house at all – your garage or barn, perhaps, but not your house. If your guests look every bit as healthy as you, at least with their clothing on, a somewhat lesser degree of caution may be warranted. (Of course, other safety concerns should be evaluated as well, including trustworthiness, weapons, possible contributions to the group, etc. Potentially transmissible diseases may be the least of your worries.) If, after five, ten, or twenty days you decide to admit them to your group, a complete history and physical is still a good idea. Unless you have medical training, you won't know everything this entails, but at least look to see if the person is breathing normally, has no rashes, and is acting normally. (See **Section 10** to learn more.) Ask about the symptoms of infection outlined earlier in this chapter. If there's any likelihood of sexual interaction at all, ask about STDs, including gonorrhea, chlamydia, syphilis, HIV, herpes, hepatitis, and venereal warts (HPV). You may want to use a medical history and physical form as a guideline. These infections may not necessarily disqualify someone from living in your home/group, but potential partners should be aware of untreated or incurable sexually transmitted diseases.

Even if the newcomers appear perfectly healthy, don't forget to check for nits (head lice). Though not life-threatening, you'll be sorry if every member of your household ends up with a head full of critters that may be difficult or impossible to eradicate. Likewise, if your own group is suffering a shared infestation (lice, scabies, fleas, bed bugs, pinworms, roundworms, fungus, etc.), you may want to apprise the newcomers of the situation.

On the other hand, your guests may not be as healthy as they had claimed or supposed. You need to decide ahead of time what your action plan will be in case someone exhibits a persistent cough, or a weeping skin wound, or prolonged diarrhea. Do you have the heart to turn them away? Though non-infectious causes of prolonged symptoms do occur, how will you discern which it is? Is there a referral center remaining open, or a doctor you might consult?

If the deciding point is not health but adequate food supplies, how much will you share? Will the companionship and having more hands to work outweigh dividing your rations? If a person is disabled and cannot contribute at all, is it your duty to help them? Difficult questions without easy answers, but best addressed before the situation arises.

This chapter has not addressed every infection you may encounter, but rather has offered general guidelines. As mentioned elsewhere in this book, protect yourself and your family by updating your immunizations to diphtheria, hepatitis A and B, tetanus, pertussis (whooping cough), polio, measles, mumps, rubella, meningitis, chicken pox, pneumonia, and influenza. Although other illness such as yellow fever, typhoid, and Japanese encephalitis are rare in the United States, immunizations are available. See the American Academy of Family Physicians recommendations at www.aafp.org/afp/2004/0701/p89.html for a list of vaccines and associated costs.

Chapter 6 – Checklist

- ☐ Update your own immunizations and those of your family or survival group, according to age. EVERYONE should have a Tdap or Td.

- ☐ Have all family/group members receive a TB test and document the result.

- ☐ Just as schoolchildren must document vaccinations and TB screening before entering a new school, consider a similar screening protocol and documentation for all your group members.

- ☐ Develop a quarantine plan and area for potential outsiders. Consider that you may need their talents, abilities, and supplies, and so may not want to turn all away.

- ☐ Develop isolation procedures for members within your group who become ill.

- ☐ Acquire a supply of disposable (or extra) dinnerware for potential guests in quarantine.

- ☐ Construct or purchase bedside commodes for your own living quarters, as well as quarantine and isolation areas.

- ☐ Develop waste disposal protocols and plans, assuming no garbage pickup or public sewer.

- ☐ Develop protocols for accepting or turning away strangers/potential group members.

- ☐ Acquire personal protective equipment: masks and gloves for everyone; face shields for potential health care providers.

Chapter 7

Animal Bites and Rabies

Infection prophylaxis and treatment

Rapid dogs, prowling coyotes, emboldened bears – oh, my!

Will we have more to worry about than our neighbor's pit bull when the American way of life screeches to a halt? Even if it's your own precious kitten that happens to pierce your skin during play, what will you do if no doctor is around to treat an infection? Does it make sense to get immunized for rabies now, while the vaccine is available? Although currently domestic animals account for the majority of animal-related injuries, will that change when starving dogs roam the streets of suburbia?

In today's western society, dog bites account for 80–90% of animal bite wounds, with cat bites coming in second at approximately 10%. According to the CDC, "4.5 million Americans are bitten by dogs each year, and one in five dog bites results in injuries that require medical attention." Children ages 5–9 are most at risk. Not surprisingly, people who have dogs living with them are more likely to be bitten than those who do not.

What will happen to the 885,000 Americans each year who require medical attention for dog bite wounds? Who will care for the 31,000 annually who require reconstructive surgery? My own nephew had his finger bitten off (or nearly so) by a friend's dog. After two surgeries his finger is still not working properly. If hand surgeons were unavailable, amputation would have been the likely outcome.

Dog bites involve the hands about 2/3 of the time, with the face involved nearly 1/3 (at least in reported cases). Bites of the legs account for most of the remainder. Cat bites usually involve the hands as well, with legs, face, and trunk effected less commonly.

This information alone is enough to say something about prevention: *keep your hands away from an angry or aggressive animal, or one who is eating, or playing roughly.* With ready medical treatment less available, prevention becomes vital.

Bite wounds include punctures, tears, scratches, and crush injuries. Of these, punctures are most likely to become infected due to the difficulty of cleaning them thoroughly and the deep deposition of bacteria and/or debris. Sharp cat teeth are more likely to cause puncture wounds than dog teeth, and are much more likely to become infected.

Cat bites almost always become infected – and *very* quickly, often within hours. I've seen patients who were bitten in the morning develop cellulitis by afternoon. I am *always* concerned about a patient who reports a cat bite on the back of the hand where infection can spread like wildfire, uncomfortably close to the underlying tendons of the hand. I always prefer to see such a patient in person, though occasionally will prescribe antibiotics over the phone in a pinch. Of course, I have patients who tell me they get scratched by their cat on a regular basis and have not become infected. Most of these are superficial scratches, which are less likely to become infected in the first place. However, since nearly every cat carries *Pasteurella multocida* bacteria, every cat bite should be considered potentially infected.

If our modern medical establishment is disrupted, it's unlikely that wound culture results will be available. On a practical note, cultures are usually not done now, anyway, unless pus is present, which is usually not the case. A typical infected cat bite reveals a few small puncture wounds with surrounding erythema (redness) of the skin and perhaps some swelling. The redness tends to spread in the direction toward the heart (up an arm or leg), following lymphatic or venous channels. Sometimes pinkness of the skin overlying a vein will outline the route of spread.

Even though cultures are not routinely performed now except in cases of significant infection, research has demonstrated which germs are likely to be present in animal bites. Dogs carry a variety of bacteria, often including the *Pasteurella* mentioned above regarding cat bites, but also *Streptococcus viridans*, *Staphylococcus aureus*, *Bacteroides*, and others.

What do you do if you or a loved one has been bitten? Assuming a typical wound, where risk of bleeding to death is not a factor, cleaning the wound is the most important first step. Use clean, soapy tap water if it is available, or sterile water or saline (salt water). Use a blunt-tipped syringe (or other device such as a bulb syringe or clean turkey baster) to gently squirt water into the wound to clean deeper tissues. Remove any visible foreign debris, such as pieces of clothing stuck in the wound. Small fragments of jagged, dangling skin may need to be snipped off.

Once the wound is clean, consider whether it should be sutured or otherwise closed.

Keep in mind that:

1. Puncture wounds should not be closed.
2. Very clean wounds that are gaping open or have a flap may heal better if they are closed.
3. Sutured wounds may develop infection more readily than those left open, especially deep wounds.
4. If a sutured wound becomes infected, it will not heal unless the sutures are removed.
5. Wounds older than 12 hours generally should not be sutured.
6. There is often no perfect answer. No matter what you do, a wound may become infected.

For a large or deep wound, or in a patient with fragile health, prophylactic (preventive) antibiotics may be advisable. *Preventive* treatment for wounds (evaluated within the first 12 hours) should be given for 3–5 days, whereas treatment of *established* infection should be administered for 7 to 10 days, using an antibiotic from the table below. Preventive treatment for puncture wounds of the hand (especially from a cat bite) is highly recommended.

What if you're bitten by a fox? A coyote? A wolf? Although little information is available regarding the exact microbes inhabiting a canine's mouth in the wild, antibiotic prophylaxis should be considered in every case, using the dog protocol (see next page).

Equally important, what about rabies? The thought of having one's brain swell to the point of death sends a chill up the spine.

<table>
<tr><th></th><th>Preferred antibiotic</th><th>Preferred alternatives**</th><th>Comments</th></tr>
<tr><td>Dog bite</td><td>Amoxicillin-clavulanate 250–500 mg 3x daily

For 3–7 days (prevention)

Or 7–10 days (treatment)</td><td>Penicillin 500 mg 4x daily

Amoxicillin 500 mg 3x daily

Doxycycline 50–100 mg 2x daily

Erythromycin**
250–500 mg 3–4x daily</td><td rowspan="2">Avoid cephalexin (due to resistant strains of Pasteurella)

Do not use doxycycline in children younger than 9 years, pregnant women, or nursing mothers (due to permanent staining of forming teeth)</td></tr>
<tr><td>Cat bite</td><td>Same as for dog bite, see above</td><td>Doxycycline or erythromycin** per above dosing</td></tr>
<tr><td colspan="4">** Many patients experience gastrointestinal symptoms when taking erythromycin. Azithromycin and clarithromycin are better tolerated and also effective. Advanced generation cephalosporins (Ceftin, Suprax, and Omnicef) are also effective, but expensive.</td></tr>
</table>

Currently human rabies is uncommon in the U.S., and is rarely a concern with domestic animals, especially those who have been properly vaccinated. In recent years in the U.S. there have been only 2–3 cases annually of human rabies, about a fourth of which were contracted overseas.[8] Encounters with bats, raccoons, and wild carnivores (including canines) are considered highest risk as of 2009, though if rabies vaccine becomes unavailable, domestic animals would be expected to become susceptible as well – not to mention people.

Does considering the possibility of pre-exposure prophylaxis seem extreme? I'd say no more so than establishing a bunker "off the grid."

Since rabies is (essentially) uniformly lethal, should you receive the rabies vaccine now, in case of future exposure? Veterinarians and veterinary students are required to receive pre-exposure prophylaxis in the form of a series of three

[8] All cases are detailed online at: http://www.cdc.gov/rabies/location/usa/surveillance/human_rabies.html.

rabies shots over the course of 3–4 weeks. Vaccination is also recommended for spelunkers (cave explorers) and travelers to rabies-endemic regions when contact with animals is possibility. Consider the 2009 case of the Virginia physician who diagnosed his own subsequently fatal case of rabies a few months after returning from India.[9]

The lowest price I have found for the pre-exposure immunization series is $513 for veterinary students, though about $750–800 is charged at travel clinics in Ohio. (The cost for post-exposure immunization is higher ($2000–7000), but this pricing probably reflects use of both the vaccine and immunoglobulin.) Unless you've been exposed to rabies, insurance is unlikely to cover the expense of pre-exposure vaccination. However, sometimes insurance will cover a vaccine if ordered through a pharmacy as a prescription, which can then be taken to your physician for administration.

If you ask your primary care physician whether you should be immunized, the answer will be "no" unless you fall into a high-risk group. (I've never even had a patient ask.) Nevertheless, you can investigate this on your own at your local health department. Your personal physician will not have the vaccine on hand in his or her office, though may be willing to order it. With a price of $225–400 per dose (plus shipping and administration costs), your doctor may require you to pre-pay, as vaccines are generally not returnable and it is unlikely your physician will have another patient waiting for the vaccine if you do not show up for the immunization. If you do get the vaccine, testing for immunity every two years is recommended, with a booster dose if necessary.

In a scarcity scenario where intensive medical treatment is not available for patients suffering from rabies (who are not likely to survive in any event), the

---

[9] "Human Rabies – Virginia 2009" online at: http://www.cdc.gov/mmwr/preview/mmwrhtml/mm5938a3.htm.

vaccine is also likely to be unavailable. If you believe society is about to collapse, now is the time for immunization. At a minimum, everyone should make sure their own pets are vaccinated, for their pets' protection as well as their own.

Exposure to a mad dog or aggressive raccoon is a clear indication for post-exposure rabies vaccine, but a scary fact is that some patients who die of rabies have had no known exposure to a rabid animal. *Any* encounter with a bat (the flying mammal variety) is reason to seek rabies vaccination. Even if you are not bitten per se, a tiny, perhaps invisible, scratch may be lethal. Consider the 2009 case of an Indiana man who died in Kentucky of bat rabies despite no known physical contact.[10]

Which animal bites are likely to carry rabies?	
Possible	Unlikely
Skunks, raccoons, bats (highest risk) Wild canines (foxes, coyotes, wolves) Pets: Dogs, cats, ferrets Most other carnivores	Small rodents (squirrels, hamsters, guinea pigs, gerbils, chipmunks, rats, mice) Rabbits and hares

Many patients are under the impression that antibiotics will prevent rabies or tetanus. Neither supposition is true. Antibiotic use is only intended to treat standard bacterial infections such as staph and strep. Though antibiotics are effective against the *Clostridium tetani* bacterium, they are not curative and do not block the bacterial toxin which causes muscle cramps and contraction, producing "lockjaw" and possibly death.

[10] "Human Rabies – Kentucky/ Indiana, 2009" online at: http://www.cdc.gov/mmwr/preview/mmwrhtml/mm5913a3.htm

Tetanus germs live in the soil and in feces, and enter the body through breaks in the skin, particularly puncture wounds which allow little exposure to air. (Tetanus bacteria thrive in low oxygen environments.) As the spores germinate, tetanospasmin toxin is excreted into the bloodstream. When this toxin binds to the nerve cells it produces painful, sometimes violent muscular contractions, often starting with the jaw and neck. When the contractions become generalized, the ability to breathe is compromised and suffocation may occur.

Is tetanus always fatal? Not under current conditions, with intensive medical care available, including tetanus antitoxin, I.V. therapy, artificial respirators, and carefully monitored medication. Per the CDC, in the U.S. there are about 40 cases of tetanus per year, primarily in under-immunized patients over the age of 60, in whom the death rate is 75% (versus 18% for younger infected individuals). However, if hospital care is unavailable, outcomes will be worse. Of treatments currently used to decrease symptoms due to *Clostridium tetani* toxin, only diazepam (Valium), morphine, and clonidine are likely to be available after a catastrophic event, and none of these can counter respiratory failure.

Has your own doctor ever treated a case of tetanus? Not likely. I haven't. So not only will treatment be a challenge, but diagnosis as well. Do you want to be your doctor's first tetanus patient, treating you with medications unlikely to save your life? The moral of this story is: **keep your tetanus vaccine up to date**. The Tdap vaccine is recommended mid-decade (i.e., ages 15, 25, 35, etc.) If you're unsure when your last vaccine was, go get one now. If it's been over 10 years, you're definitely due. Even if it's been over 5 years an update wouldn't hurt. And take your parents and grandparents with you – they're the ones most likely to die if they become infected.

Chapter 7 – Checklist

- ☐ Update your pets' rabies (and other) immunizations.
- ☐ Consider whether the rabies vaccine is appropriate for you and your family.
- ☐ If you have received the rabies vaccine, consider whether to have a rabies titer performed and the vaccine updated.
- ☐ Stockpile amoxicillin-clavulanate or other appropriate antibiotics per text regarding animal bites.
- ☐ Update your own tetanus vaccine, and that of your family.
- ☐ Safeguard your house against raccoons, bats, dogs, and other critters. Seal off porches, attics, barns, and outbuildings.
- ☐ Teach your children and family to avoid putting their hands or face near any animal, including your own pets.
- ☐ Procure supplies for wound irrigation: sterile water or saline, and blunt-tipped syringe.

Chapter 8

Respiratory Infections and Symptoms

Cough, wheeze, sinus infection, runny nose

Cough

Your 8-year-old daughter has been awake all night coughing. She's burning up with fever and is breathing too fast. Morning brings no relief and she refuses to eat. She says her chest hurts. Does she have pneumonia? Should you carry her five miles to a doctor – if there is one? Will your whole family get sick? Should you use your precious stock of antibiotics?

Such scenarios will arise. Watching a suffering child is hard on anyone, but are you helpless without a physician?

Having a seasoned mother or grandmother on hand would certainly be advantageous, but knowledgeable grannies seem few and far between in this age of the nuclear family. To help you in your decision-making process, here's a systematic approach a doctor (and mother of four) would take if presented with such a patient.

Cough plus fever equals infection (99+% of the time). But first, what sort of infection? Other important questions to consider include:

- Is the cough serious or simply a matter of post-nasal drainage?
- Is the rapid breathing caused by the fever or the infection?
- Is the child in danger of dehydration?
- Does the patient have underlying asthma or other lung disease?
- How rapidly did the illness come on?
- Have other family members been sick, and if so, have they recovered?
- Has the child been immunized against pertussis (whooping cough) and influenza?
- What illnesses are prevalent in the community?
- Is there a history of travel outside the community, or exposure to someone outside the community?

Does the situation appear to be an emergency? When confronted with potentially life-threatening situations, doctors are taught: first, take your own pulse. Rarely is something so urgent that you don't have time to think a situation through analytically.

Most respiratory infections are **viral**, so this is the default answer until proven otherwise. In the current day and age, antibiotics are dispensed like candy in order to (hopefully) get a person well a day or two sooner, a practice that must end when supplies are limited.

Though a coughing patient presents many diagnostic possibilities, one way to categorize the symptom is whether it's originating from the **upper airway** or the **lower** (above the neck or below). Even a terrible-sounding cough may merely be from drainage, or a tickle in the throat. Coughs coming from the lower airway are often accompanied by wheezing or rattling, and are generally of more concern.

To determine this, first observe, does your child have a runny nose? Can you see a river of mucus (snot) draining down the back of the throat? Does she clear her throat often? Can she tell you that she feels mucus draining? A yes answer to any of these indicates the cough is likely from the upper airway, as in a cold. (Of course, a child could have a drainage cough and a chest cough at the same time, but this is unusual. For chest coughs, see below.)

There are two approaches to a cough caused by drainage: dry it up or thin out the mucus. Antihistamines (diphenhydramine, cetirizine, chlorpheniramine – all OTC antihistamines) will decrease the amount of secretions and therefore decrease the cough. Alternately, using an expectorant such as Mucinex (guaifenesin) will make the mucus more watery, similar to saliva, which tickles the throat less. If one approach doesn't work, the other can be tried.

If the cough seems to be coming from the chest, put your ear to your child's back. You don't need a stethoscope to hear wheezing or rattling, especially in a child. Rattling is usually heard more on inspiration whereas wheezing generally occurs with expiration. Hearing any abnormal sound in the chest confirms the lower airway is involved. (One exception: sometimes mucus draining from above travels down the bronchial tube far enough to produce a rattle or cough. If the rattle disappears when the throat is cleared, this is probably the case.)

The most common cause of a chest cough with rattling or wheeze is **acute viral bronchitis**. (Viral influenza causes a dry chest cough, generally with little or no rattling.) With bronchitis, the wheezy congestion is usually bilateral (involving both sides of the chest). Viral pneumonia is usually bilateral as well.

Hearing rattling or wheezing on one side only is more suggestive of bacterial pneumonia (see below). Rales, a fine crackling sound (like rubbing a clump of hair between your fingers), often accompany pneumonia.

A chest cough is much more common in any patient with underlying asthma (or COPD in an adult). Even a simple cold might result in chest congestion in an asthmatic patient, requiring more frequent use of an asthma inhaler.

Chest coughs are treated a little differently than drainage coughs. Antihistamines are generally avoided, to prevent trapping of thick mucus within the bronchial tubes. (There is an exception to every rule, and sometimes antihistamines are helpful for a chest cough as well.) Expectorants which thin the mucus make it easier to cough out accumulated secretions. Bronchodilators may help open the airway, and decrease cough as well as wheezing.

Bronchodilators for Cough and Wheezing	
Mild – Moderate	Strong
Caffeine	Albuterol (Rx)
Phenylephrine (Sudafed PE)	Ipratropium (Rx)
Vicks VapoRub	Primatene Mist (epinephrine) (OTC)
Pseudoephedrine ("real" Sudafed)	Aminophylline
Ephedrine (Ephedra/ma huang)	Corticosteroids (delayed action)

Beware that bronchodilators may produce other effects within the body including rapid heart rate, elevated blood pressure, anxiety, jitteriness, irregular heartbeat, and possibly heart attack or stroke. For this reason ephedrine-containing products were banned in the U.S. for treating weight loss and colds, although Primatene Tablets remain available for asthma relief.

If a patient is getting worn out from coughing, or can't rest, or is developing a sore chest, then a cough suppressant is in order. (Note – a *productive* cough is often a good thing. This is how secretions are cleared from the lungs and bronchial tubes. You don't want to suppress a productive cough altogether.) The over-the-counter cough suppressant dextromethorphan (the "DM" in Robitussin DM) is typically prescribed for both adults and children. As discussed in **Chapter 30**, honey may work as well, especially in children. (Do not give to children under 12 months due to the concern for infant botulism.) Narcotics are stronger cough suppressants, as in Robitussin with Codeine, however these are rarely necessary. It takes only a small dose of codeine to suppress a cough – a quarter pill of a Tylenol #3 or Vicodin is effective.

Coughing is sometimes improved by slowing the breathing via decreasing a fever. Fever increases the metabolic rate, which in turn increases the respiratory rate. Lowering the body temperature slows both the heart rate and respiratory rate, and may thereby decrease respiratory irritation, leading to reduced cough. Hopefully you've stocked up with a 500-pill bottle of Tylenol (acetaminophen). Motrin or aspirin decrease fever as well, but aspirin is best avoided in children who may have influenza, due to the risk of Reye's syndrome (swelling of the liver and brain, often fatal).

Assuming you've tried some of the above suggestions, what next? Keep your hands off the bottle of amoxicillin, at least for now.

Is this illness viral? As I already said, the default answer is yes. Respiratory illnesses that sweep through a family are typically viral (at least in the U.S. at this time), as are those with a rapid onset (within a few to several hours). Viral illnesses are usually at their worst within a few days of onset. The period of highest contagion is also early on, often before a person shows definite symptoms of infection, hence the ease of transmitting infection. When only a single person in a community becomes ill, this is more suggestive of a bacterial infection. Keep in mind, though, that a child in a community of adults may not have developed the resistance to respiratory viruses that adults have, and hence may develop a cold when no one else does so.

The two most common types of bacterial infections to be aware of are: 1) **secondary bacterial infection**; and 2) **unilateral bacterial infection.**

School-aged children and healthy adults are primarily at risk for bacterial infection that sets in on the tail end of a viral infection. In such a situation the patient may seem to be improving, then suddenly (or gradually) worsens. Mucus that was once clear begins to turn green or yellow. Discolored mucus does not always indicate bacterial infection, however. (American doctors overuse this criterion all the time to justify giving antibiotics.) Other signs of a **secondary infection** include a cough that begins to deepen or become productive or painful, a fever mid-way through an illness rather than at the beginning, increased difficulty breathing, and a general deterioration in the overall condition of the patient.

A person's overall condition is probably the most important consideration. In someone who is feeling better but happens to have a worse cough, it is not necessary to jump to antibiotics just yet. A secondary bacterial infection may clear on its own in a healthy individual. If a person's overall condition is good, observing his or her symptoms over several days may reveal improvement. If further significant deterioration occurs, antibiotics are probably indicated. Appropriate antibiotics to consider include amoxicillin, cephalexin or other cephalosporin, the tetracyclines, sulfa drugs, or, in certain cases, a fluoroquinolone antibiotic, such as ciprofloxacin, Levaquin, or Avelox. Most any of the inexpensive antibiotics should be effective against common respiratory bacteria except for nitrofurantoin or metronidazole. As a general rule, cephalexin, amoxicillin-clavulanate, ciprofloxacin, and the other fluoroquinolone drugs should be reserved for resistant or serious infections.

Babies and the elderly are at greater risk of a unilateral bacterial infection, that is to say, **pneumonia**, especially children under the age of 1 year, or any adult old enough to seem a bit feeble. Pneumonia is most often caused by aspirating food or microbe-infested mucus, which becomes trapped in one lung, triggering localized infection. Accumulated fluids clog up the alveoli (air sacs) in the lung, preventing oxygen absorption and carbon dioxide release. If the fluids cannot be removed, a patient may literally drown in his own secretions. Sometimes the infection enters the blood stream, causing sepsis and death. (Although bacterial pneumonia usually starts in one lung, it may occur bilaterally, which can make it difficult to differentiate from viral pneumonia clinically, that is, without laboratory testing or X-rays.)

When listening to the lungs, the affected side usually demonstrates wheezing or rattling, whereas the unaffected lung sounds clear. If breathing is shallow, you may not be able to detect the difference from side to side. Sometimes breath sounds are diminished on the infected side, especially if fluid surrounds the lung (pleural effusion). The patient may complain of one-sided chest pain, particularly on deep inspiration or while coughing. Occasionally a patient may exhibit no respiratory symptoms, but rather simply feel weak or sick, which may make the diagnosis a challenge.

Before the age of antibiotics, **chest percussion** was commonly employed in the treatment of pneumonia, to loosen the phlegm. This is still done for cystic fibrosis patients. The therapist's (or parent's) hand is cupped and clapped against the chest rapidly and firmly enough to rattle the mucus loose, but not so strongly as to produce bruising or pain. For a patient with pneumonia, the entire chest – front, back, and sides – should be percussed several times daily.

Get your pneumonia vaccine today!

This is a good time to reiterate the wisdom of receiving a pneumonia vaccine, which should be considered *now* for:

- any person over the age of 65
- *anyone* with COPD, asthma, diabetes, or other chronic disease
- any patient with a history of pneumonia
- smokers, ages 19–64
- infants and children, ages 2 months to 5 years

Up to this point, we've mostly been avoiding the use of antibiotics, but for a one-sided **pneumonia**, especially in a sick-looking individual, they *should* be used. (Some patients with so-called "walking pneumonia" exhibit classic signs of a unilateral pneumonia on physical examination, but don't actually look or feel particularly ill. These patients *may* not require antibiotics – occasionally watchful waiting may be appropriate.) A baby, feeble adult, or someone with underlying asthma or COPD who exhibits chest rattling or wheezing should be treated, especially if they are worsening. In adults, amoxicillin, cephalexin, doxycycline, trimethoprim-sulfamethoxazole, or a fluoroquinolone is usually effective. In children, amoxicillin, cephalexin, or Augmentin (amoxicillin-clavulanate) are good choices.

By two to three days on antibiotics you should see some improvement; if the situation is worsening or is no better by three to four days, the antibiotic should be switched to one from a different antibiotic class. Five days of treatment may be sufficient in an otherwise healthy adult, but 7–10 days may be necessary, particularly in a debilitated or chronically ill individual. Cough may linger weeks longer than the actual pneumonia, but as long as the overall condition is improving, as determined by careful reexamination, antibiotics may be discontinued per the above protocol.

What about your 8-year-old daughter with cough, fever, chest pain, and rapid breathing?

Her symptoms, especially the chest pain and rapid breathing (tachypnea), are suggestive of pneumonia and she should be treated as such, although it is still possible she is suffering a viral infection, including influenza (see below). In an adult, a pulmonary embolism (blood clot to the lungs) should also be considered, although fever would likely be less prominent.

Influenza is a special case of a respiratory virus because, currently, we *do* have antiviral medications that shorten the course of the disease (Tamiflu is most commonly used). Typical influenza comes on fairly rapidly, usually within a day or two, with symptoms of a dry cough, fever, body aches, and often headache. For this prescription antiviral medication to be effective, it needs to be started within 48 hours of the onset of symptoms, so the decision must be made more quickly than with some other respiratory infections. If you have Tamiflu available to you for use, the question arises as to who should be treated. Unless a pandemic occurs with a lethal strain, Tamiflu should probably be restricted to those at greatest risk of dying, i.e., those with underlying heart or lung disease, or overall frailty. Though typical influenza may make a young adult wish they were dead, it is rarely fatal (except for certain strains).

Tamiflu Dosing Recommendations for Influenza A and B	
Treatment of Influenza Treatment should be started within 2 days of onset of symptoms	**Prevention of Influenza** Treatment should be started within 2 days of exposure and continued until exposure is past
Ages 13 years through adult: 75 mg twice daily x 5 days **Children ages 1 through 12 years:** 10 mg/ pound twice daily x 5 days (Maximum: 75 mg per dose)	**Ages 13 years through adult:** 75 mg once daily x 10 days to 6 weeks **Children ages 1 through 12 years:** 10 mg/pound once daily x 10 days to 6 weeks (Maximum: 75 mg per dose)
Tamiflu is supplied in 75 mg capsules for adults, as well as 30 mg and 45 mg capsules and (6 mg/mL) oral suspension for pediatric use. However, the adult capsules may be opened and the powder divided (and mixed with a small amount of sweet liquid) to achieve the proper pediatric dose.	

Difficult choices may face you. Assuming a limited supply, should Tamiflu be given to a 90-year-old patient or reserved for the eventuality of a younger, currently uninfected person developing influenza, perhaps someone with asthma? Or should you treat an 80-year-old (with useful skills) rather than a 40-year-old (who has been nothing but a drain on your resources)? These are not only ethical, but practical decisions as well, which should be considered before the need arises.

Beyond pneumonia, a bigger concern for many patients with a fever and significant cough is **dehydration**. People tend to eat and drink less when they're coughing all the time. Additionally, with a higher temperature, fluids are lost from the body more quickly, especially in babies and young children. Elderly patients may have a full-blown case of pneumonia, but not exhibit a fever. Also, thirst is often an inadequate drive for sufficient fluid intake. A more reliable measurement of dehydration is body weight. A 100-pound adult who loses 5 pounds of body weight is mildly dehydrated. A 20-pound baby losing a single pound is equally dehydrated (see **Chapter 2**). Unless you are able to provide intravenous rehydration, you'll have to insist that the patient ingest more fluids than they will spontaneously desire, which may be difficult to achieve.

As discussed, humans at the extremes of age are more susceptible to pneumonia. In a feverish, wheezy, rattling baby I would tend to start oral antibiotics sooner (though again, many of these illnesses are viral). But if the baby deteriorates and is unable to take medication by mouth, the odds of I.V. hydration and antibiotics being available are slim to none in a post-Armageddon scenario. The elderly also succumb more easily, but may exhibit few specific symptoms. I have seen elderly patients with pneumonia who exhibited no cough, no chest pain, no shortness of breath, no fever. Sometimes the only apparent symptom is deterioration in overall status, or a worsening of dementia, or loss of appetite.

Age discrimination is likely to occur when supplies are limited, and every situation will pose different decision points. On the one hand, an elderly person may be an invaluable fount of practical knowledge, or may provide the emotional stability for a family, or may be as healthy as a fifty year old. On the other hand, an octogenarian may contribute little to a group and drain valuable resources, leaving younger people (unnecessarily) vulnerable. Treating an older person for pneumonia will require at least a 5-day supply of most antibiotics – and often longer, since few patients will have the opportunity to jumpstart their treatment with I.V. antibiotic therapy.

Wheeze

> *You've heard that sound before, but not coming from your own lungs. Sure, your father always sounded like his chest was full of crud, but he smoked two packs a day. And once or twice you saw your nephew use some sort of asthma inhaler. Now you've got it. Your chest is tight, it's hard to breathe, you cough every time you try to breathe deeply, and you make a strange raspy sound when you exhale. What does it mean? Pneumonia? Emphysema? Pleurisy?*

In a person without a history of asthma or COPD (chronic bronchitis or emphysema), wheezing is a sign of acute lower respiratory tract narrowing or obstruction, usually from infection, although allergy, inhaled foreign body, and chemical irritation are also possible.

Wheezing occurs as the airways narrow. The same amount of air your body always requires must now pass through this constricted bronchial tube, but at an increased speed to make up for the decreased diameter. Just like playing a flute, air passing through a narrow passage will cause a whistling or wheezing sound – at least until so little air can pass that no sound is made. Hence, sometimes a soft wheeze is more serious than loud wheezing, especially if breathing is rapid or labored.

Wheezing and Geometry

Remember high school geometry? The area of a circle is πr^2.

If r, the radius of the airways, is cut in half, the cross-section of the bronchus decreases by three-fourths. What seems like a little narrowing may result in significant respiratory obstruction.

The most common cause of wheezing in an otherwise healthy individual is the so-called chest cold, or acute bronchitis. Even though acute bronchitis is usually caused by a virus – a good 90% of the time – doctors prescribe antibiotics for several reasons:

- Patients believe they're sick enough to demand them.
- Patients are unhappy if they later worsen and require further medical attention
- Doctors aren't always convinced themselves, despite the data
- Testing to confirm a viral infection is too inconvenient or expensive
- Doctors want an excuse to make patients happy
- Although symptoms generally resolve by 3 weeks, both patients and doctors expect more rapid resolution of symptoms
- Although non-antibiotic treatments reduce symptoms, they may cost more or have other side-effects

Despite all this, a rational post-Armageddon approach to the chest cold accompanied by wheezing is to follow what we already know: avoid antibiotic use for acute bronchitis in otherwise healthy individuals.

As with every rule, there are exceptions. Otherwise *un*healthy individuals are more susceptible to secondary bacterial infections, especially those with COPD, diabetes, and asthma. Giving antibiotics early in the illness when symptoms are at their worst sometimes prevents a case of respiratory distress or pneumonia. In general, though, antibiotics should be reserved for situations where the development of pneumonia is likely, or where the airway is severely compromised, or where the patient's condition is deteriorating. Clearly this requires on-going careful assessment of the patient.

So if not antibiotics, what does help?

Of the traditional therapies, cough suppressants (see above) are useful for dry coughs, since repetitive coughing irritates the airways, sometimes causing further narrowing and increased wheeze. Over-the-counter decongestants are useful for a mild case (caffeine, pseudoephedrine, phenylephrine, Vicks VapoRub.) *Ephedra* (ma huang), an herbal remedy now banned in the U.S., is also effective, but may cause rapid heartbeat, nervousness, or palpitations. (Primatene Tablets contain ephedrine, a derivative of *Ephedra,* and remain available behind-the-counter for relief of broncho-constriction due to asthma.) For a more severe case, a short round of corticosteroids will relieve symptoms within a few days (3–10 days of prednisone 40–60 mg daily with food, or a Medrol Dosepak).

Short-acting metered dose inhalers are another option. The same inhalers used for asthma or COPD will help open the bronchial tubes. It's unlikely your doctor will prescribe an albuterol inhaler for stockpiling to a person with no current or prior history of wheezing, but you can purchase Primatene Mist without a prescription. Although doctors essentially *never* recommend this medication, it is effective at relieving broncho-constriction short-term (up to a few hours per dose). Why don't doctors prescribe this epinephrine inhaler? For one thing, it's more likely than prescription inhalers to cause side-effects such as rapid heart rate, jitteriness, and tremor. More importantly, asthmatics may treat themselves when they should be seeking professional medical care. As a result they may end up in the emergency room or worse yet, dead. (Of course, if you're reading this book, you are thinking of future emergency situations when professional care may not be available.) Since epinephrine may also be used for severe, acute, allergic reactions (anaphylaxis), having it available seems prudent.

Runny nose and sinus infection

> *Your nose is dripping again, and the familiar pressure is building in your forehead and cheeks. Every time you yawn, your ears pop, and you've been clearing your throat for a week already. You're sure it's a sinus infection. After all, your doctor always gave you antibiotics before. If you don't take some now, will you ever get well?*

As a general rule (at least in modern America), patients would rather hear that they have a sinus infection than a virus. After all, a sinus infection resolves with antibiotics, doesn't it? Who wants to waste a trip to a doctor to be told it's only a cold?

Sinusitis means inflammation of the sinuses around the nose and eyes. Typical symptoms are nasal congestion, drainage, and pressure or pain in the face – either in the forehead, cheeks, around the nose, or behind the eyes . . . or all four, if you're unlucky.

Sinusitis does not necessarily indicate a bacterial infection requiring antibiotics. What does that mean, anyway, "requiring" antibiotics? Is sinusitis a life-threatening condition?

The strictest definition of the "need" for antibiotics would be a situation in which a patient would die without them. We may want to narrow the definition to exclude those situations where antibiotics are necessary to live, but on their own do not suffice to effect a cure. One such example would be a bullet wound to the gut. With fecal bacteria contaminating the abdominal cavity, life-threatening infection is inevitable. Yet without surgery to repair a lacerated colon, antibiotics alone will not remedy this situation. It would be unwise to use your precious store of antibiotics on a person who is going to die anyway.

The next level of "need" for antibiotics is where withholding them may lead to serious, likely long-term disability or pain. An untreated prostate infection probably won't be fatal, but can lead to long-term misery. Depending on pain tolerance, dental infections may fall in this category (though extraction is a better answer). A COPD patient may cough for months without antibiotics – or may never clear up. An infection in the foot probably won't be lethal, but if the bacteria reach the bone, the result may be permanent pain or the need for amputation.

The third level of "need" is where the use of antibiotics *may* significantly shorten the duration of an illness that often has a good chance of resolving on its own – eventually. Sinusitis and middle ear infections fall in this category (and sometimes the next).

A final category of "need" is using antibiotics to *possibly* improve symptoms a day or two sooner than otherwise. This is the case with many of the upper respiratory infections doctors treat nowadays, including a large number of sore throats.

Writing this, I realize there are many who believe they *must* take an antibiotic for sinus symptoms no matter what I say. If you're in this group, you'd better stock up now with a lifetime supply of amoxicillin.

What doctors usually call a **sinus infection** typically starts with a **common cold** (and often remains simply a common cold with sinus pressure as a symptom). Colds can cause sinus pressure, allergies may do so as well, changes in barometric pressure or altitude may yield similar symptoms, and certainly a true sinus infection may result in sinus pressure. When patients (and doctors) say "sinus infection," the implication is a bacterial infection, though viral involvement of the sinus cavities is much more frequent.

When I started in medicine decades ago, the diagnosis of "sinusitis" was much less common. A cold was a cold. People expected it to take a week or two to resolve. Times have changed, and now we all not only want instant access to information, but instant healing as well. Though antibiotics do not guarantee rapid healing, people believe they do, and if one doctor won't prescribe what a patient wants, the next one likely will.

Let's compare **sinusitis** to another example, that of an **abscess**. An abscess is an enclosed pocket of infection (much like a pus-filled sinus in some ways). Antibiotics will not cure an abscess (at least not one larger than pea-sized) because the blood supply is only on the outside of the abscess, hence the antibiotic circulating through the blood does not penetrate far enough to kill the germs within. The cure for an abscess is to lance it. Once the pus drains, antibiotics are not needed. Of course, many doctors are too chicken not to prescribe an antibiotic in addition to lancing an abscess, especially if they won't have the opportunity to follow up with the patient.

A true sinus infection is a mucopus-filled sinus cavity (mucopus = mucus mixed with pus). Like an abscess, the blood circulation is only at the periphery of the infection, with poor penetration into the interior of the sinus. In modern times, a CT scan or sinus X-ray is used to diagnose a pus-filled sinus, which looks white on an X-ray. An older diagnostic test (a skill which doctors would need to reacquire) is trans-illumination of the sinus cavity. A bright light can pass through an air-filled cavity more readily than through a pus-filled cavity. Using antibiotics to treat a pus-filled sinus may be reasonable, depending on the misery and underlying health of the patient, but is neither always necessary nor effective.

But is a pus-filled cavity the only illness that causes sinus pressure? No. The sinuses are lined with a mucus membrane, similar to the interior of the nose. Everyone has had their nose plug up to the extent they cannot breathe through one side or the other. The lining of the sinus cavities can swell an equal amount, and cause the sensation of sinus pressure. Such swelling may be caused by allergies, barometric or altitude changes, chemical irritation, colds, other viruses, as well as true bacterial infection. Relieving the swelling is often effective in alleviating the sensation of pressure. Also, decreasing the swelling opens the air passages, thereby allowing mucus to drain more easily.

Decongestants are the mainstay of opening the airways. Pseudoephedrine remains the most effective and may be purchased without a prescription, though you will have to sign for this medication. Short-acting and long-acting forms are available. Sometimes doctors prescribe oral corticosteroids to decrease swelling of sinus passages (prednisone 40–60 mg daily for 3–10 days). Over-the-counter

Afrin provides near-immediate relief of nasal congestion, but does not penetrate well into the sinuses. Sometimes using Afrin short-term will jumpstart the effectiveness of pseudoephedrine. When a mucolytic (expectorant, guaifenesin) is added to this regimen, the accumulated mucus is thinner (waterier) and thus able to drain more easily.

I know many of you are thinking, "That won't work for me. If I don't take an antibiotic, I'll have a sinus headache for month."

You may be right. So if your supply of antibiotics is unlimited, go ahead and take some. But if you only have enough to treat a few rounds of illness, I suggest you put up with your headache (for a week, or two, or three) and reserve your potentially life-saving antibiotics for a potentially life-threatening situation.

If you do decide to treat a sinus infection with antibiotics, what should you use and how long should you treat? Interestingly, one study showed three days of a sulfa drug was as effective as ten, though physicians sometimes treat for as long as a month or more. You cannot necessarily rely on relief of symptoms as your gauge for when to discontinue antibiotics. Even if all the bacteria are killed, your body may take another week for symptoms to resolve. Most doctors prescribe an antibiotic for 7–14 days, which is usually effective. Keep in mind, though, that what you're calling a sinus infection could easily resolve within 14 days on its own anyway.

Amoxicillin is most commonly prescribed (but is probably the least effective; many infections that seem to respond may well have cleared up without antibiotics). Other choices include the same antibiotics as for other respiratory infections, i.e., doxycycline, trimethoprim-sulfamethoxazole, azithromycin, ciprofloxacin, cephalexin, amoxicillin-clavulanate, clarithromycin,

Levaquin, or Avelox (in approximate order of increasing strength).[11] Don't waste your strongest drug on a non-life-threatening infection.

How long should you wait before deciding to treat sinusitis with an antibiotic? In a healthy person *without* underlying chronic illness such as asthma or COPD, I'd suggest waiting three or four weeks, or even longer *if* the condition is not deteriorating. In a person *with* underlying lung disease or someone prone to pneumonia, I would observe carefully for a week, or perhaps longer, only starting antibiotics if the condition worsens. There are some patients who do well to begin an antibiotic at the first sign of a cold, for example, an oxygen-dependent patient who ends up in the hospital every time he or she contracts a virus. However, will such a patient survive the demands of a post-Armageddon world?

Lastly, what should you do about a **simple runny nose** that is not a sinus infection? Usually a drippy nose is caused by a cold virus or allergies, though even a change in temperature or eating spicy foods may trigger rhinorrhea (runny nose). Antibiotics are only useful for nasal drainage if a bacterial infection is present – but how would you determine this? The most common criterion that is used is when clear nasal drainage becomes *progressively* more yellow or green over several weeks, especially if accompanied by additional symptoms, such as increasing sore throat, ear ache, or fever. However, this is not an absolute indicator and even if a bacterial infection is present, antibiotics are not always mandatory. Nasal irrigation alone may suffice to rinse the majority of microbes away, and a healthy immune system can often overcome a mild bacterial infection.

---

[11] Erythromycin is sometimes prescribed for sinusitis, but is frequently poorly tolerated and probably no more effective than amoxicillin. It remains a consideration for penicillin-allergic patients.

In general, rhinorrhea (runny nose) should be treated symptomatically. Antihistamines decrease the volume of secretions. Interestingly, certain antihistamines work better for specific causes of runny nose. The non-sedating antihistamines Claritin, Allegra, and Clarinex work much better for allergies and vasomotor rhinitis than they do for runny noses caused by viral infections. Of these, both Claritin and (more recently) Allegra are available over-the-counter as inexpensive generics. At some pharmacies, the same strength of these medicines is still covered by prescription, at a lower cost than the over-the-counter product. Cetirizine, belonging to another class of non-sedating antihistamines, works well for both allergies and colds. The sedating antihistamines diphenhydramine and chlorpheniramine also work well for any cause of runny nose.

Other options to dry up a runny nose

Atrovent nasal spray, a prescription that is effective with as-needed use

Singulair, for preventing runny nose in allergic rhinitis, as well as asthma

Pseudoephedrine, a decongestant which induces dryness in some patients

Nasalcrom, an over-the-counter nose spray for preventing allergic rhinitis, similar in effectiveness to the nasal corticosteroids (but much cheaper)

Nasal corticosteroid sprays, available only by prescription and relatively expensive (although Flonase now comes in generic)

Nasal irrigation, using a neti (netty) pot (1 tsp. salt in 1 pint lukewarm water) – see video at University of Wisconsin School of Medicine and Public Health at http://www.fammed.wisc.edu/research/past-projects/nasal-irrigation#video

Drying of nasal secretions is also a side-effect of other medications not aimed primarily at the nose, especially antidepressants, nausea drugs, and muscle relaxers.

As discussed, when nasal secretions continue week upon week, becoming increasingly discolored, a secondary bacterial infection *may* be present. In patients with underlying lung problems such as asthma, beginning an antibiotic at this point is reasonable if the patient has a history of bronchitis or pneumonia. If the patient is generally healthy and there are no other symptoms present, continuing to treat symptomatically is preferable when supplies are limited.

One last comment on the isolated runny nose: if the drainage seems to be coming from one side only, and especially if a very foul odor is present, you may be dealing with a **foreign body in the nose**. Children especially are prone to inserting various objects in the nostrils, which get stuck and block the flow of mucus, resulting in a localized "cesspool." The treatment of a foreign body in the nose is to remove the offending object. Antibiotics may disguise the problem for awhile but will not resolve the situation. You probably won't be able to see the bead or other object without a strong light and a pair of tweezers. It also helps to hold the nostril open with a small speculum (or possibly a small pair of pliers).

Although strictly speaking **ear infections**, **sore throats**, and **mouth infections** do involve the respiratory system, they will be addressed separately in the following chapters.

Chapter 8 – Checklist

Items to include in your medical supplies:

- ☐ Antihistamines: diphenhydramine, cetirizine, chlorpheniramine, loratadine
- ☐ Expectorants: Mucinex or Robitussin, or generics of the same
- ☐ Cough suppressant: honey, dextromethorphan, codeine
- ☐ Decongestants: caffeine, pseudoephedrine, phenylephrine, Vicks VapoRub
- ☐ Bronchial inhalers (preferably albuterol by prescription, otherwise OTC Primatene Mist)
- ☐ Steroids: Medrol Dosepak (methylprednisolone) or prednisone
- ☐ Antibiotics: penicillin, amoxicillin or ampicillin; Augmentin; cephalexin, erythromycin or azithromycin, doxycycline or tetracycline, ciprofloxacin, trimethoprim-sulfamethoxazole
- ☐ Antipyretics for fever: Tylenol (acetaminophen), aspirin (avoid in children), ibuprofen
- ☐ Antivirals: Tamiflu for influenza; acyclovir for herpes
- ☐ Stethoscope and possibly an otoscope
- ☐ Peak flow meter to assess breathing impairment and improvement
- ☐ Wind-up LED flashlight
- ☐ Neti pot, salt, and water for nasal irrigation

Immunizations to protect against respiratory infections

- ☐ Have every family or group member receive an annual influenza vaccine. Those 65 and older should receive the high-dose flu vaccine.
- ☐ Have all eligible family members receive the pneumonia vaccine.
- ☐ Make sure everyone has received the Tdap tetanus update, which also protects against whooping cough.
- ☐ Babies, toddlers, and school-age children should all be immunized diseases that often include a respiratory component, including measles, mumps, rubella, *Haemophilus influenzae* B, chicken pox, and possibly meningococcus.

Chapter 9

Sore Throat, Sore Mouth, Sore Lips

Viral pharyngitis, mono, strep throat, thrush, herpangina, herpes simplex

"Daddy, my throat hurts," your feverish toddler whines, unwilling to leave his sickbed. No one else is sick – not yet, anyway. Should you treat him now, before everyone else comes down with whatever he has? What exactly does he have, anyway? Is it strep? Could it be mono? Which is more dangerous? Could he die without antibiotics?

Sore throat

No one is a stranger to a sore throat. An adult may choose to wait it out, but when it comes to your kids, who wants to take a chance? The real question in identifying the cause of a sore throat is whether special treatment is required, i.e., antibiotics (or occasionally steroids or surgery). Nearly any other treatment is merely a matter of comfort, that is, helping you feel better until your natural immunity kicks in, thus ridding the body of infection. Even the use of antibiotics for strep throat is rarely life-saving, so why do doctors bother to prescribe them? Is strep truly lethal untreated?

Nowadays, when political health reform is the major medical concern, the treatment of sore throat is almost "cookbook" medicine. Consider this scenario:

your 5-year-old son was up all night with a terrible sore throat, fever, and swollen glands. In the morning you take him to the doctor, where you wait an hour or two holding your sick child, trying to isolate yourself from other patients with who-knows-what sorts of illness. At last you see the physician, who performs a quick exam and a rapid strep test. The test is positive, your child gets a prescription for amoxicillin, you're happy to have a cure in hand, and your doctor is relieved to be able to move on without trying to convince yet another worried parent that antibiotics are not effective for viral infections.

But what if the power grid collapses and there's no physician in your neighborhood? Can the nurse up the street check your child for strep at home? What if an epidemic of diphtheria has emerged? How will you know? Should you give your child your only supply of penicillin . . . or save it in case of future pneumonia?

What would a doctor do? *Tag, you're it now* . . . what would you do when no professional is around?

Diagnosis and treatment of sore throats does involve more than the knee-jerk prescribing of antibiotics. Though you may not notice this happening, in the above scenario a doctor is actually asking him- or herself the following questions:

1. Is it likely a common virus?
2. Could it be strep?
3. Should I consider mono?
4. Could it be anything else, especially something potentially serious?

In a post-catastrophe situation, treatment will be decided primarily on symptoms and physical examination. Based on this assumption, here is the essence of what you need to know.

First, most sore throats are actually **viral pharyngitis**, and therefore do not require antibiotics. Even nasty-looking cases of tonsillitis (with exudates, or pus, on the tonsils) are commonly caused by viruses. Unfortunately, there is no foolproof way to tell the difference between a virus and strep throat by symptoms alone. However, there are clues to help you decide. A mild sore throat in conjunction with other cold symptoms is usually viral. Laryngitis (or hoarseness) occurring with a sore throat is nearly always viral. Throat irritation caused by post-nasal drainage or a cough is often viral. Sore throats without a fever are usually viral.

Signs a sore throat is likely viral (and requires no antibiotics)	
Presence of: laryngitis or hoarseness cough other cold symptoms	**Absence of:** fever swollen glands pus on tonsils

Americans want quick relief and often demand antibiotics, attributing their recovery to the medication, when likely they would have improved anyway. Most viral sore throats begin to improve within several days, and nearly always by a week. . . or two.

The exception to this is **infectious mononucleosis** (mono), which is also caused by a virus, but symptoms can persist for months. In young children (under the age of 10 or 12) mono usually acts like any other virus, and is often asymptomatic. Adults over the age of 30 are presumed to have had mono whether or not they've ever displayed symptoms. Typically, mono is a concern in teenagers and young adults, who may start with a "normal" sore throat, fatigue, and fever, but with symptoms persisting well beyond a week, sometimes leading to prolonged tiredness and a general feeling of unwellness that lasts for several weeks to a few months. Even mono requires no antibiotics, though occasionally if the throat is extremely swollen, steroids are useful in decreasing the swelling (prednisone, 40–60 mg daily, with food, for 3–10 days). Mono usually causes swollen glands in the sides of the neck (and often up the back of the neck). A third of patients have puffiness around the eyes. In many cases the illness reaches its peak within the first week or two, then gradually subsides. About 95% of patients recover from mono without any specific treatment. (Note – up to 1/3 of patients with mono also have strep (see below), which is difficult to prove without lab testing. Still, don't overlook symptoms of both.)

However, a person who continues to decline beyond the second week should be evaluated for additional problems. If respiratory symptoms continue to worsen, indicating the possibility of a secondary infection, a trial of antibiotics may be helpful. Some mono patients develop enlargement of the liver or spleen, which may cause abdominal tenderness. Trauma to the abdomen may cause these swollen organs to rupture (potentially lethal), hence the advice for patients with mono to avoid contact sports and similar rough activities. In an Armageddon setting, finding a surgeon to perform emergency repair of a ruptured spleen seems unlikely, so protecting one's organs from injury is essential.

Although viral sore throats are most common, **strep throat** is what strikes fear in a parent's heart. (Strangely, most parents don't quite know what they're afraid will happen.) Typically, a patient with streptococcal pharyngitis will have a fairly bad sore throat accompanied by fever and swollen neck glands. The throat may look terrible, with beefy red tonsils coated with white spots, or conversely, may appear barely irritated. Sometimes children will complain of a stomachache or headache rather than a sore throat. Two clues which make strep much more likely are 1) a rash, usually on the abdomen, that feels dry, like fine sandpaper, and 2) tiny red spots on the roof of the mouth. A patient with laryngitis (hoarseness or losing the voice) or a cough probably does not have strep throat.

Using the Centor Criteria for Strep Throat

There are 4 Centor criteria for the diagnosis of strep throat:

1. fever
2. NO cough
3. tender, swollen neck glands (anterior adenopathy)
4. pus (exudate) on the tonsils

If all 4 criteria are present, Group A beta-hemolytic streptococcus is likely.

Per the CDC, do not treat with antibiotics unless at least 3 criteria are met (unless testing has documented strep – but don't even check for strep unless at least 2 criteria are present)

In children the use of these criteria will over-diagnose strep throat.

What's the big deal about strep throat anyway? The symptoms are not necessarily worse than those of a virus, and most people get over strep throat without antibiotics, even though it is a bacterial infection! For those who do take antibiotics, the typical recovery period is only a day or two shorter than for those who do not.

The main concern has been **rheumatic fever**, an inflammatory and/or immunologic disorder triggered by a preceding group A Streptococcal infection (such as strep throat). Rheumatic fever can cause joint pain, fever, and most importantly, permanent heart valve damage or even death. Treatment includes long-term antibiotic treatment (for months to years) and sometimes heart valve replacement. Clearly, in an Armageddon situation neither of these options may be viable – so perhaps best to prevent the problem in the first place.

But is it preventable? The answer is yes, at least to a degree. Taking an appropriate antibiotic lessens the risk by about 50%.[12]

But how high is the risk anyway? Certainly if the odds were 50:50 that you would die from untreated strep throat, you'd want to take antibiotics. But what if the likelihood of rheumatic fever were closer to that of winning the lottery?

Fortunately, the incidence of this dread disease has declined over the past several decades. According to the CDC's Summary of Notifiable Diseases, United States, 2008, there were approximately 100 cases of rheumatic fever reported annually between the years 1985 and 1994, with a high of 1738 in 1977, at which time the U.S. population was 220,000,000, yielding an incidence of approximately 0.0008% (1738 cases/220,000,000 Americans/year). If taking antibiotics only decreases the risk of rheumatic fever by 50%, the untreated incidence might be double this, or 16 per million population. According to a recent article in the Journal of the American Medical Association[13] there are an estimated 7.3 million doctor visits annually for sore throats. Clearly if only 100 to

[12] Other sources say the risk is virtually eliminated by taking antibiotics.
[13] Antibiotic Treatment of Children with Sore Throat, JAMA. 2005;294(18):2315–2322. doi: 10.1001/jama.294.18.2315

1738 out of 7 million people with a sore throat develop rheumatic fever, the risk is quite low, at least in the United States. In developing countries the risk remains higher.

Another way of looking at the question is this: how many patients with strep throat must be treated with antibiotics to prevent one case of rheumatic fever? In an outbreak half a century ago it was estimated that 50–60 patients would need to be treated to prevent one case of rheumatic fever. Currently the number is probably in the thousands – or possibly much higher.

Does it make sense to treat a thousand cases of presumed strep throat (or perhaps many more) to prevent one case of rheumatic fever? In this day and age, where a round of antibiotics is $4 or less, perhaps so – currently doctors treat all cases of presumed or proven strep throat with antibiotics to decrease the likelihood of rheumatic fever weeks or months down the road. (Of course, a good number of patients with strep throat do not see a physician and so not all strep is actually treated.)

But if antibiotics become worth their weight in gold, is this approach reasonable? Should you use (squander?) your limited supply of medicine to possibly prevent a disease with less than a 1 in 1000 chance of occurring? You will have to decide yourself, based on your supply of medicine and conditions at the time. Of course, when little Susie is burning up with fever and moaning with a sore throat, emotion may rule the day.

This raises the next question, could a sore throat be something else? Could it be serious in the short term, perhaps in some other way?

The other serious but rare illnesses associated with a sore throat are **peritonsillar abscess** and **meningitis**. These diseases would be very difficult for a layman to assess, but in general would give the picture of a patient who is getting worse and worse – fever, headache, increased pain, possibly vomiting, drowsiness, or other mental changes. In such a case, strong antibiotics are worth a try (Augmentin, Ceftin, Suprax), but better to find a physician if at all possible. (Currently such a patient would be hospitalized and administered intravenous antibiotics.) One other cause of sore throat seen primarily in adults is **oral gonorrhea**, contracted through oral sex (see **Chapter 12** on STDs).

Most practicing doctors (in the U.S.) have never seen a case of **diphtheria**, though this disease would eventually re-emerge if immunizations were no longer an option. Diphtheria remains endemic in developing countries where widespread vaccination is difficult to achieve. Travel to, or unvaccinated visitors from, endemic areas are the most likely routes of spreading diphtheria.

Currently babies are immunized against diphtheria with every DPT vaccine, and adults receive a booster with each tetanus shot. (Update yours now with a Tdap if you haven't done so already.) A sore throat caused by diphtheria features a grayish exudate or membrane (coating of pus) on the tonsils or throat, and very swollen neck glands. The throat tissue bleeds if the membrane is wiped away. Although currently a case of diphtheria would be treated with an antitoxin as well as antibiotics, the antitoxin would not likely be available if the health care system collapses. Treating with penicillin (or erythromycin) for 14-days should (hopefully) be effective. Just as your doctor would, educate yourself regarding diagnosing this condition by searching the Web for images of diphtheria.

In summary, what is a reasonable approach to the post-Armageddon patient with a sore throat?

1. Do not administer antibiotics in a person who is only mildly ill.
2. If a cough or laryngitis is present, be confident the cause is viral.
3. If a bad sore throat, fever, and perhaps headache, a rash, or spots on

the roof of the mouth occur, it may be strep, but this does not necessarily require antibiotics either – be confident the risk of rheumatic fever is quite low (currently 1 in 1000 or less). The decision to administer antibiotics is not an emergency – waiting even a week to treat will not increase the risk of rheumatic fever. You have time to weigh your options.

4. Observe the patient for worsening symptoms – most sore throats are improving by two or three days. Even if not, as long as the patient is not worsening, antibiotics are probably not required. In a teenager or young adult, consider mono – which usually resolves without treatment as well (and is not improved with antibiotics).
5. In a patient weakened by other illness, such as significant asthma, *do* administer antibiotics if the person's condition is deteriorating.
6. Reserve your supply of antibiotics for life-threatening conditions, such as pneumonia and other illnesses discussed elsewhere.
7. If you do decide to use antibiotics for a sore throat, the following are among the best choices: penicillin, amoxicillin, amoxicillin-clavulanate, cephalexin, erythromycin, azithromycin, and clarithromycin. Treatment for five days is probably sufficient, although a 10-day treatment course is usually recommended.

Tongue, lips, gums, and cheeks (buccal mucosa)

Back to our patient . . . your two-year-old daughter, who hasn't eaten in days. Her neck glands are swollen and she has blisters on her lips and tongue. She'll barely take a sip of water. Is this strep or something else?

Many patients, both young and old, confuse infections of the mouth with infections of the throat. Everyone's heard of a sore throat, but what about a sore mouth? The tongue and inside of the cheeks (buccal mucosa) are rarely involved in acute respiratory conditions, at least not in a painful way. Certain infections (strep, measles) may cause red spots on the palate, but these do not hurt.

However, there are a few oral problems worth mentioning that do cause discomfort or concern: thrush, herpes simplex, herpangina, aphthous ulcers, and geographic tongue.

Almost the only infection that regularly involves the tongue is **thrush**, a yeast infection that occurs when the normal flora (normal germs) in the mouth is altered, or when the immune system is not functioning properly. This occurs most frequently after a round of antibiotics or corticosteroids, but is also seen in otherwise healthy infants and in adult denture wearers. Thrush usually begins with soreness of the tongue, along with a little redness. Eventually the tongue and sometimes the inner cheeks are coated or spotted with white, cottage-cheesy-looking matter. Prescription antifungal medicines, such as nystatin oral suspension (swish a half teaspoon around the mouth and swallow, 4 times daily) or Mycelex Troches (dissolve 1 in mouth, 5 times daily), are effective in clearing the infection. However, once the cause of thrush is removed, this overgrowth of yeast will usually resolve on its own. Denture wearers can usually prevent thrush by removing their dentures nightly and cleaning them thoroughly.

An old-time but effective over-the-counter remedy for thrush is gentian violet, a purple antifungal dye that will stain the lips and skin for a few days (and anything else it touches as well). The 1% and 2% solutions are available from pharmacies or online for $5 to $10. A single application is usually sufficient, but may be repeated after several days if needed. Simply swab the gentian violet all over the tongue and inner cheeks. The same medication may be used topically for vaginal yeast infections as well. Repeat the application in 5–10 days if symptoms have not completely resolved.

Two conditions often confused with thrush are simple **dry mouth** and **geographic tongue** (benign migratory glossitis). Dry mouth is often caused by medications (antidepressants, antihistamines, diuretics) or simply breathing through the mouth due to nasal congestion. Brushing the tongue or using chlorhexidine rinse will help a dry or coated tongue. When a patient complains of an odd pattern on the tongue, faintly resembling a map, this is likely geographic tongue. The cause is unknown and the map-like patterns may change from day to day. Geographic tongue is benign and requires no treatment. Sometimes it is a little uncomfortable, and rinsing the mouth with salt water or mouthwash may be comforting, but probably does not speed healing. It resolves in days to weeks on its own.

Whereas the above conditions cause minor discomfort, the next three may cause true pain, sometimes mimicking a sore throat when the posterior tongue or inner cheeks are involved.

Of these, **aphthous ulcers** (or aphthous stomatitis, canker sores) are probably the most common, those painful white ulcers that occur on the inside of the cheeks, the gum line, or around the edges of the tongue. These are not contagious and the cause is unknown. No specific treatment is necessary, although patients do obtain relief through the use of Aphthasol, Kenalog in Orabase, viscous lidocaine, topical Maalox, or over-the-counter teething gel.

Aphthous ulcers are often confused with oral herpes, which occasionally causes intraoral lesions, but primarily occurs on the outer mouth. **Herpes simplex** causes cold sores or fever blisters on or around the external lips, sometimes extending as high as the cheeks or nose. The lesions start as red bumps, blisters, or small pustules that develop into blisters that may ooze and crust over. These lesions may be painful (especially the first outbreak), and patients sometimes claim they can feel the sores coming on even before they break out. About half the adult population has herpes simplex type 1 in their systems, whether they know it or not. The sores tend to erupt during times of physical or emotional stress, including with colds or fever, hence the name. Oral herpes is contagious upon contact with the infected area (including self-inoculation), via kissing, sex, or simple touching.

Acyclovir is a prescription antiviral medication used to treat or prevent cold sores. It is available as an ointment or a capsule. Although younger people may be emotionally traumatized by the presence of a cold sore, treatment is primarily a cosmetic issue. Before the availability of antiviral medication, I never saw a patient develop a serious consequence of oral herpes, although this is theoretically a possibility (for example, herpes encephalitis). In my estimation, oral herpes is not worth worrying about at the end of the world as we know it, though others may feel differently. Generic acyclovir is inexpensive and most doctors are willing to prescribe long-term supplies for patients with recurrent eruptions. Treatment is most effective if started within the first few days of an outbreak (acyclovir dosage: 200 mg 5x/daily for treatment; 400 mg 1–3x/daily as prevention).

Finally, **herpangina** is a condition seen primarily in toddlers, but sometimes occurring in school-aged children and even adults. Herpangina can resemble a terrible case of canker sores. The inside of the mouth may be covered with scattered shallow white ulcers, much like the aphthous ulcers described above. However, herpangina is caused by a virus, generally one of the Coxsackie group A viruses. Antivirals used for herpes virus are not effective; neither are antibiotics. Treatment is symptomatic: acetaminophen for fever, headache, sore throat, and mouth pain, with attention to avoiding dehydration. Teething gel may offer some relief. Herpangina clears up on its own in about a week without treatment.

As for your 2-year-old daughter mentioned earlier, she has herpangina and is fine in a week.

Dental infection

In a post-Armageddon world (without dentists) the answer to dental infection will be either 1) suffering or 2) tooth extraction. Antibiotics can buy time, however, and often tone down an infection to tolerable levels. First-line antibiotics choices are penicillin, amoxicillin, or erythromycin. Other effective options are Augmentin, cephalexin, azithromycin, or clarithromycin.

Best answer: get your teeth in top shape now.

Dental problems and treatments are addressed in greater detail online at: www.armageddonmedicine.net.

Also, download "Where There Is No Dentist," free online at: http://www.hesperian.org/publications_download.php

Chapter 9 – Checklist

Items to include in your medical supplies:

- ☐ Tongue blades (or spoons) to depress the tongue to examine the pharynx (throat)
- ☐ Mirror and examination light (wind-up LED or solar-powered)
- ☐ Steroids, antibiotics, anti-yeast meds, pain relievers, teething gel – per text
- ☐ Gentian violet antifungal dye; gauze to make swab
- ☐ Antivirals: acyclovir or Valtrex
- ☐ Chlorhexidine oral rinse

Actions to take:

- ☐ Download the free book "Where There Is No Dentist" free online at http://www.hesperian.org/publications_download.php.
- ☐ Have all family and group members obtain needed dental care.

For the health professional, consider stockpiling:

- ☐ Rapid strep kits and rapid mono kits
  Traditional strep culture supplies
  Cotton swabs, tongue blades, appropriate antibiotics
  Microscope, stains, and supplies to do manual CBC and differential

Chapter 10

Ear Infection and Ear Pain

Otitis media, otitis externa, infected cysts, shingles, neuropathy, parotitis

For the second night in a row your child is burning up with fever and refusing to eat. The first night she cried for hours. The second, you cry along with her in frustration and fear. You'd take her to the ER – if there was one. You think it's her ear but just aren't sure. Should you use ear drops? Does she need an antibiotic? Is there any other way to make her feel better?

Ear pain

Ear pain, like dental pain, can make it difficult to focus on anything else. Relief becomes the only objective. Fortunately, despite the severity, ear pain is rarely a true emergency for the vast majority of both children and adults.

If you or your child complains of ear pain, the first decision point is whether the problem is in the ear canal, the middle ear, or possibly the throat, glands, skin, jaw, or nerves. Ear infections fall primarily into two types: **external ear infection** (otitis externa) and **middle ear infection** (otitis media). The treatment varies according to the part of the ear affected. **Ear lobe infections** are often tender, but not painful in the same way as otitis, and are very uncommon in children (except at the site of piercings). A **sore throat** or **swollen neck glands** can masquerade as ear pain, so it's always worth checking. In middle-aged and older adults, **shingles** and other **nerve irritations** must be considered. The hinge of the jaw sits right in front of the ear, and inflammation of the joint may cause local pain (**temporomandibular joint dysfunction,** or TMJ). Sometimes inflammation of the mumps gland in front of the ear (**parotitis**, or **parotiditis**) will cause ear pain.

Otitis externa

Otitis externa (external ear infection or swimmer's ear) involves only the ear canal, that is, the ear external to the ear drum (tympanic membrane), as opposed to internal structures. Ear canal infections are usually caused by minor trauma, such as a scratch in the ear canal or over-cleaning with Q-tips, or by a change in the pH (acid level) of the ear canal due to the presence of water. Always remember that earwax protects the ear canal. It is rarely necessary to remove excessive earwax, unless it is obstructing one's hearing significantly.

How can you distinguish an external ear canal infection from a deeper infection? The key elements are appropriate history, tenderness, discharge, odor, swelling, and lack of fever or cold symptoms. Often the patient gives a history of swimming or water in the ear. Thorough questioning may reveal the use of fingernails, hair pins, Q-tips, toothpicks, or other instruments to clean or scratch the ears. On exam, the ear is often quite tender to touch or on movement (wiggling the ear). Sometimes the ear feels wet, has a watery discharge, or perhaps an odor. The ear canal may become swollen, preventing the insertion of a Q-tip (which patients should not be using anyway). Typically this type of ear problem produces a significant amount of tenderness, and touching, pulling, or pressing on the ear increases the original pain. In contrast, middle ear infections generally cause little or no tenderness of the external ear structure.

For a mild swimmer's ear (external ear infection) simply leaving the ear alone may result in a cure. Do not insert swabs, or fingernails, or bobby pins, or anything else into your ear. For worse symptoms, a 50:50 mix of white vinegar and water dropped into the ear three or four times daily helps to reestablish the proper pH (acid level) of the ear, which promotes healing. If this is ineffective, prescription Cortisporin Otic Suspension is usually effective, but this medication may not be in your medicine chest. A reasonable alternative for moderately severe to severe symptoms would be a brief course of oral steroids (adult dose: 40–60 mg of prednisone daily for 3–4 days) in conjunction with topical application of the vinegar solution mentioned above.

Oral antibiotics are unlikely to be effective for a swimmer's ear, but infections inside the ear canal caused by trauma may respond to an oral antibiotic such as cephalexin (250–500 mg 3–4 times daily), trimethoprim-sulfamethoxazole DS (one tablet twice daily), or ciprofloxacin (500 mg twice daily) for five to ten days.

If the ear canal is full of debris or pus (which you won't be able to tell unless you have some way of looking, say with an otoscope), irrigating the ear gently with a 50:50 mix of white vinegar and warm water may be helpful. Keep in mind that this may increase discomfort in an already painful ear. It is not recommended if a middle ear infection is suspected, especially if the ear drum may be perforated. Blood or mucus (snot) coming from the ear is often a sign of perforation. Ear irrigation is best avoided in the great majority of cases.

Otitis media

The type of ear problem parents dread most is the middle ear infection. Who can bear to watch a feverish child moaning with pain? For those who've never experienced it, a middle ear infection can hurt as badly as a severe toothache, kidney stone, or even labor pains.

Ear infections of this type can occur alone, but commonly are a consequence of an upper respiratory infection causing congestion of the nose and eustachian tube. The normal ventilation of the middle ear is blocked, trapping bacteria between the ear drum and blocked eustachian tube. Fluid and/or pus accumulate, causing infection and putting pressure on the sensitive ear drum. This pressure is what causes much of the pain associated with a middle ear infection. As the pressure builds, the pain increases. Once it has reached its maximum, the tissues undergo no further stretching, and the symptom of pain recedes.

Eustachian tube dysfunction (ETD, or blocked eustachian tube) can cause similar but usually less severe ear pain, and without fever. In this case, the ventilation of the middle ear is again blocked, but infection does not occur. Rather, the trapped air is reabsorbed into the blood stream, putting a negative pressure on the ear drum, sucking it in (as opposed to outward pressure with otitis media). This causes a blocked sensation, much like that experienced with a change in altitude. ETD can occur alone, but occurs more commonly with colds and nasal allergies, and treatment is aimed at the underlying congestion.

For the past several decades, antibiotics had been considered mandatory for middle ear infections. Before the age of penicillin, however, lancing a bulging ear drum was standard treatment. This is a lost art among doctors about 60 years of age and younger, except among ENT (ear, nose, throat) specialists. Currently it is recognized that neither antibiotics nor lancing is required for a typical middle ear infection. For most adults and children, such infections will resolve on their own in an otherwise healthy patient, with antibiotics, lancing, and ear tubes reserved for persistent, recurrent, or severe infections.

This doesn't mean you must simply stand by and watch your child suffer. Pain relief is the goal of treatment in the first few days of illness. It's also another way to confirm the diagnosis. A more serious illness, such as meningitis, will not improve significantly with acetaminophen or ibuprofen. If the pain does not improve at all with either of these OTC medications (or a combination of both), and especially if the patient is growing sicker in other ways (cough, headache, vomiting, mental changes), seek professional attention if available. Many patients obtain significant relief by applying heat in the form of a hot water bottle or hot compresses. Avoid sleeping on a heating pad, which may cause serious burns, roasting your skin like a slow-cooker.

But what do you do if no doctor can be found? For a child or adult who appears seriously ill with an ear infection, a round of antibiotics is in order. Not knowing what microorganism is responsible, choosing an antibiotic that kills most common bacteria is desirable. Appropriate antibiotics for childhood ear infections include cephalexin, azithromycin, clarithromycin, trimethoprim-sulfamethoxazole, and in adults, perhaps ciprofloxacin. (Primary care physicians often use amoxicillin or erythromycin for initial treatment, but these may work little better than placebo.) Other choices include Augmentin, Omnicef, Ceftin, doxycycline, penicillin, tetracycline, and injectable Ceftriaxone. Oral antibiotics are generally used for 5 to 10 days. Although the pain should be relieved by then, the plugged feeling due to a swollen eustachian tube may persist for a few weeks. Usually no medication is required to relieve the swelling, although decongestants such as over-the-counter pseudoephedrine and/or Afrin nasal spray can be helpful.

Occasionally the pressure from a middle ear infection will cause the ear drum to burst on its own, which may relieve the pain to a great extent. Visualize the process more as a pimple popping than an explosion. The ear drum is stretched thin, sometimes to the point where the weakest part gives way, allowing the built-up fluid (blood-tinged mucus or pus) to escape (which may be confused with the fluid that drains from an external ear canal infection). Avoid irrigating an ear when this may have occurred, as you don't want to force water into the middle ear. In most cases a perforated ear drum will heal, just as the small incision from lancing an ear drum heals. For most adults and children, a middle ear infection that ruptures the ear drum will resolve without antibiotics.

It's always worth checking the throat and neck glands when a patient complains of ear pain. Sometimes an inflamed throat will feel like an earache rather than a sore throat. (For more on sore throats, see **Chapter 9**.) Likewise, swollen glands in the neck can be perceived as ear pain. Often an ear infection will cause the neck glands (lymph nodes) on the same side to swell and/or become tender.

When ear pain is mild and intermittent, especially when it is associated with yawning or swallowing, the problem is usually eustachian tube dysfunction (ETD) rather than infection. Your ears may pop or feel plugged, as on an airplane or travelling through the mountains. ETD often accompanies a cold or sinus infection, and responds well to pseudoephedrine. It does not require antibiotics unless it persists beyond several weeks, or is associated with a worsening or persistent respiratory infection.

Miscellaneous causes of ear pain

Other common causes of ear pain are **pimples** (small **abscesses**) in the ear canal and **scratches** of the ear, usually caused by bobby pins or fingernails. These generally heal on their own, and respond well to heat, ibuprofen, and acetaminophen. If symptoms persist, the ear drops and/or antibiotics mentioned above may be helpful.

Some people, especially those with a current or prior history of pierced ears, develop **cysts** in the ear lobe, which can become infected. A cyst alone will feel like a bump or knot, which rarely hurts unless it becomes infected. As with abscesses, lancing, not antibiotics, is the cure for an infected cyst (though sometimes antibiotics do resolve a tiny lesion). An infected cyst may also rupture, and thereby resolve the infection without medical intervention. Applying moist heat several times a day can speed this process along.

Inflammation or infection of the mumps gland (parotid gland, salivary gland), which sits at the angle of the jaw in front of the ear, sometimes causes ear pain. Again, antibiotics are rarely needed for **parotitis** (also called **parotiditis**). OTC pain meds, warm compresses, and warm salt-water mouth rinses are helpful.

In an adult, ear pain may also be caused by **shingles** (varicella zoster virus) in or around the ear, or an irritated nerve (**trigeminal neuralgia**). Shingles causes a localized, often painful rash resembling chicken pox (small red bumps that turn into blisters). Antiviral medication (acyclovir or Valtrex) may be helpful (see **Chapter 13** for details of treatment). The pain of trigeminal neuralgia is usually one-sided, often sporadic, typically stabbing or lancing, and can be quite severe, requiring narcotics. Daily antidepressant (amitriptyline and others) or anti-seizure medications (gabapentin, Lyrica) can decrease the level of discomfort over time. If significant pain persists beyond 3 to 7 days, seeing a doctor is a good idea. If none is available, the good news is that even these problems resolve on their own, sooner or later.

In summary, although ear pain can be severe, even if you do nothing at all, the problem has a good chance of resolving without medical intervention. Avoiding known triggers for ear infections is only sensible and will prevent many a problem: don't use Q-tips, fingernails, or bobby pins in your ears; keep your ears dry; avoid piercing the ears. Pain medications, decongestants, local heat, and patience help lessen the discomfort, with antibiotics reserved for severe or persistent infections.

Chapter 10 – Checklist

Items to include in your medical supplies:

☐ Otoscope with washable specula (consider LED light); batteries or power supply

☐ Hot water bottle (for relief of ear pain)

☐ Bulb syringe or large syringe for ear irrigation

☐ Hydrogen peroxide and white vinegar

☐ #11 scalpel or similar knife for lancing cysts

☐ OTC decongestants: Sudafed, Vicks, Afrin

☐ Prescription oral antibiotics per text

☐ Prescription topical antibiotics (Cortisporin Otic Suspension)

☐ Pain medications: OTC Tylenol, ibuprofen, naproxen and prescription tramadol and/or narcotics.

☐ Prescription gabapentin for treatment of chronic pain conditions (post-herpetic neuralgia or trigeminal neuralgia)

Chapter 11

Gastrointestinal Infection and Symptoms

Viral gastroenteritis, traveler's diarrhea, *C. diff*, diverticulitis, *Giardia*, worms, cholera

Your brother is the last to arrive, returning from south of the border shortly before the last flights were cancelled. Communication is down and curfew has been imposed. Fortunately, you have plenty of food, water, and firewood. Everyone is healthy and enjoying the camp-like atmosphere. Though you're not sure about the outside world, your little group is safe and secure . . . until, on the third day after his arrival, your brother falls ill.

Up all night with nuusea and diarrhea, he lies in bed, thoroughly miserable. The Tylenol you offer affords minimal relief from his fever and sweats. Suddenly things appear less certain. Though he's your brother, should you have turned him away? What do you do now?

Breaking protocol, even for a relative, may threaten your entire group's security. (Don't miss **Chapter 6** regarding quarantining new arrivals.) Given the likelihood of contagion, and though the damage may already be done by having exposed the entire group, your first step should be to isolate your brother from the others. Once this has been accomplished, the cause of his illness may be considered. Your brother may not be contagious, but at this point you have too little information to make a determination. The default answer is that he *is* contagious until proven otherwise.

Turning toward the differential diagnosis (that is, the various diagnoses that can cause a specific problem), under ordinary circumstances a simple stomach virus tops the list of suspect illnesses (at least in the U.S.) **Viral gastroenteritis** is currently by far the most common cause of acute nausea, vomiting, and/or diarrhea. Additional symptoms may include headache, fever, loss of appetite, gas, abdominal pain, and sometimes respiratory symptoms. Give it a day, or two, or three, and your own immunity kicks in, attacking the virus and ridding your body of disease. Occasionally symptoms will persist as long as a week or two, with gradual improvement. Staying hydrated is the most important consideration (see **Chapter 2** for a home rehydration therapy recipe). Anti-emetics (nausea drugs, such as meclizine) may be required to help keep fluids down and prevent dehydration. For viral gastroenteritis, loperamide (Imodium) is often useful to decrease the fluid loss and discomfort of diarrhea. Both these medications are available over the counter (or even cheaper by prescription) and should be included in your medical supplies.

But is this viral gastroenteritis? Can a doctor really tell just by looking?

Not actually. In coming to a diagnosis, physicians factor in patient history, physical exam, lab tests (if available), and most importantly, the likelihood of certain diseases. Could this be **cholera**? Perhaps, but it is exceedingly rare in the United States given our current sanitation standards. Cholera may become a consideration when trash pick-up ceases and sanitary conditions decline. Cholera is not likely to emerge this soon after a crisis (more on this later).

Could his illness be due to something else then, **food poisoning** perhaps? This question points to the importance of obtaining a complete medical history. For a person with nausea and diarrhea important questions to consider include:

- Was the patient exposed to others with a similar illness?
- If so, what was the course of their illness?
- Did the patient eat any suspect or unusual foods? If so, what?
- Given a history of travel, what diseases are common in areas a patient has visited?
- Has the person taken any medication?
- Has the person visited a hospital or other health care facility?
- Does the patient have a prior history of the same illness?
- Does the patient have a family history of a similar illness?

Your brother has just returned from "south of the border," a vague geographical description. Anyone traveling outside the U.S., or from one country to another, may pick up a strain of bacteria foreign to their digestive system that results in traveler's diarrhea. **Traveler's diarrhea** is usually due to an unfamiliar strain of *E. coli*, though *Shigella*, and *Campylobacter* infection are also common. Unless you have a clinical microbiologist or infectious disease specialist among you, you will have no clue as to which organism is present. (Your doctor wouldn't know either without laboratory facilities.)

Upon further questioning, your brother says, no, he's never had this illness before, nor has anyone in his family. There were, however, others he met while traveling who had developed similar symptoms, though the natives didn't seem to be susceptible. This raises the odds of his problem being caused by one of the bacteria listed above. Everyone knows antibiotics kill bacteria. Should you use your precious stockpile of ciprofloxacin or Zithromax (azithromycin) to help him? *One thing's for sure – you don't want to get what he's got.*

As with many medical situations, there is no single, simple answer. You must weigh all the available information and make the best informed decision you can. For the most part (about 90% of the time) traveler's diarrhea resolves without antibiotics within 5 days. Perhaps 10% of patients will have symptoms lasting a week or longer (and rarely up to a month – perhaps 2%). *Not* using antibiotics is a reasonable option (especially if you don't have any). In an Armageddon scenario, antibiotics should be reserved for life-threatening conditions.

Can traveler's diarrhea be life-threatening? Rarely. In a patient with bloody diarrhea or a high fever, the risk increases. Such a patient should probably be treated if symptoms persist beyond a few days or are worsening. If antibiotics are to be used for traveler's diarrhea, current recommendations are ciprofloxacin 500 mg or norfloxacin 400 mg twice daily for 3–5 days. Trimethoprim-sulfamethoxazole has been used in the past (1 DS tablet twice daily), but is less effective due to bacterial resistance. An over-the-counter alternative is Pepto-Bismol (bismuth subsalicylate), 1 fluid ounce (or two 262 mg tablets) every 30 minutes for up to eight doses per day, for 1–2 days, as needed. Bloody diarrhea that does not respond may be due to *Campylobacter*, which may require erythromycin (250–500 mg 3x daily for 5 days, though erythromycin may cause diarrhea in and of itself) or azithromycin (1000 mg in a single dose).

Another consideration is other members of your group. Are they all in good health? Anyone with diabetes, colitis, or in frail health in general is at greater risk of dehydration. Sometimes treating the index case will stave off spread of a contagious disease. However, in this case, the group has already been exposed, at least to a degree. Should you treat everyone then? Though there is no perfect answer, watchful waiting is probably the best answer for the group as a whole. If they develop symptoms later, they could be treated later. Traveler's diarrhea is not especially contagious, and is acquired through ingesting contaminated food or water. You should develop a consensus among your group regarding the treatment plan, based on your members and available supplies. For the index case (your brother), because a single dose of antibiotics is often effective, treating with one dose of ciprofloxacin 750 mg orally (one and a half of the 500-mg tablets, which may be split) or 500 mg of levofloxacin is reasonable. If this doesn't resolve his symptoms within a day or two, or if he develops bloody stools, a single 1,000-mg dose of azithromycin can be offered.

> *The group decides they would rather deplete their ciprofloxacin stock by two pills than run the risk of having to treat more people later. Upon offering the precious remedy you are surprised by your brother's reply, "I already took that for a week."*

Don't waste time on recriminations. When in misery a sick patient rarely thinks to offer all the information they might possess. You're the doctor now. You're supposed to figure it out. You should have asked this question before. (It's on the list.)

So what does this mean? It's unlikely he's suffering from traveler's diarrhea if he already took ciprofloxacin, though a resistant organism is possible. Have we ruled out food poisoning yet? Could he have eaten something that caused an infection?

Food poisoning is caused by toxins (chemical poisons) produced by bacteria. In some cases, the toxin was already present in the food (meaning the bacteria had already had the opportunity to multiply within the food, as may occur when leaving potato salad out in the sun all afternoon). This sort of food poisoning occurs shortly after eating, within 1–6 hours. Clearly this is not the current situation. The other type of food poisoning occurs 12 to 72 hours after the suspect food is ingested, after the bacteria have reproduced within the colon.

But food poisoning, like traveler's diarrhea, usually resolves on its own, and 7 days of ciprofloxacin (500 mg twice daily) would treat most cases. Still, resistant organisms (including *Campylobacter*) occur, and may require the use of erythromycin or azithromycin.

Botulism is a specific type of food poisoning likely to become more common when home canning becomes more popular, and causes neurologic symptoms as well as nausea and vomiting. It is dealt with in a separate chapter (see **Section Seven – Selected Conditions**).

You confer as a group and decide, again, that you would rather part with a limited amount of antibiotics than run the risk of treating more people later. Whether it's food poisoning or traveler's diarrhea, you hope a 1,000-mg dose of azithromycin does the trick.

Since your brother is still nauseated, you insist he take a dose of meclizine an hour before administering the large antibiotic dose. No sense having him vomit up medicine worth its weight in gold (or at least silver).

Now it's watch and wait. Your brother keeps the medicine down and falls asleep. You hope by morning he's feeling better. The group is becoming angry and is talking about putting him out. Better one person die than everyone. It's day 3 already and they decide they'll give him two more days to recover – unless someone else gets sick first.

As the designated contact person, you enter his sickroom at dawn. A terrible odor greets you. "I couldn't help it," your brother says, indicating the stains on the bed sheets. "I think I'm dying."

Any hospital nurse can make the diagnosis now. The stench of C. *diff* is practically wafting up from the page. Your brother may be right – he *might* die without treatment.

C. diff, or *Clostridium difficile*, colitis occurs almost exclusively in people who 1) have been exposed to other ill patients (especially those in hospital or extended care facilities); or 2) those who have previously taken antibiotics for some other diagnosis, such as a respiratory or skin infection. The antibiotics kill off the normal flora (good germs) in the bowel, leaving only resistant bacteria, which can thrive and take over (but only if they are already present within the gut). *C. diff* produces a toxin that causes diarrhea, often with abdominal cramping and fever. When present in large numbers, *C. diff* bacteria lend the stools a characteristic, offensive odor somewhat different than that of normal diarrhea. The offending bacteria must be eradicated (or at least subdued) in order to relieve symptoms.

The traditional treatment of C. *diff* infection is oral metronidazole (500 mg, 3–4 times daily for 5 to 10 days). Although I did just say that C. *diff* is caused by taking antibiotics, it is also cured by this unusual antibiotic that doctors reserve for very specific infections. (Oral vancomycin is also effective but much more costly and I have not recommended it for stockpiling.) *C. diff* colitis is one situation when you do *not* want to slow down the diarrhea by using Imodium, in order to allow the infection to be transported out of the body as quickly as possible.

What if you don't have metronidazole on hand? Without treatment, an elderly, debilitated patient is likely to succumb to C. *diff* colitis. However, a younger, otherwise healthy individual may be able to overcome it on their own. I imagine this happens now and then in the community, in persons who have a relatively mild case and do not seek medical care. Personally, however, I have not seen a documented case of spontaneous remission. (It is difficult to document if the patient does not seek treatment.)

Recently attention has been given to an alternative treatment, namely fecal transplant, or trans*poo*sion. Yes, it's just what it sounds like: the transplantation of feces from one person to another (see **Chapter 30** on **Herbal Therapy and Other Natural Remedies**). Currently the focus of fecal transplant is on those patients with recurrent or persistent C. *diff* infection, but it could also be used in someone with a first-time occurrence. Hopefully you're not gagging as you read. Details of fecal transplantation are given in the above-referenced chapter.

> *As for your brother, you treat him with a week's worth of metronidazole, he recovers, no one else becomes ill, and he proves to be a vital, contributing member of your community.*

Thus far we have covered the common infectious causes of acute nausea, vomiting, and diarrhea: viral gastroenteritis, traveler's diarrhea, food poisoning, and C. *diff* colitis. A few other conditions merit discussion as well.

In people middle-aged and older, **diverticulitis** is another common cause of diarrhea, often associated with abdominal cramping, nausea, and sometimes fever or bloody, maroon-colored stools. Diverticulitis is infection of small pouches along the intestine (diverticuli) that bubble out as weakness in the intestine as we age, much like tiny internal hernias. Food particles and bacteria may become trapped in these pouches where infection can propagate. Some patients are convinced that seeds (or other hard, small food items which don't digest well) bring on their symptoms. Although not well-supported by medical research, avoiding popcorn, nuts, sesame seeds, etc. may be prudent in the patient with recurrent diverticulitis, especially when emergency treatment is unavailable.

The symptoms of diverticulitis may come on quickly, or "simmer" a few weeks before causing sufficient distress to induce a patient to see a doctor. Quite often patients attribute their symptoms to ordinary diarrhea or a stomach virus to start. When their symptoms don't resolve as expected, they seek medical care.

Typically a patient's abdomen is at least mildly tender, though may be quite tender, more commonly toward the left side, but either side is possible. This is, admittedly, not very specific. Additional treatable causes of abdominal tenderness should be considered, including urinary tract infection, pelvic infection, and all the conditions mentioned above. (I say treatable causes because certain problems, such as perforated colon or intestinal infarct, will simply be fatal without surgical care.)

In the modern era, patients who visit an emergency room will likely have a CBC (blood count), stool hemoccult test (looking for blood in the stool, which often occurs with diverticulitis), and possibly a CAT scan performed. You will likely have none of these tests at your disposal. In a person without another reason for infection (travel, food poisoning, antibiotic use, urinary symptoms), the diagnosis of diverticulitis should be considered in anyone about 40 years of age or older who presents with (usually left-sided) abdominal pain, tenderness, diarrhea, and possibly fever.

The bacteria involved in diverticulitis are the same ones that are found in the intestine; therefore antibiotics that kill these germs are prescribed. Sometimes a single antibiotic such as Augmentin (500 mg three times daily) or Avelox (400 mg once daily) is effective, although I prefer using combination therapy of either TMP-SMX DS or ciprofloxacin 500 mg twice daily, plus metronidazole 500 mg 3–4 daily. (Patients on metronidazole must avoid alcohol or run the risk of serious vomiting.) Continuing the antibiotics for 3–4 days after symptoms have resolved is a good idea. Keep in mind that if you use only a single antibiotic, a *C. diff* infection may emerge, necessitating the use of metronidazole anyway.

Lastly, one infection I rarely see and one I've never encountered: giardiasis and cholera.

Giardiasis is fairly common in the United States, but not among my own patient population. Still, I look for it in anyone who has persistent or chronic diarrhea. Now and then I find it. Each year about 19,000 cases are reported to the CDC (see www.cdc.gov) but no doubt many, perhaps most, go unreported. Giardiasis causes both acute and chronic diarrhea, though as many as half of infected people have no apparent symptoms (making it all the easier to spread). It is the most common human protozoal infection in the U.S., occurring throughout the continent, but more so in northern states. Children under age 10, and adults ages 35–44 show the highest incidence of infection, which peaks in summer months, coincident with summer recreational water use.

The *Giardia lamblia* flagellate protozoal infection is spread primarily via contaminated water sources or occasionally food, as well as by close person-to-person contact. As few as 10 cysts may result in infection. With sanitation a great concern with the demise of modern society, allowing your children to swim in a community lake may be risking infection. Pets *may* be a reservoir for the infection, but this is unproven.

How will you know if you or your children have giardiasis? You probably won't, at least not at first. If acute diarrhea develops, it may clear within a few days or a few weeks. Symptoms may come on gradually after an incubation period of 1 to 3 weeks, or hit all at once. Initially diarrhea caused by giardia should be treated like an intestinal virus (since it acts like an intestinal virus). Attention to prevention of dehydration is vital, but since fever and vomiting are uncommon, replenishing fluids orally is usually possible.

However, if symptoms (cramping, gas, nausea, loss of appetite, frothy or greasy diarrhea, weight loss) persist beyond a few weeks, empiric treatment for giardiasis should be considered. Unless you have a skilled biologist, doctor, or lab tech on hand, you will not be able to make a certain diagnosis. Under the microscope, an examination of liquid stool may show motile trophozoites or possibly cysts.

The only effective antibiotic likely to be in your survivor's medical kit is metronidazole, which is effective at a dose of 250 mg given three times daily with food for 5–7 days. Other antibiotics, such as penicillin, do not kill *Giardia lamblia*, so don't bother. Alternative treatments include tinidazole (2 gm once), nitazoxanide (500 mg twice daily for 3 days), furazolidone (100 mg four times daily for 7 days), albendazole (400 mg daily for 5 days), and paromomycin (500 mg three times daily for 7 days). Of course, it is unlikely you will have these on hand, and your doctor is unlikely to prescribe them for stockpiling. Albendazole, however, is used as a de-wormer for sheep and cattle and might be considered if no human therapy is available.

Speaking of albendazole, let's take a detour and worm our way over to helminthic infections (**worms**). Most of us in America take it for granted that we don't now and will never have worms. This may change when sanitation becomes an issue. Albendazole, mentioned above, is also useful for pinworms and roundworms (400 mg as a single dose), the most common worms encountered in the U.S. **Pinworms** are those tiny, short (quarter-inch) worms that cause rectal itching, especially at night. "Starving maggots" is a vivid descriptor. Pinworms are spread person to person, especially among young children who don't wash their hands after wiping, or who scratch their bottoms, then return to play with other children. All close contacts with an infected individual should be treated, since both asymptomatic infection and re-infection are common.

Roundworms are much longer, reminiscent of earthworms, but with a more substantial consistency, and the potential to attain lengths of over a foot! The life cycle begins when eggs, present in contaminated food, are ingested. The larvae hatch in the small intestine, make their way into the bloodstream, are carried to the lungs, then back to the GI tract, where they mature into worms. *Now here's the gross part:* the diagnosis is usually made when adult roundworms wriggle out the mouth, nose, or anus. One such experience is probably enough to convince you of the desirability of treatment. Other symptoms of roundworms include non-specific abdominal pain, intestinal blockage, and malnutrition. Again, since many infections are asymptomatic (. . . at least to start with), treating all close contacts is advisable lest the horror be repeated.

Humans are also subject to various other helminthic infections, including tapeworms, whipworms, and flukes. You can't be expected to become an expert on every possible infection. Fortunately, albendazole is effective for a variety of intestinal worms. Since albendazole can be obtained (for veterinary use) without a prescription, you may want to have this on hand and use it for any worm infection you experience.

Returning to giardia, will simple chlorination sterilize drinking water contaminated with *Giardia lamblia* organisms or cysts? Probably not. Filtration using an absolute 1 micron pore size is effective, as is boiling water for about 1 minute (3 minutes for elevations above one mile). Young mothers need to think about how they'll be dealing with the diaper situation. With disposables a thing of the past, appropriate washing of both diapers and hands is essential. While stocking up on bleach is a good idea, a kettle to boil diapers should be considered.

And now for the real killer: **cholera.** Most American doctors have never seen a case of cholera, myself included, but Armageddon may change that.

Cholera is exceedingly rare in the U.S. with only about 7 cases reported annually between 2003–2007 (per the CDC). But how quickly can this change? The aftermath of the January 2010 earthquake in Haiti sheds some light on the question. Again per the CDC, Haiti had not had a cholera epidemic in at least a century. But with the crowded living conditions and poor sanitation, as of October 21, 2010 an epidemic had been identified. By six weeks later 91,770 cases had been reported, 43,243 of whom had been hospitalized – this from a country a little smaller than my home state of Ohio!

If cholera is just another diarrheal disease, what's the big deal? Won't a little Imodium and Gatorade put things to right? Is a 2–3% case-fatality rate something to worry about? What would you say if you knew it could kill you within two hours? In Haiti, of those who died, the median time to death was a mere eight hours after onset of symptoms.

The CDC thought the problem important enough to provide an entire training manual free, online as of January 2011. You can access the 50-page **Haiti Cholera Training Manual: A Full Course for Healthcare Providers** online at: http://www.cdc.gov/haiticholera/pdf/haiticholera_trainingmanual_en.pdf.

Here are a few highlights from the manual:

1. Without laboratory examination to detect the *Vibrio cholerae* bacterium (a gram-negative rod), the diagnosis must be made clinically (according to symptoms only).
2. Transmission occurs through contaminated water or food (not person to person). Contamination of water with feces from infected individuals is the usual cause, although the organism can live in warm coastal waters as well.
3. Profuse watery diarrhea may rapidly produce dehydration, electrolyte loss with muscle cramping, acidosis, vomiting, and death.
4. Although this is a bacterial infection, the mainstay of treatment is oral (or I.V.) rehydration therapy. If using I.V. fluids, Ringer's Lactate is preferred.
5. Moderate to severely ill patients should receive antibiotic therapy to help decrease diarrhea volume and duration (doxycycline 300 mg x 1 dose; or azithromycin 1 gm x 1 dose; or tetracycline or erythromycin 500 mg 4x daily for 3 days)
6. Avoid anti-diarrheal medicines, which may prolong cholera infection.

With the above reference available free, there is little reason to go into detail here. The main point is to have oral rehydration therapy available and to administer it liberally, as much as one liter per hour if fluid loss is excessive. Again, weighing the patient if at all possible is the best way to determine if fluid replacement is adequate. Cholera is a secretory diarrhea, meaning it will cause diarrheal fluid loss far beyond the amount of fluids normally ingested. The diarrhea may be so severe as to make it difficult for the patient to reach the bathroom. A hole cut in a cot, with a collecting pan underneath, is one solution to uncontrollable diarrhea.

Prevention of spread is vital. As a caregiver, you certainly don't want to become infected. Hopefully you have several boxes of disposable gloves available, or at least a pair of Playtex gloves. Hand-washing is essential to limiting spread of the disease – especially to yourself.

We've covered viruses, bacteria, food poisoning, worms, and giardiasis – most of the common gastrointestinal infections you're likely to encounter. What have we missed? A few more acute infections to consider include:

1. **Acute hepatitis** – which may cause nausea, weight loss, right-sided abdominal pain, jaundice, and occasionally death. Acute hepatitis is usually viral, but antiviral treatment is ineffective. The answer is to get vaccinated *now* against hepatitis A and B. No vaccine is available for hepatitis C.
2. **Appendicitis** – causing lower abdominal pain (usually right-sided), fever, and nausea. Without surgery, the appendix often bursts, spewing infection into the abdominal cavity, which is generally fatal. If surgery is not an option, your only hope may be to try antibiotics

(same as those used in diverticulitis, see above), though the odds of this working are slim.

3. **Urinary tract infections** (see next chapter)
4. **Female infections** (see **Chapters 12** and **24**)
5. **Gallbladder infections** – causing upper abdominal pain, fever, and bloating. These are often associated with **gallstones**. Small stones can pass on their own, large ones cannot exit the gallbladder, but mid-size stones may get stuck in the ducts, causing back-up of digestive juices, sometimes resulting in death. If you're worried about TEOTWAWKI and know you already have gallstones, you'd best have your gallbladder removed. Symptoms of gallbladder infection (cholecystitis) include severe abdominal pain, usually in the right upper abdomen, along with nausea, vomiting, fever, and sometimes jaundice (yellowed skin and/or eyes). The pain of gallbladder infection usually comes on within hours, as opposed to days as in the case of hepatitis. A large or high-fat meal may precipitate symptoms. Of note, cholecystitis actually means inflammation of the gallbladder, with infection being only one cause. Many gallbladder attacks subside on their own within 12–18 hours and do not require antibiotics. If symptoms persist, antibiotics may be warranted. Hopefully, administering an anti-nausea drug such as meclizine (25–50 mg) first may allow the patient to tolerate oral antibiotics (3rd-generation cephalosporin, Augmentin, cephalexin, ciprofloxacin, or TMP-SMX plus metronidazole), although often when a patient is vomiting, I.V. antibiotics are necessary (3rd-generation cephalosporin plus metronidazole).

Although other infections exist, the above delineates the most common that occur in generally healthy individuals. Patients with chronic liver disease, inflammatory bowel disease, diabetes, chronic kidney disease, and immune-deficiency diseases may be prone to unusual or difficult to treat infections, which are beyond the scope of this book.

Chapter 11 – Checklist

Items to include in your medical supplies:

- ☐ Medications:
  Pepto-Bismol, liquid and tablets
  Meclizine for nausea and Imodium for diarrhea (both available OTC or Rx)

- ☐ Chlorine bleach

- ☐ Absolute 1 micron water filter

- ☐ Cotton diapers and kettle to boil them in

- ☐ Prescription oral antibiotics, as listed, including metronidazole

- ☐ Veterinary albendazole (available OTC)

- ☐ Hydration supplies: salt, sugar, fruit juice, and water for oral rehydration solution
  Ringer's Lactate solution, along with tubing and supplies, for I.V. hydration

- ☐ Disposable or reusable plastic gloves

Actions to take:

- ☐ Print out and store with your medical supplies:
  Haiti Cholera Training Manual: A Full Course for Healthcare Providers online at: http://www.cdc.gov/haiticholera/pdf/haiticholera_trainingmanual_en.pdf.

- ☐ Immunize you and your family against hepatitis A and B

Chapter 12

Urinary and Reproductive Infections

Bladder, kidneys, STDs, prostate

Less than a week since the grid collapsed your new bride begins to complain of lower abdominal pain. She's been a little nauseated and her period is a day or two late. Now her back is starting to hurt and she's lost all interest in sex. By the third day you begin to worry something's really wrong, but it's twenty miles to the nearest doctor – if he's even in. Do her symptoms point to a specific diagnosis?

As always, the first thing to do is obtain a complete history. Doctors would look for the most common causes first, always keeping in mind less frequently encountered situations.

The two most common causes of lower abdominal pain with accompanying nausea are bladder infections and intestinal viruses. Other conditions to consider include kidney infection, pelvic infection, sexually transmitted diseases, early pregnancy, and all the conditions covered in the previous chapter.

An intestinal virus causing lower abdominal pain would probably have diarrhea as a symptom as well. Lacking this, we should focus our attention first on urinary conditions.

Cystitis (bladder infection) is exceedingly common in women of all ages. Is your wife having burning on urination, other pain with urination, malodorous urine, or frequent urination? She might have been too modest to mention these typical symptoms. However, some women simply don't experience them, especially elderly women, who may just "feel bad" or seem confused.

Honeymoon cystitis is a special case of cystitis related to recent onset of (or increased) sexual activity, once reserved for the honeymoon period. The mechanics of sexual intercourse allow the introduction of local (skin, vaginal, fecal) bacteria into the female urethra and bladder, often resulting in infection. With treatment options likely to be limited, it behooves all sexually active women to make sure they empty their bladder after vaginal sexual intercourse.

Visually inspecting the urine is a good idea, though this may or may not be helpful. Totally clear, normal-smelling urine may still be infected, although cloudy malodorous urine is more suspicious. The appearance of the urine is as related to fluid intake as it is to infection, with clear urine often reflecting large fluid intake, and a darker color a sign of more concentrated urine. Dark or pink urine may also reflect the presence of blood, a sign of infection, kidney stones, or menstrual bleeding.

You may want to purchase the same colorimetric urine testing strips doctors use, such as Multistix 10 SG, which will detect the presence of blood, white blood cells, and nitrites, all indicators of infection. They are available online (Amazon and elsewhere) and perhaps in your local pharmacy, 100 strips for under $40. Kits with fewer test strips are also available, but per-test cost is much higher. The official shelf-life of these chemical test strips is only a year or two, but if stored as directed, they may be stable for several years.

The fortunate patient with cystitis *does* have burning or painful urination. I say fortunate because these patients have an "early warning system," and thus can begin treating themselves at the first sign of infection. If symptoms are caught right away, sometimes fluids alone can flush the infection out of the system. Drinking a gallon of water a day may prevent the need for antibiotics. I have seen patients cure themselves this way. Cranberry juice seems to help some, but not all, urine infections, depending on the type of bacteria present. There is little harm in trying, although I would not suggest putting off antibiotic use for more than a few days, especially if symptoms are worsening.

However, many patients do require antibiotics, especially those who are prone to recurrent infection. In this case, the combination of drinking extra fluids plus early antibiotic treatment often prevents a more serious condition from developing. Whereas one or two doses of antibiotics may suffice with early treatment, a more established infection may require 5, 7, 10, or more days of antibiotic therapy, a concern when supplies are limited.

How will you know which germ is present and which antibiotic to use? You won't without culturing, which is unlikely to be available. Therefore, treating with an antibiotic that is known to kill typical urinary bacteria is advisable. There is no set length of treatment. If symptoms are gone in 24 hours, there's little to be gained by finishing a 7-day course of antibiotics; three days usually suffices, or sometimes even one. First-line antibiotic choices are nitrofurantoin, TMP-SMX, and amoxicillin (especially in children and pregnant women). Second-line choices are ciprofloxacin, Levaquin, or Augmentin. Cephalexin is also often effective, as are most other cephalosporins.

For women with recurrent bladder infections causing severe burning, laying in a supply of over-the-counter Azo is a good idea. Azo is a lower dose of the same medication doctors prescribe (Pyridium, phenazopyridine). Keep in mind that although Azo provides rapid relief of symptoms, it is not curative, and only hides the infection until antibiotics kick in.

> *Your wife admits to a little burning on urination, and thinks she remembers having a urinary infection once before. You decide to try a sulfa drug, TMP-SMX DS, twice daily. By the third day of antibiotics, though, she's no better, even with plenty of fluids. In fact her abdomen is more tender, and her nausea and back pain are perhaps a little worse. Did you choose the wrong antibiotic? Could something else be wrong?*

There's no sense blaming yourself. The sulfa drug is a reasonable choice, but it doesn't appear to be working. What does this mean? Perhaps she has a resistant urinary infection, but maybe the diagnosis is wrong. Does it make any difference if this is a kidney infection instead of a bladder infection?

Most cases of cystitis don't cause back pain – but some do. Most bladder infections don't cause significant nausea and fever – but some do. However, these symptoms do point toward the possibility of a kidney infection, a potentially serious situation. Kidney pain is normally felt in the flanks (or sides), typically just below the ribs in the back. Tapping on the kidneys usually produces more tenderness than palpating (pressing) does. Pounding lightly over the kidneys with the fleshy part of the fist is effective for identifying kidney tenderness in most patients. Untreated or insufficiently treated bladder infections often progress to kidney infections, although sometimes kidney infection occurs without apparent bladder infection.

Fortunately, the same antibiotics that work for bladder infections work for kidney infections. Whether or not your wife has tenderness over her kidneys, a change in antibiotics to a second-line drug is the next step.

Since you have more Augmentin on hand than any other of the second-line medications, you start your wife on 500 mg three times daily. She's able to keep the first seven doses down, but her nausea seems to be worsening, and by the third day she's actually vomiting. Not only that, but the lower abdominal pain actually seems worse, and now she admits to a vaginal discharge. You start to worry about dehydration and ponder a trip to the distant doctor, but without communication, you still have no idea if he's there. Why isn't she getting better? Does she need I.V. antibiotics? Could she die without them?

By now a kidney infection due to a susceptible organism should be improving, at least a little. Could the problem still be due to resistant urinary bacteria? That is certainly possible. But before jumping to that conclusion, let's return to the history.

With the primary source of pain just above the pubic bone, you need to consider the pelvic organs as well. Could your wife be pregnant? Could the nausea be morning sickness? She said her period was a day or two late. Has it started yet? No? Why not? Does she have a history of irregular periods? No? Was her previous period normal?

Assuming your wife's period has not yet come (now making her about a week overdue), the question of pregnancy arises. But at five weeks gestation, even if an ultrasound machine were available, it is unlikely to detect either a normal or ectopic (tubal) pregnancy. An over-the-counter pregnancy test should be accurate at five weeks gestation, but odds are, you don't have one. (Add OTC pregnancy test kits to your list of supplies.)

Perhaps a little more history is in order.

Your wife said she was a virgin when she married you, and you believe her. You both want children, but aren't sure how soon. You figure, if it happens, it happens. But could your wife be on birth control? When you ask, she admits to starting the pill on the first day of her last period. And yes, she's somehow still taking them, despite her vomiting.

Breathe a sigh of relief. One problem down. The odds of pregnancy in a person consistently taking birth control pills are very low. However, amenorrhea (lack of a period) is not uncommon, especially in women who've just started birth control pills.

How about some questions for you? Were you also a virgin when you married her? Is there any possibility you've transmitted an STD (sexually transmitted disease)?

No, you blush, you were not a virgin. Once your previous girlfriend was diagnosed with chlamydia and advised you to be treated as well, but lacking symptoms yourself, you chose not to, and decided to use condoms instead. You've still never had symptoms. Surely you're not to blame for your wife's illness.

Maybe, maybe not. But pelvic infection due to *Chlamydia trachomatis or N. gonorrhoeae* can cause every symptom your wife is experiencing. Whereas **gonorrhea** will likely make itself known in both men and women, **chlamydia** can linger without symptoms for months to years. It can be spread from partner to partner, sometimes resulting in symptoms, sometimes not.

How can you tell if your wife has a urinary infection or pelvic inflammatory disease? The next step a physician would take is to perform a pelvic exam. You can do a limited one yourself.

To perform a limited pelvic exam, after obtaining permission from your wife (or patient), insert your index and third finger of your dominant (preferably gloved) hand into the vagina. If lubricant is unavailable (don't forget to stock KY), wet your hand first to lessen friction. Gently feel for the cervix, a rounded structure which has the consistency of the end of your nose. While applying gentle pressure to the side of the cervix, try to move it from side to side a little. With a urinary infection this should produce little if any pain. With a pelvic infection, it often causes significant discomfort (as would having sex).

As you withdraw your hand, observe any discharge clinging to your glove. Clear or white mucus is normal (the same material as when blowing your nose). Yellow or green is abnormal and may indicate a bacterial infection. A thick white discharge is often a sign of yeast infection, especially in a person who's been on an antibiotic several days already.

(Note – sometimes a thick white discharge is merely the accumulation of vaginal cells that have been shed, similar to a sunburn that has peeled. Without other symptoms, such as itching, burning, or local irritation, no treatment is necessary.)

Your wife permits the exam, but nearly jumps off the bed when you touch her cervix. You notice both a thick white discharge and some yellow mucus on your gloved hand.

A person can certainly have a yeast infection *and* a bacterial infection at the same time. If she's also having vaginal itching, she probably does have a yeast infection, which will likely worsen if she takes additional antibiotics. But a yeast infection "never killed anyone" (not quite true, but close), whereas an untreated pelvic infection potentially may.

Still, with all the vomiting, can you get your wife to hold down another antibiotic?

She's willing to try, though she's still quite nauseated. She wonders if the Augmentin may have caused the vomiting.

Good chance it did. Augmentin is preferably given with food, but even then, the clavulanate component of the pill often causes GI upset.

Per the 2010 CDC guidelines, outpatient treatment of pelvic inflammatory disease ideally consists of two concurrent antibiotics for 14 days: 1) ofloxacin (400 mg twice daily) or levofloxacin (500 mg once daily); plus 2) metronidazole (500 mg twice daily). Ciprofloxacin (500 mg twice daily) is much less expensive than ofloxacin or levofloxacin and may be an effective substitute, but resistance is a concern, as is also true of doxycycline (100 mg twice daily) and azithromycin (1000 mg in a single dose – possibly repeat in 4 to 7 days).

Since the introduction of levofloxacin (Levaquin) and moxifloxacin (Avelox), ofloxacin (Floxin) is little used, at least in my community. Levaquin and Avelox remain brand-name only and are quite expensive (about $150–200 for about 10 days of treatment). However, Avelox is effective as monotherapy, that is, without the metronidazole. Floxin runs about $65 for the same quantity, but ciprofloxacin costs as little as $4 (hence its overuse, and hence the bacterial resistance). The checklist at the end of this chapter includes a Web site with a free 116-page download outlining numerous other treatment options, as well as management of all common STDs.

Fortunately you have ciprofloxacin and metronidazole on hand. Though your wife gags a bit, she is able to keep both down. By the third day, she's starting to feel a little better, and after a week feels back to her normal self (except for vaginal itching). Should you take the same drugs yourself? And what about her yeast infection?

Men with chlamydia (or women with minimal or absent symptoms) should take one of the regimens above, *but* generally don't require the metronidazole. Inexpensive treatments include ciprofloxacin, doxycycline, and azithromycin; more expensive but effective options include ofloxacin, Avelox, and Levaquin. Metronidazole may be added if a one drug alone is ineffective.

As for yeast, it is a bothersome but not life-threatening symptom. The OTC anti-yeast or antifungal creams (Monistat, Gyne-Lotrimin, Mycelex) are certainly effective. Gentian violet, a purple dye (OTC), is usually curative in a single topical application applied to the vagina and surrounding tissues.

Next, suppose rather than your wife, your father complained he was having frequent urination with a little burning. He's not running a fever, but is getting up at night to urinate, and sometimes feels he can't empty his bladder completely. Should you again suspect a simple bladder infection or chlamydia?

The answer to this question depends somewhat on the age of your father. Any man over the age of about 50 is likely to be suffering from a chronic prostate problem. Younger men may have an acute (or chronic) prostate problem, a urinary infection, or an STD.

Starting with the older generation first: although they, too, could acquire any of the sexually transmitted diseases under discussion, they're usually having less frequent sex and with fewer partners, so the risk is greatly diminished. But what they do experience is the gradual enlargement of the prostate, which presses on the urinary tract, causing obstruction or irritation. Not all urinary symptoms are due to infection. A slowing of the urinary stream that comes on over the course of years, so gradually that it is barely noticed, is usually an enlarged prostate without infection, or **benign prostatic hypertrophy**. Antibiotics won't improve this condition unless there is concurrent infection. Of the OTC meds available, saw palmetto is the only one likely to help, and even then it takes months. The alpha-blockers Flomax (tamsulosin), Hytrin (terazosin), and Cardura (doxazosin) can help more quickly, within days to weeks, but do require a prescription. Any middle-aged or older man experiencing chronic urinary symptoms should ask their physician about stockpiling one of these alpha-blockers. At a minimum, lay in a lifetime supply of saw palmetto, an herb which slows the growth of the prostate, which continues throughout life. Proscar and Avodart are prescription drugs that accomplish the same thing (probably more effectively), but at a much greater expense ($30–130/month).

Urinary symptoms that come on more rapidly, over days to weeks, may signify a true prostate infection. Naturally you may not know for sure whether infection is present – doctors don't necessarily know either. We often prescribe a therapeutic trial of an antibiotic to see if it helps. Antibiotics useful for **chronic prostate infections (chronic prostatitis)** include ciprofloxacin (500 mg twice daily) (or Levaquin 500 mg daily, or Avelox 400 mg daily, both expensive), TMP-SMX DS (one twice daily), or doxycycline (100 mg twice daily). Sometimes other antibiotics work, including Augmentin or cephalexin. Improvement should be noted within about 10 days of use. If the antibiotic hasn't helped at least a little by then, it probably isn't going to do so. If antibiotics do help, they should be continued at least two weeks, though up to a month may be needed for ciprofloxacin, or even longer for TMP-SMX DS or doxycycline.

Chronic prostatitis is a good example of a condition where you'll want to weigh the pros and cons of using your antibiotic supply. Although the condition is uncomfortable, it is seldom life-threatening, and often recurs. You could end up using more antibiotics for this aggravating condition than it would take to treat 3–4 cases of life-threatening pneumonia. If you're a patient suffering from recurring chronic prostatitis, you should take it upon yourself to acquire your own supply of antibiotics, as it would be unfair to expect others to share with you in the quantity that you would need to effect relief (which is unlikely to be permanent). Although usually indicated for prostatic enlargement, rather than chronic prostatic infection, surgical removal of the prostate is another option, which could be considered a pre-Armageddon fix.

With your father in his early 40s, you doubt an enlarged prostate is the cause. Perhaps it is a simple bladder infection after all.

There's no such thing as a simple bladder infection in men. Any infection is considered complicated. The default answer is that it is not a bladder or kidney infection, unless the man has some underlying condition, such as an anatomically abnormal bladder, urethra, or ureters, which would probably reveal itself before the age of 40. Those few men who contract bladder infections should be treated with the antibiotics listed above for female cystitis, but for a minimum of five days, although 7–10 is probably better.

If not bladder infection, then what could it be? Again, more history is required.

Perhaps your father has swelling of the epididymis, a tube running behind the testicles. **Epididymitis** causes swelling, pain, and tenderness in the scrotum, usually on one side. Younger men (under age 35) tend to contract sexually-transmitted infection (see chlamydia and gonorrhea, below), whereas older men generally have non-sexually transmitted epididymitis (requiring 10 days of ofloxacin 300 mg twice daily, or levofloxacin 500 mg daily. If these are unavailable, ciprofloxacin 500 mg or doxycycline 100 mg twice daily may work.) The discomfort of epididymitis is usually enough to make a person willing to risk their antibiotic supply. Non-treatment may result in infection of the testicles, infertility, and/or abscess formation.

No, he checks himself and finds no tenderness around the scrotum or testicles. Is there anything else this could be? It's really not all that bad, he says, just annoying. Maybe the infection spread from the cold he's been treating for a week.

No, that wouldn't be the case, but now you have another clue: he's been treating himself for a cold. Cold medications containing antihistamines and/or decongestants are a common cause of urinary symptoms in men. Occasionally they shut off the bladder altogether, which can be an emergency requiring catheterization or even surgery.

> *You advise your father to lay off the multi-symptom cold medicine and within three days, his symptoms have resolved completely. You feel like a genius – or at least a real doctor. For a moment you're glad you're the go-to man. But then you see your brother approaching.*
>
> *Impressed that you've helped your father, he wonders if you can help him as well. "It kind of burns when I pee," he says. "Maybe I have what Dad had."*

But having read this chapter, you know he does not. In a young man, burning on urination is caused by an STD until proven otherwise. A doctor probably would check the urine, but you may not have that option available. Might as well go for the gold and ask him about STDs.

STDs – sexually transmitted diseases – practically a ho-hum occurrence in the ER, but often emotionally devastating to the persons involved. From the perspective of an experienced physician, anyone having sex with someone other than a virgin (and how do you know for sure?) should expect to encounter a sexually transmitted disease sooner or later – it's like having sex with whomever your partner had sex with, and whomever they did, and so on down the line. Oh, what a tangled web we weave.

Sometimes a sexual partner will share knowledge of diagnosed STDs, so that all affected parties may be treated, but this often gets lost in the shuffle and with so many asymptomatic infections, many patients go untreated. Unfortunately, someone down the road may develop serious symptoms from the same organism that has caused no symptoms in another. It's playing with fire if you expect to be one of the luckier ones. Condoms help – IF they're used from the beginning EVERY SINGLE TIME – which rarely happens.

So what causes burning on urination? Certainly chlamydia, gonorrhea, and trichomonas do. Herpes and HPV are possible as well, though less likely. How can you sort them out?

Two easy questions are helpful: is there any discharge from the penis and are there any visible sores or bumps?

Yes, he's seen a few bumps along the shaft of the penis, and there's a little one right at the tip. Ah, good, you think. Genital warts.

And you're probably right. But STDs often run in pairs, and genital warts caused by the **human papilloma virus (HPV)** don't usually cause burning on urination. They might, if one were growing inside the urethra, blocking the flow of urine, but this is fairly uncommon. One good bit of news is that visible warts are usually caused by strains of HPV that don't cause penile (or cervical) cancer.

Treatment of small warts is easier than that of large warts, though when treating, it's hard to know if you've identified them all, since tiny warts are essentially invisible to begin with. If the warts aren't enlarging, you might even want to leave them alone, as long as the risk of transmission is minimal (i.e. –

you are celibate, or use condoms ALL the time). Given enough time (often years), genital warts sometimes resolve without treatment.

If the lesions are enlarging or spreading, you'll probably want to treat them. In normal times, this is best done by a professional or with a prescription product, which your doctor is unlikely to prescribe for stockpiling unless you already have the disease. Condylox and Aldara are most commonly dispensed (and are rather expensive). Otherwise, possible over-the-counter remedies to consider are the same ones used for common warts, that is, freezing devices or acid-containing formulations. Look in the "foot" or "skin" aisle at the drugstore, or ask the pharmacist. Any of these treatments may cause soreness when used on tender skin, so better to go slowly and err on the side of under-treatment. You can always treat again if needed, 7–14 days later.

Back to your brother. In addition to bumps, are there any sores?

No, not currently. He thought he had some once, but decided it must have been where the zipper on his jeans had rubbed. Nothing to see now, though.

Friction *might* produce sores on the penis, but he may have had herpes ulcers and not known it.

Genital herpes is caused by one of the herpes simplex viruses, usually Type 2, but sometimes Type 1. The virus lives in the nerve roots and sometimes breaks out periodically, appearing as small blisters reminiscent of cold sores or chicken pox. Because the nerves are involved, the sores are typically quite painful, and because blister fluid may contain millions of viral particles, the active lesions are quite contagious. Unfortunately, herpes is also contagious even before the rash appears, thus making sexual spread more likely. If one partner has it, the other partner is considered infected by default.

Since the infection cannot be cured (though symptoms can be improved), is it worth treating herpes at the end of the world as we know it? Maybe. At Wal-Mart ninety of the 200-mg acyclovir capsules run only $10. That many could last a month or a decade, depending on the number of outbreaks. Acyclovir can be used either preventively (200 to 400 mg, 1–3 times daily – use the lowest dose which proves effective for a particular patient) or as treatment at the first sign of an outbreak (200 mg five times daily for 7–10 days). Most people don't get monthly outbreaks, but if they did and were treated for each one, this would amount to 35–50 capsules per month (possibly only 20–50% as many as preventive therapy would require). If your doctor is willing to prescribe hundreds of pills in advance, perhaps the price is worth it.

The most sensible use of acyclovir at TEOTWAWKI may be for infected expectant mothers in the last month of pregnancy. Although in women with recurrent genital herpes the risk of transmission to the newborn is only about 1%, the consequences can be devastating. Taking acyclovir 200 mg 4–5 times daily in the weeks leading up to delivery is known to decrease the chance of herpes outbreak at the time of childbirth, thus theoretically minimizing the risk of transmission.

As for your brother, perhaps he had herpes in the past, or perhaps his jeans did rub him sore. Or perhaps he has a single blister just inside the urethral opening of the penis. One thing about herpes, outbreaks tend to occur in the same area. Again, more history is in order.

Did he have urinary burning with his single episode of penile sores? No. How long has he had this burning, anyway? He's had a little burning on most days for a few months. Any discharge of pus from the penis? He blushes and says no.

In a patient with herpes, burning on urination would tend to be episodic, as with the rash of herpes. This doesn't fit. With gonorrhea, symptoms tend to come on fairly quickly, and usually produce enough discharge that a patient would notice. This leaves two likely suspects for his symptoms: chlamydia and trichomoniasis. Without a microscope or lab available, this would be difficult to differentiate, especially in men. Some, but not all, women with trichomoniasis experience a malodorous yellow-green vaginal discharge, but this is also non-specific. Lacking known exposure to a specific infection, the best approach may be to treat one or the other problem, and if this fails, then treat the other.

Treatment guidelines for common STDs

Trichomoniasis	Metronidazole 2 grams orally as a single dose, OR Metronidazole 500 mg twice daily for 7 days, OR Tinidazole 2 grams orally as a single dose.
Chlamydia	Azithromycin 1 gram orally as a single dose, OR Doxycycline 100 mg twice daily for 7 days.
Gonorrhea	Cefixime 400 mg as a single dose PLUS either a 1-gm single dose of azithromycin, OR doxycycline 100 mg twice daily for 7 days

Don't forget to treat partners of infected patients.

For a comprehensive guide to the treatment of sexually transmitted diseases, download the CDC's free 116-page **Sexually Transmitted Diseases Treatment Guidelines, 2010** at http://www.cdc.gov/std/treatment/2010/STD-Treatment-2010-RR5912.pdf, which also covers syphilis, chancroid, granuloma inguinale, lymphogranuloma venereum, hepatitis, HIV, and treatment options in special populations.

You decide to treat your brother with a week's worth of doxycycline. He clears up and tells everyone you're smarter than any doctor he's ever known.

Chapter 12 – Checklist

Items to include in your medical supplies:

- ☐ Antibiotics for urinary infections and STDs, per text
- ☐ Anti-yeast creams (Monistat, Lotrimin, Mycelex) or gentian violet antifungal dye
- ☐ Antiviral medication: acyclovir 200 mg capsules
- ☐ Urinary test strips: Multistix 10 SG or equivalent
- ☐ OTC pregnancy tests
- ☐ Condoms (and possibly other birth control devices)
- ☐ OTC phenazopyridine (Azo) for short-term relief of urinary burning
- ☐ Cranberry juice or pills, or dried cranberries, to treat mild urinary infections
- ☐ Exam gloves and lubricant (KY or equivalent)
- ☐ OTC wart treatments (freezing device and/or acid-containing preparations)
- ☐ OTC saw palmetto to retard growth of the prostate
- ☐ Prescription alpha-blockers for chronic prostatic symptoms

Actions to take:

- ☐ Download and print CDC's free 116-page **Sexually Transmitted Diseases Treatment Guidelines, 2010** at http://www.cdc.gov/std/treatment/2010/STD-Treatment-2010-RR5912.pdf

- ☐ Immunize you and your family against hepatitis B

- ☐ Consider immunizing your children against human papilloma virus.

SECTION FOUR

Skin Conditions

Chapter 13

Common Skin Infections and Rashes

Infections, inflammations, and irritations

The line is long as neighbors and friends arrive for sick call. Though by now you feel confident treating rhinitis, bronchitis, colitis, and cystitis, you dread seeing yet another rash. Lumps and bumps, scales and nails, white spots, red spots, purple, brown, and black spots – is there any way to make sense of it all? Should you just give up and try the shotgun approach – a cocktail of steroids, antibiotics, and antifungal medications for everyone?

What you need is a way of categorizing the many rashes you will encounter. This may be done by location, by appearance, by accompanying symptoms, by prognosis, or by cause. By the end of this chapter, you'll have a handle on how to treat the most common problems.

Probably the most useful system for the layman to categorize rashes is according to appearance, distribution, and symptoms. Blistering rashes have different causes than flaky ones. Localized dermatitis is more likely to be a chemical irritation than is a generalized rash. Itchy spots suggest allergies or immunologic reactions, whereas those without itching point to other etiologies.

A good place to start is with what a patient would say. When experiencing a skin problem, patients usually complain, "I have a rash on my ____" (fill in the blank). Occasionally they add that it itches or hurts. Beyond that, the physician typically has to guide the conversation, inquiring into likely possibilities based on the appearance and history of the problem. A single chapter on rashes cannot cover the full spectrum of clinical dermatology, but it can review the diagnosis and treatment of perhaps 75% of those likely to be encountered. We'll take the approach that common things occur commonly, and leave the zebras for another time.

Most rashes are more of an irritation or cosmetic concern than a serious health problem, but people worry about rashes because they are so easily apparent. More important, though, is the overall condition of the patient. Is he running a fever? Any difficulty breathing? Does he have a stiff neck? Maybe too tired to eat? Don't forget to ask about more than the skin and to do at least a quick physical exam. Generalized symptoms may indicate an internal problem such as meningitis, a systemic allergy, strep throat, or a blood or other disorder. Fortunately, except for strep throat, these are uncommon.

In the short run, people worry about skin infections or infestations. In the long run they worry about cancer. Except for melanoma, even without treatment most people would outlive skin cancer, so let's begin with infections where you can truly make a difference.

Bacterial skin infections

Of the serious conditions, **cellulitis** is probably the most common. Cellulitis is infection of the skin and underlying soft tissues, usually caused by staph or strep bacteria. Untreated, the infection may spread via the circulation or lymphatic channels, eventually causing blood infection (poisoning) and possibly death. Fortunately cellulitis is curable with oral antibiotics most of the time.

Cellulitis typically occurs on the extremities, though it may appear anywhere on the body. The arms and legs are most prone to minor injury, such as abrasions, bug bites, cuts, and scrapes. Cellulitis appears as an isolated area of pink or reddened skin, usually only barely elevated, and usually with a fairly smooth border, though the shape may be somewhat asymmetric. Bacteria enter the skin and begin multiplying, causing the body to react by sending white blood cells to the area. This inflammatory response as the immune system attempts to fight the infection causes redness, swelling, warmth, and sometimes pain or pus. Pruritus (itching) is not normally seen with cellulitis except in the healing phase.

Sometimes an entry point is visible, such as a bee sting or splinter, a scratch or irritation. Other times, cellulitis seems to start "out of the blue." However, on careful questioning or examination, an imperfection in the skin nearby may be found. Athlete's foot may be a portal of entry for cellulitis of the leg; dishpan hands may allow bacteria to enter a small crack, then travel upwards, causing cellulitis in the arms. Occasionally a respiratory infection will lead to cellulitis of the face.

Cellulitis usually starts small, and then enlarges. The initial lesion may be so tiny or nondescript that it goes unnoticed. Minor infection may be resolved by the body's own immune system. By the time an infection grows to a few inches across, however, most people become concerned, and few put off seeking care once the rash has spread several inches.

As the skin is stretched, it often appears a little shiny. The color may vary from slightly pink to bright red. In darker-skinned individuals this may be more difficult to discern. Feeling the rash for warmth or mild elevation may help delineate the borders of the infection. Pressing on the area (palpation) may elicit complaints of mild to moderate tenderness. It is probably a good idea to wear gloves; certainly you should do so if any blood or other body fluid is present, or if your own skin is not intact, or if you cannot wash your hands immediately after touching the rash.

An **infected skin wound** is not quite the same as cellulitis, but may be treated much the same. Infected wounds usually exhibit redness at the edges, sometimes pus or yellowish scabs, as well as increased tenderness, warmth, and perhaps a little swelling. If the infected wound has sutures in place, they should be removed. Germs living on sutures are not killed by antibiotics circulating through the blood stream, and so serve as a source of on-going infection. Except for very mildly infected superficial wounds (which should respond to topical bacitracin or mupirocin), infected wound edges will not grow together anyway, and need to heal from the inside out.

If you suspect cellulitis, outline the visible or palpable border with a ballpoint pen. This is a good way to determine later if the rash is expanding or improving. A local reaction to a bee sting or bug bite may have the same appearance as cellulitis, but usually comes on more quickly and isn't likely to spread after about 24 hours, even in a sensitive individual. Untreated, cellulitis is very likely to continue spreading. Even with antibiotics, the affected area may enlarge a little beyond the outlined borders during the first 24 hours of antibiotic therapy, though generally not more than a centimeter or so (less than half an inch).

Fortunately, almost all cases of cellulitis respond well to oral antibiotics. Penicillin, amoxicillin, and ampicillin are NOT effective (most of the time). Augmentin (a combination of amoxicillin and clavulanate) used to work in nearly 100% of patients, though with the emergence of methicillin-resistant *Staph aureus* (MRSA), it is not quite as reliable. Good antibiotic choices for cellulitis (and other skin infections) include Augmentin (250–500 mg three times daily) or cephalexin (250–500 mg three to four times daily). If one of these is ineffective, switching to (or adding) trimethoprim-sulfamethoxazole (one DS tablet twice daily) or doxycycline (50–100 mg twice daily) may be helpful, as these antibiotics usually are effective against MRSA. Occasionally a strain of *Pseudomonas* bacteria will cause cellulitis, particularly in the diabetic patient. If none of the above antibiotics are working, switching to ciprofloxacin or Levaquin may resolve the infection. Of these, currently only Cipro comes as a generic (ciprofloxacin), which is quite inexpensive. In general, the erythromycin drugs (including clarithromycin and azithromycin) are not advisable for skin infections, but may work in a pinch for a mild infection (particularly in a penicillin-allergic patient) if other options are unavailable.

How will you know if the antibiotic is working? In the first day of treatment, the redness may not decrease, but neither should it increase more than a little, not expanding over about a quarter inch or so beyond the outlined borders. By the second or third day the reddened area should be distinctly smaller. If this is not the case, switching to or adding a second antibiotic is a consideration. To cure cellulitis generally takes at least five days of treatment, and often longer. In times of antibiotic scarcity, I would treat at least five days, continuing medication for two or three days beyond clearing of the redness, for up to about 10 days. If the infection hasn't resolved by then, a different antibiotic should be tried, generally one from a different class. Often the reddened area remains a little darkened after a bout of cellulitis. It is not necessary to treat until this dusky appearance resolves, which may take a few weeks.

Classification of Common Antibiotics

Type	How they work	Examples
Cell wall antibiotics	These work by disrupting the synthesis of the bacterial cell wall (not present in humans).	**Cephalosporins** Cephalexin, cefuroxime, cefixime **Penicillins** Penicillin, ampicillin, amoxicillin,
RNA inhibitors	These interfere with bacterial RNA and thereby inhibit bacterial protein synthesis.	**Lincosamides** Lincomycin, clindamycin **Macrolides** Erythromycin, azithromycin, clarithromycin **Tetracyclines** Tetracycline, doxycycline
Cytoplasmic membrane disrupter	These act like a detergent, altering the permeability of the cytoplasmic membrane.	**Polypeptides** Bacitracin, colistin, polymyxin B
DNA inhibitors	These inhibit the bacterial DNA enzymes and prevent DNA replication.	**Quinolones** Ciprofloxacin, levofloxacin, moxifloxacin
Folate inhibitors	These inhibit folate synthesis, which is required for nucleic acid synthesis. Without folate, bacteria are unable to divide.	**Sulfonamides** Trimethoprim-sulfamethoxazole, silver sulfadiazine, sulfasalazine, trimethoprim
Toxic free radicals	Disrupts DNA and protein.	Metronidazole

To prevent a recurrence, it is important to make sure the skin remains intact. Treat any athlete's foot as discussed below. Avoid over-washing of the hands, or exposure to insects, thorns, and other sources of injury.

One other potentially dangerous infection is an **abscess**. An abscess often begins much like cellulitis, but as the body fights the infection, a collection of pus forms, like a big pimple, but much deeper. As the skin and surrounding tissues are stretched, pain becomes more pronounced, sometimes reaching the unbearable stage. At this point, the abscess may burst on its own, relieving the pressure and much of the pain simultaneously. This is not a bad thing – in fact, it is often all that is necessary for the infection to resolve.

Strictly speaking, an abscess does not require antibiotics (though most doctors are too chicken not to prescribe them, and patients are afraid not to take them). Once the abscess has an "escape route," the body can take over from there. If an abscess hasn't popped on its own, lancing it may be required, using a #11 scalpel, or perhaps an X-Acto or similar knife, preferably after anesthetizing the overlying skin with 1 or 2% lidocaine. Try to determine how deep the infection is and numb the patient accordingly – through the overlying skin and subcutaneous tissue. It is not necessary to numb the inside of an abscess. If the patient feels a cutting sensation, not merely pressure, stop and inject a little more lidocaine. If you don't have anesthetic, you can still lance an abscess, but work fast. Cutting quickly is more merciful than slowly sawing your way through sensitive tissue.

An abscess must be "ripe" before it is lanced, that is, the collected pus should feel like a small water balloon under the skin (fluctuance). If you happen to lance an abscess before it has formed a fluid pocket, little harm is done. The infection now has a potential route of escape, and is unlikely to build up further, but an antibiotic may be advisable (see cellulitis, above). The incision should be long enough to allow all the pus to escape, at least a quarter inch or so (one cm). Large abscesses require longer incisions, at least a third to half the diameter of the lesion. You may have to cut deeper than you initially suspect to reach the pus (a few millimeters for a small abscess, up to a centimeter or two for a larger one).

A word of caution – sometimes when lancing an abscess the pus spurts out (even a foot or more), so having some gauze or a towel handy to protect yourself is a good idea. Also, be prepared for a nasty odor. I try to collect the pus with gauze, and then ball it up in my gloved hand as I remove my gloves, sealing the offending contents in first one inverted glove then the other, which works quite well and limits the spread of unwanted germs.

After the pressure is released and the flow of pus has stopped, press gently around the edges of the incision to encourage more to escape. When the abscess seems to be empty, irrigate the open wound with sterile (or at least clean) water or saline.

It is often difficult to tell the difference between an abscess and an **infected sebaceous cyst.** Sometimes with a cyst you can identify a small, clogged, central opening, like a blackhead, though this is not always apparent. Often the patient can tell you that a small bump was present for months or years before it suddenly enlarged and grew painful. The treatment is much the same as an abscess, except for two things: the cyst may be compartmented, and the contents may be different. If a cyst/abscess does not seem to collapse fully after lancing, try using a #11 scalpel or a hemostat to open the fibrous tissue between compartments. This may require poking around a bit, but you do want to evacuate the area completely. An infected cyst will likely yield pus, but also sebaceous material, a pearly white goo of variable consistency (from creamy to almost solid), which is often the clue to whether the lesion is an abscess or a cyst. Again, try to evacuate the area completely, but realize that eventually the cyst may recur, since this procedure does not remove the lining that produces the sebaceous material. Patients usually don't care, and are grateful for the immediate relief.

The incisions are not sutured shut, but left open and allowed to drain. It is important that the wound not seal itself over, which allows fluid to re-accumulate, starting the process all over again. A large abscess that has been lanced may require the patient to pull the edges apart periodically. Inserting a small drain may be necessary to keep a lanced abscess open. One quick way to make a drain is to cut a strip of material from a sterile glove (say, about one cm wide and several cm long). This can be inserted into the wound (to its full depth), leaving a "tail" protruding from the wound, which should be taped to the adjacent skin, to prevent early dislodgement. Drains commonly fall out within a day or two, but if they haven't by two or three days, they may be removed.

Any sharp utensils should be immediately disposed of in a hard plastic bottle, such as a bleach bottle. If saving the contaminated knife is prudent in times of scarcity, washing it thoroughly with clean, soapy water, then soaking it a few minutes in a 10% bleach solution should be adequate sterilization.

With today's abundant supply of clean water, I often advise my patients to soak an abscessed area in warm water for 20 minutes, 2–3 times a day (and clean the tub or basin afterward to prevent spread of infection). This keeps the edges from sticking together, and helps drain any residual pus. If abundant water is not readily available, applying wet compresses will accomplish much the same thing. Showering is also fine, allowing the spray to rinse the wound directly. Expect the wound to drain a little for up to several days. Keep the area covered with gauze smeared with bacitracin ointment until the drainage has ceased.

* * *

With the worst of the common skin infections now behind us, we can move on to less serious conditions.

Impetigo is the prototype of a (usually) minor skin infection. Young children often get it on their face or extremities, but occasionally on the torso as well. Scabby lesions or golden-yellow crusty sores that don't heal as expected are commonly impetigo. It's common knowledge that small cuts or abrasions should heal within a few days. When the sore continues on and on, or if it spreads or becomes oozy, impetigo (or other bacterial infection) is often the culprit. Such infections may or may not begin with underlying trauma, such as an insect bite or a scratch.

Impetigo and other superficial bacterial infections are generally caused by the same germs that cause deeper skin infections, i.e. staph and strep, and therefore they respond to the same antibiotics listed above for cellulitis. However, for small patches of infection, a topical antibiotic is worth a try. Bacitracin is available inexpensively over the counter, as is Triple Antibiotic Ointment (which contains neomycin, a medication that can cause a poison ivy type rash, so better to avoid it). Bactroban (mupirocin) or Altabax (retapamulin) are usually effective, but are available only by prescription. However, your doctor might write you a tube if you ask. I have not used Silvadene cream (silver sulfadiazine) or other topical silver preparation for impetigo, but theoretically it should be effective. Impetigo is contagious not only to other people, but to other parts of one's own body, so keep the affected area covered, wash your hands or wear gloves when applying the medication, and treat any new areas that may pop up. Any treatment that seems to be working should be continued for a minimum of three days, and more likely five to seven. If no progress is observed by two or three days, a change to a different topical antibiotic may be in order, or switching to an oral preparation.

Another possible remedy is a dilute bleach bath, on the order of chlorinated swimming pool water (1/2 cup household bleach in 40 gallons of bath water). This has been shown to improve atopic dermatitis in patients who react to skin bacteria, though I've found no specific studies regarding impetigo. Although unavailable in the U.S., fusidic acid is also effective against impetigo.

Blistering rashes

Blistering rashes cause much concern and sometimes pain, but are rarely life-threatening. The most common blistering rashes include chicken pox, shingles (varicella zoster), herpes simplex (oral and genital), and poison ivy or poison oak (see **Itchy Rashes**). Of these, chicken pox is the only one that will affect the entire skin surface in an otherwise healthy individual. Other pox-related and blistering rashes exist, but are relatively rare.

The rash of **chicken pox** (varicella) starts as small red spots, either flat or slightly elevated, that develop into small blisters within a few days. Most people age 20 years or older have experienced and/or seen a case of chicken pox. Younger folks are less likely to recognize the lesions, since the introduction of the chicken pox vaccine several years ago. If you haven't had chicken pox or the vaccine yet, now is a good time to be vaccinated. Chicken pox is caused by a virus, and so antibiotics are not helpful unless the open sores become secondarily infected. In such a case, one or more of the pox would become larger and redder, possibly with yellow or green pus rather than the typical clear blister fluid. If topical bacitracin is ineffective at improving a localized bacterial infection, the oral antibiotics mentioned above under "cellulitis" should do the trick.

Chicken pox often causes a fever in addition to the rash, along with a general feeling of unwellness, and sometimes a headache or body aches.

Unfortunately, it is probably most contagious the first day or so, often before the diagnosis is certain, and remains contagious until all the lesions are scabbing over, usually about a week or two. Oral antihistamines and topical Calamine lotion are effective at relieving the itch.

Only rarely does chicken pox cause a serious condition requiring hospitalization, far less than 1 case in 100. Almost everyone gets over chicken pox without medical intervention. Although the medications listed below for shingles are somewhat effective if given early in the course of chicken pox, I would reserve these antiviral drugs for the very ill. Unfortunately, although the rash and other symptoms disappear, the virus lies dormant in the body for the rest of one's life. Occasionally it reactivates in a specific nerve and causes the rash of **shingles** (varicella zoster). The most typical presentation of this is a band of reddened bumps and blisters (vesicles) half-way around the torso. However, shingles may appear anywhere on the body. The individual spots resemble chicken pox, but the rash is localized to the distribution of a specific nerve root. When it occurs on or near the eye, it can be serious and should be treated with acyclovir or similar antiviral drug to prevent permanent corneal scarring.

What concerns people most about shingles is the pain during and after an episode, and the fear of contagion. Because the virus lives in the nerve roots, when it reactivates it causes nerve irritation and pain. Some people have very little discomfort, or only a little itching. Other patients complain bitterly of the pain both during and after an episode. Occasionally the pain is present for several days before the rash emerges, making the diagnosis difficult to ascertain. People cannot catch shingles from an exposure to an affected person, but people who've never had chicken pox can catch the disease. Like chicken pox, the period of contagion lasts until all the lesions are scabbing over, about a week or two.

Older people are much more susceptible to shingles and are currently advised to get the shingles vaccine. Most have not yet done so, primarily due to cost concerns and availability. For patients over age 50, especially anyone with chronic illnesses, undergoing shingles vaccination now is advisable, even at a cost of nearly $200 for the immunization (which insurance may cover). The vaccine does not eliminate the occurrence of shingles altogether, but does decrease the risk by about 50%, while also reducing the risk of post-herpetic neuralgia (lingering pain after shingles) by about two-thirds.

Management of shingles

If an antiviral drug is going to be effective for shingles, it needs to be started very early in the course of the disease, generally within 72 hours of the onset of the rash. In times of scarcity, reserving treatment for those with lesions near the eyes is a reasonable consideration. The least expensive medication is acyclovir (800 mg five times daily for 7–10 days). Other choices are Valtrex (valacyclovir) 1,000 mg or Famvir (famciclovir) 500 mg, either medication three times daily for a week, or twice daily in those with poor kidney function.

In the years before antiviral drugs were available, corticosteroids were often used for shingles, and still remain an alternative. They will not hasten healing of the rash, but may decrease the pain afterwards. One treatment option is prednisone, 30 mg daily for 1 week, 15 mg daily for the second week, and 7.5 for the third.[14]

[14] See Management of Herpes Zoster (Shingles) and Postherpetic Neuralgia (Am Fam Physician 2000;61:2437–44,2447–8.)

The pain may require narcotics, though many patients respond to OTC NSAIDs such as ibuprofen or naproxen, or even simply Tylenol (acetaminophen). Other possible treatments for post-herpetic neuralgia include capsaicin cream, lidocaine patches (Lidoderm), or low-dose antidepressants such as oral amitriptyline, nortriptyline, imipramine, or desipramine. Again, these treatments do not cure anything. They are only useful to decrease the level of pain. Anyone who can live reasonably comfortably without these treatments should probably do so when medical supplies are limited.

The other two common blistering rashes are **herpes simplex** (Types 1 and 2) and **poison ivy**. Poison ivy will be discussed later under "Itchy Rashes."

Most people can recognize a cold sore, that is, **oral herpes**. Cold sores, also known as fever blisters, appear as a blistered or crusted lesion on or about the lips. They are often quite painful, and patients may complain of a tingling in the area before the rash appears. Sometimes clusters of cold sores erupt as high as the nose or cheeks. (The painful white ulcers that occur inside the mouth are not generally caused by herpes.) Again, like chicken pox, herpes is contagious until all the lesions are crusted over.

Genital herpes may occur anywhere on the external genitalia and surrounding areas, or within the vagina, or even urethra. External lesions appear as red spots or blisters, which are often painful. Internal lesions may or may not hurt, and often cause a little discharge or bleeding.

Although oral herpes is usually Type 1 and genital herpes usually Type 2, this makes no difference in treatment. The same antiviral drugs used for shingles are effective at decreasing symptoms of herpes and possibly limiting contagion, but at a much lower dose than that needed for shingles (see **Chapter 12**). However, there is no cure for herpes. Under times of stress (physical, hormonal, or sometimes emotional) the rash is likely to recur. If antiviral drugs are in scant supply, which is quite likely at TEOTWAWKI, it makes little sense to treat this condition in the average patient.

If one half of a sexually-involved couple has genital herpes, the other is assumed to be infected, whether or not symptoms have ever occurred. Abstinence, or monogamy with a monogamous partner, is the only answer to preventing further spread of herpes. No medical cure has appeared on the horizon, so practicing safe sex is the only real answer (and condoms are not always effective). For additional specifics, see **Chapter 12**.

Fungal rashes – mold and yeast

I love fungal rashes. They're so very irritating yet so easy to cure (in most people). Patients hate the itch and appearance, especially when the rash occurs in the private parts, i.e., around the genitals or under the breasts. Quite often they've tried some cream or other before they seek treatment, possibly the correct one – but give up too soon. Knowing a few "tricks of the trade" will help the layman treat most fungal and yeast rashes effectively.

When the skin is dry and intact, fungal and yeast organisms have trouble taking hold. However, when the skin is moist and slightly abraded, as in skin folds, they grow like crazy. Likely locations for this **moist type of fungal or yeast rash** are between the toes, in the armpits, under the breasts, in the groin area, the diaper area, and any other skin fold.

Usually a healthy body can resist invasion by these organisms, but under special conditions, anyone can succumb to a yeast or fungal infection. Probably the most common situation where this occurs is after taking an antibiotic, which kills off some of the "good bacteria" (normal flora), allowing the unfriendlier types to flourish. A person who develops a sore mouth, perhaps with a white spotty coating, after taking an antibiotic has **thrush** (a yeast infection in the mouth) until proven otherwise. If, at the same time, they experience a rash in a warm, moist area, it is likely yeast or fungus as well. Itching or vaginal discharge that occurs after taking an antibiotic is typically an overgrowth of yeast (**yeast vaginitis**, or **candidiasis**).

Skin that stays moist too long is also a breeding ground for yeast and fungi – sweaty feet, wet diapers, and the area under drooping breasts are common examples. Also, both fungi and yeast love sugar. Recurring yeast infections may be a sign of new-onset or uncontrolled diabetes.

Moist yeast and fungal rashes usually start with itching and redness, much like a simple diaper rash. At this point, keeping the area clean and dry is all that may be required for the body to heal. In the next stage the skin starts to break down, developing superficial sores or weeping skin. Sometimes open sores develop, especially wherever friction occurs. Occasionally yeast rashes become secondarily infected with bacteria, which may require antibiotics in addition to yeast medication (see bacterial skin infections, above, and yeast treatment, below).

The other type of fungal rash is the dry variety. Ringworm (or tinea corporis) and the dry type of athlete's foot are most common. **Ringworm** causes round or oval spots which are usually dry, slightly pink, and sometimes itchy. The rash commonly occurs on the extremities, though may appear anywhere. With time, the center of the spots often clears, leaving a ring-like lesion. **Athlete's foot** between the toes is usually the moist variety, but when it occurs on the soles of the feet, it appears as a dry, flaky, cracked, or peeling rash that may or may not causing itching. This type of foot fungus is quite common in older patients, especially those with diabetes or thick, yellow fungal-infected toenails. Jock-itch is another fungal (or sometimes yeast) infection, that can be either the wet or dry type.

Over the years I've seen patients make the same mistakes over and over when treating yeast and fungal rashes. They dab on a little medicine now and then, when they think of it. Or they use the medicine until the rash is half gone, then quit. Or they stop the antifungal treatment while still taking an antibiotic.

Treating a fungal skin infection is not rocket science, nor does it necessarily require a physician, but knowing a few fundamentals will make it more likely that your treatment will succeed.

Having the right diagnosis is a good place to start. In medical school doctors are taught to scrape any scaly rash and examine the debris under a microscope, searching for fungal elements. In current practice, this is seldom done, especially since the CLIA laws took in-office lab testing out of the hands of many physicians. (Dermatologists may perform the test more frequently than family docs do.) Likewise, a sample of a vaginal discharge or other body fluid could be examined for evidence of yeast, fungal, or even bacterial infection. Doctors are not the only ones capable of performing such a test – biologists, high school science teachers, veterinarians, cytotechnologists, or anyone interested in developing the skill could become adept at microscopic examination if they desired and had the correct equipment.

Microscopic examination is not performed as often as it could be for three more reasons: 1) the history and physical often yield the correct diagnosis; 2) it's quicker to skip the test; and 3) a trial of medication is both inexpensive and usually effective, plus it offers very little risk if the diagnosis happens to be wrong.

Assuming the rash you want to treat is a yeast or fungal rash, using an over-the-counter antifungal preparation is usually effective. Lotrimin or Gyne-Lotrimin (clotrimazole) and Lamisil (terbinafine) cream are my first choices, though Tinactin (tolnaftate) and miconazole also work. Using any of these twice a day until the rash appears to be gone PLUS one week is usually sufficient. For people taking an antibiotic, the cream should be continued about a week after the antibiotics are discontinued. For diabetics, it will be difficult to eliminate a yeast or fungal rash unless one's blood sugar is well-controlled. For people with the dry type of athlete's foot in a moccasin-type pattern (soles and sides of the feet), who also have fungal infection of the toenails, the rash may persist indefinitely or recur frequently unless the nail infection is also cured.

At TEOTWAWKI treating **toenail fungus** will be a very low priority. Fungal-infected nails become thick, yellow, brittle, and difficult to trim. Even now, treatment is effective only about half the time using strong oral medication, and the problem is usually more of a cosmetic issue than a medical one. Investing in a good set of nail clippers (or even wire cutters or similar tools) may be a better idea than trying to eradicate the fungus. On the bright side, a recent study showed that applying Vicks VapoRub to fungal nails at least once daily for several months worked as well as prescription medication.[15]

Anyone who has a foot fungus should assume their shoes are contaminated. Treating shoes with an antifungal foot powder is currently an option, though I usually advise people to discard their old shoes and buy new ones. In times of scarcity, disposal may not be an option. If you are prone to foot fungus, you may want to stock up now on white cotton socks which can be bleached, and good shoes that allow your feet to breathe rather than sweat.

---

[15] Novel Treatment of Onychomycosis Using Over-the-counter Mentholated Ointment: A Clinical Case Series. *J Am Board Fam Med.* 2011;24(1):69–74.

Sometimes doctors use a steroid cream to decrease the itching and inflammation caused by a fungal or yeast rash, or to improve the appearance more quickly. The only steroid cream available over the counter is 0.5 or 1.0% hydrocortisone. Although these are not very strong, they would come in very handy for multiple problems, so stocking up on this inexpensive medication is a good idea. There is little reason to purchase the lower strength, as neither is strong enough to cause or mask a serious problem.

If the steroid cream *does* seem to work especially well, it raises the question of whether the underlying rash is actually caused by a fungus, or is simply an inflammation or irritation. One way to know the difference is to treat a single area with the antifungal only. If it makes no difference by a week or two, perform the same experiment with the steroid cream alone, or try both medications concurrently on separate areas. When doctors aren't sure which sort of rash they are treating, they often use both creams, a shotgun approach disdained by purists, but patients are glad when the problem resolves, regardless of which medication actually did the job.

Occasionally doctors use prescription antifungal medications for prolonged, persistent, or deep-seated fungal rashes. These medications were previously quite expensive, but now terbinafine costs as little as $4 for a month of treatment. Anyone prone to this sort of fungal infection may want to consult their physician about stocking up now.

Intertrigo

Intertrigo is redness and irritation of the skin as it rubs together at skin folds, and as such is easily confused with yeast infections. Also, a simple irritation may become secondarily infected with yeast or bacteria, and so it may be difficult to tell the difference. There is little if any harm in accidentally treating intertrigo with an antifungal medication (which is unlikely to help if there is no infection involved).

Keeping the affected area dry and avoiding friction are usually sufficient to resolve simple intertrigo. Using a hair dryer (on the affected area) and wearing cotton clothing may help. Occasionally doctors advise OTC 1% hydrocortisone cream. Stronger steroids (some of which cost as little as $4) may improve the condition more rapidly, but require a prescription. If using a cream, the area must still be kept dry. I rarely recommend an ointment, which is greasier, though if this cuts down on friction, it may be effective. Sometimes zinc oxide ointment (diaper rash cream) is useful as a barrier against perspiration. Other patients do well with Pinxav or Bag Balm (udder cream). If none of these measures work, the rash my indeed be caused by yeast, and may be treated with the agents discussed previously.

Acne

Is a pimple the end of the world? Some would think so. This topic is for the teenagers who still care about blemishes as society collapses around them.

Although taking daily oral antibiotics is a common treatment for **acne** at the current time, it shouldn't be in times of scarcity. A few tubes of prescription Retin-A (tretinoin) might be worth stockpiling, if you can afford a few hundred bucks. Save the doxycycline for serious problems.

What I would recommend is stocking up on the readily-available OTC products which contain benzoyl peroxide or salicylic acid, the active ingredients in most topical acne products (even the expensive ones like Proactiv). Clearasil, Dermalogica, Neutrogena, Oxy, Persa-Gel, Stridex, University Medical, and

Zapzyt acne products all contain benzoyl peroxide as the active ingredient. The primary thing to remember with every acne medication is that none of them cure active zits, rather, they all work by preventing new pimples from forming, and therefore must be applied daily to all acne-prone areas. The above products work best on facial acne (which I'm assuming everyone can recognize); acne which occurs on the chest or back is less likely to respond.

Although I find many herbal remedies recommended in the lay literature, scientific evidence to support their use is limited. However, Oregon grape root, tea tree oil, *Saccharomyces*, and basil may be effective for mild to moderate cases according to the authors of **Botanicals in Dermatology: An Evidence-Based Review**, available online at: http://www.medscape.com/viewarticle/723144_2. If you've tried something and it works, great. Otherwise, general principles of skin health may keep your acne at bay. If you have dry skin, avoid over-washing, and use a gentle soap (if any). If you tend toward oily skin, daily cleansing, perhaps using witch hazel, is important. Either way, eating a healthy diet, exercising regularly, and avoiding makeup will help optimize the appearance of your skin.

Rosacea

Adults middle-aged and older who have acne-like eruptions on their nose and/or cheeks usually have **acne rosacea** rather than acne vulgaris (teenage acne). Sometimes instead of pimples, the cheeks look bright pink or appear to have small broken blood vessels. Rosacea is mostly a cosmetic issue, although some people develop eye involvement, with redness, crusting, and irritation. Topical metronidazole or azelaic acid is today's treatment of choice (both are prescription only), but any traditional acne medications as described above may be effective. The rare patient with eye involvement may benefit from daily tetracycline (500 mg, 1–2 times daily) or doxycycline (50–100 mg daily).

Rather than worry about treatment, focus on prevention. Avoid common triggers for rosacea which include any form of excess heat (sun exposure, indoor heating, hot baths), wind, alcohol, spicy foods, emotional stress, or changes in humidity, temperature, medication, foods, (or anything else you're aware of that triggers the rash).

Flaky rashes

Whether people will worry about **dandruff** at TEOTWAWKI is debatable. Personally I'd be more concerned about a supply of shampoo. Unless a person is suffering from psoriasis with its endless flaking, using the currently available OTC dandruff shampoos is usually sufficient. Both Selsun (selenium sulfide 1%) and Nizoral (ketoconazole 1 %) shampoos are essentially half-strength versions of the prescription products. Selsun does make other products for dandruff containing either pyrithione zinc or salicylic acid as the active ingredient, which may relieve an irritated scalp. Before stockpiling a case, you may want to try them all now to decide which works best for you.

Cradle cap, a thick, flaky, waxy accumulation on the scalp, is seen primarily in newborns. Nizoral shampoo is also useful for this condition, but since cradle cap is in no way harmful, I'd simply suggest waiting until the infant outgrows the problem, which will take a few weeks to several months. Put a bonnet on the baby if you don't like the appearance.

Psoriasis is a chronic inflammatory dermatitis that produces plaques of reddened, irritated skin, overlain with thick silver or white flakes. It often occurs on the scalp, the back of the elbows, and over the kneecaps, in a symmetric pattern, but may occur anywhere on the body. Psoriasis may produce itching, though usually this is not intense. Sometimes the disease causes swelling and pain in the joints, or pitting and thickening of the fingernails.

Psoriatic dermatitis is a highly annoying problem, but not life-threatening. There are numerous treatments but no cure. A patient could stock up on strong prescription cortisone creams, some of which are quite inexpensive, but you'll need a lifetime supply. (Both betamethasone and triamcinolone generics are available for $4/tube.) Methotrexate is quite effective, but doctors are unlikely to prescribe sufficient quantities for any type of stockpiling, especially when blood monitoring is unavailable. Although taking oral steroids may yield short-term improvement, psoriasis almost always rebounds to a state as bad as or worse than it was to start with.

One of the easiest treatments for psoriasis is sun exposure (or indoor tanning). In temperate climates, psoriasis is usually worse during the winter months when clothing blocks what little sun is available. In summer the disease improves on sun-exposed skin. Keeping the skin well-hydrated is also useful, but over-bathing and strong soaps should be avoided. Applying a thick coating of a gentle skin cream immediately after showering may help relieve cracking, itching, and flaking.

Of the herbal remedies known to be of some benefit, topical salicylic acid (from white willow bark) can help remove hyperkeratotic scales. Once these scales have been removed, dithranol (derived from the bark of the araroba tree) may be applied to help decrease inflammation. Plant-derived psoralens may decrease the formation of scales. Oregon grape root, *Mahonia,* avocado oil, and indigo naturalis have all been shown to be superior to placebo when applied topically.

Itchy rashes

Although a little itching (pruritus) is quite common with any flaking or blistering rash, the itch is a secondary feature. In this next set of rashes, itching is frequently the primary complaint. Patients may not like the appearance of the rash, but the itch is what drives them to the doctor.

Eczema (atopic dermatitis)

Eczema, or **atopic dermatitis**, is a problem with which I am intimately familiar. It comes in many varieties, sometimes masquerading as dry skin, a fungal infection, or allergy. Although eczema acts like an allergy, it is not. My favorite description of atopic dermatitis is "an itch that rashes" (as opposed to a rash that itches.) Whereas I may absentmindedly notice a few mildly itchy bumps in the crease of my elbow, upon scratching the area, many more erupt in a maddening cycle of unquenchable itching. Many a patient has resorted to running very hot water over the affected area, or applying alcohol, or simply slapping the skin – the inflicted pain is more bearable than the itch. NOT scratching is, therefore, the first step in the treatment of this bothersome rash.

Eczema is actually a layman's term for atopic dermatitis, and may refer to other types of eczematous dermatitis. It is not always possible to distinguish one dry, itchy, or flaky rash from the other, and sometimes one rash leads to the other. For example, dry skin may lead to eczema. For the purposes of this book, I will use the term eczema to refer to atopic dermatitis.

As mentioned, eczema is not an allergic condition, though it often acts like one. It is an immunologic condition of unknown cause. However, many patients are aware of certain chemicals, plants, foods, or conditions that make their rash worse. Eczema is also common among atopic individuals, that is, those with allergies or asthma. Within a family group, some individuals may have eczema, allergies, asthma, or any combination thereof.

Eczema tends to be symmetric, but is not always so. Common areas are the creases of the inner elbows, behind the knees, and behind or around the ears. Among infants, facial eczema is fairly common, and appears as dry, sometimes pink, irritated skin, usually on the cheeks. The buttocks of adults and children are sometimes involved.

Patients often scratch themselves raw. Experience has taught me that using a hair brush inflicts less damage than sharp fingernails. The hot water treatment, which I've tried, yields only temporary relief, and tends to bring out more bumps. I'm not recommending either, just relating how desperate patients are for relief from the itch, which may lead to anxiety, depression, or insomnia.

Fortunately, it is possible to improve, if not cure, the condition in almost every case.

The first step is to avoid as many triggers as possible. I wouldn't dream of holding a cat. Strong detergents are a no-no. Some patients must avoid milk products; others must shower immediately after mowing the grass to rinse off the offending irritants. Anything that causes an itchy, runny nose can make the skin itch as well, then scratching causes the rash to emerge. So DON'T SCRATCH . . . echoes of my father's voice from decades ago.

Patients with eczema also do well to use little, if any, soap on susceptible areas, and to avoiding perfumes, skin creams, and bath gels. Keeping the skin moisturized is important, but make sure to use a mild product without dyes or perfumes. What so-called moisturizers actually do is seal in moisture via a thin coating of oil. The best time to apply skin cream is immediately after showering, when the skin is supple and thoroughly hydrated. Vaseline Intensive Care is a nicely formulated cream, but something as simple as Crisco, lanolin, or even Vaseline will work. Though these sound greasy, if you apply a very thin layer of warmed product to warm skin, this should not be a problem.

Beyond avoiding triggers and using moisturizer, what else can be done? The mainstay of medical treatment of eczema is topical steroid creams. For a mild case, the over-the-counter 1% hydrocortisone will do (which is also appropriate for babies and facial eczema). For a worse case, a stronger steroid cream will be necessary, several of which are available for as little as $4, including betamethasone, fluocinolone, and triamcinolone. Stock up now by asking your doctor for a long-term supply. For $10 you can get up to three 45- to 80-gram tubes, enough for at least a few years for most patients. Although these tubes will have expiration dates of only a year or two in the future, they will likely be good for several years beyond the imprinted date. I personally have used topical steroid creams a decade out of date with good success.

In addition to steroid creams, oral antihistamines are useful in lessening the itch. Most antihistamines are now over the counter at modest prices, including Claritin (loratadine), Zyrtec (cetirizine), Benadryl (diphenhydramine), Chlor-Trimeton (chlorpheniramine), and most recently Allegra (fexofenadine).

One additional concern is infection of traumatized skin. Staph and strep bacteria are the most common culprits, and may require oral antibiotics if careful cleansing is not sufficient. *Infected* eczema is often redder than the ordinary irritation, and may become oozy. Effective antibiotics include cephalexin, erythromycin, Augmentin, and perhaps doxycycline or sulfa drugs.

Severe eczema may require expensive immune-modulating drugs for remission, but neither the drugs nor appropriate monitoring are likely to be available at TEOTWAWKI.

Though I have neither used nor prescribed herbal treatment for eczema, and though many products are advertised for this use, is there any research to support herbal therapy? According to a scientific review article (**Botanicals in Dermatology: An Evidence-based Review)** many creams have been evaluated in atopic dermatitis.[16] The botanical preparations shown to be *in*effective for atopic dermatitis include creams containing witch hazel, chamomile, sea buckthorn, black seed oil, and borage oil. Evening Primrose oil also has no proven efficacy.[17] Creams containing the following ingredients showed some improvement in the rash of eczema: St. John's Wort, Oregon grape root, and licorice. Of products given orally, oolong tea, traditional Chinese medicine, and Japanese Kampo medicine were found to be useful.

Poison ivy, poison oak, poison sumac (rhus dermatitis)

I include **poison ivy** here because it is every bit as itchy as eczema and is treated similarly. Less than a second of exposure to any part of these plants may produce a rash and itching that continues for weeks. Prevention is key, starting with learning to recognize those plants native to your area.[18] Using a topical product containing quaternium-18 bentonite lotion (Ivy Block) prior to an expected exposure may decrease the risk of reaction.

The rash of poison ivy begins as red bumps, clusters, or streaks that then turn to blisters containing clear fluid, anywhere from 24 hours to two weeks after exposure. The rash may not break out all at once, and so patients often think the reaction is spreading; however the blister fluid is NOT contagious and the rash

---

[16] **Botanicals in Dermatology: An Evidence-based Review** Am J Clin Dermatol. 2010;11(4):247–267, online at: http://www.medscape.com/viewarticle/723144.

[17] See http://www.aafp.org/afp/2009/1215/p1405.html.

[18] See http://en.wikipedia.org/wiki/Poison_ivy and http://en.wikipedia.org/wiki/Poison_sumac for pictures and maps of poison plant distribution.

appears only on skin where contact with the plant has occurred. For most people, the rash is intensely itchy, though some seem to experience no itching at all. Once exposed to any of these plants, you have a maximum of twenty minutes (more likely ten) to wash the urushiol oil from your body and prevent the rash from developing. Unfortunately, this is rarely possible.

Once the rash has developed, the same steroid creams and antihistamines used to treat eczema are helpful in treating poison ivy (see above). A severe case of poison ivy may require oral steroids. I often prescribe prednisone 60 mg daily for 3 days, then 40 mg for 3 days, then 20 mg for 3 days. Although the rash will improve greatly within 2–3 days, stopping the oral steroids that quickly often leads to a recurrence. Beware of burning poison ivy – the smoke may cause a widespread reaction, including airway swelling, if inhaled.

Does jewelweed prevent or treat poison ivy? Many swear by this herbal remedy. Yet in the scientific literature there have been few studies. However, one study done at the Pennsylvania State University College of Medicine concludes the answer is no.[19] Still, if it works for you, I can't argue with success.

Contact dermatitis (metal allergy)

Poison ivy is one kind of **contact dermatitis**. The other common type is metal allergy. Skin that has been exposed several times to certain metals, primarily nickel, can become sensitized, reacting with redness, itching, and blistering. The treatment is primarily prevention via avoiding exposure. Some people use a coating of clear nail polish on their jewelry to avoid contact with the metal although this, too, causes an allergic rash in sensitive individuals.

[19] See Treatment of poison ivy/oak allergic contact dermatitis with an extract of jewelweed, *Am J. Contact Dermat*. 1997 Sep;8(3):150–3, online at http://www.ncbi.nlm.nih.gov/pubmed/9249283.

If a rash from metal allergy does occur, removing the offending metal (earrings, rings, bracelets, watches, belt buckles, etc.) will allow the area to heal within a few weeks, perhaps with the aid of a steroid cream (see Eczema, above). Also, certain medicines are known to cause contact dermatitis, including Benadryl cream and neomycin (in Triple Antibiotic Ointment – doctors recommend Bacitracin antibiotic ointment instead to avoid this problem).

Other plant allergies

Of more concern is the likelihood of reactions to other plants in an era when people may begin experimenting with whatever botanicals are available.

Plant chemicals may cause rashes in at least four ways:

1. Immediate contact reactions, whether chemical or allergic
2. Allergic reactions to ingesting the plant – hives, anaphylaxis, gastrointestinal
3. Allergic rashes when botanical use is combined with patient sun exposure
4. Delayed allergic reactions, such as poison ivy

Sun spurge is known to cause an irritant dermatitis. Burning bush and garden rue may cause photosensitization, making a person more susceptible to sunburn. Blistering skin rashes *may* occur to a varying degree when a person using the following botanicals is exposed to sunlight: bergamot oil, giant hogweed, celery, parsnip and parsley. Plants that may cause an allergic contact dermatitis rash similar to that of poison ivy include arnica, marigold, propolis, tansy, fever few, yarrow, elecampane, chamomile, citrus peel oil, and tea tree oil.

If a reaction occurs following use of any botanical, avoiding that plant will usually resolve the problem within 2 to 4 weeks. Cross-reactions with similar plants are possible. For more information, consult the World Allergy Organization at www.worldallergy.org.

Hives (urticaria)

Urticaria, or hives, is among the itchiest of rashes, and is sometimes associated with other allergic symptoms. When hives occur along with difficulty breathing, this may be anaphylaxis, a potentially life-threatening allergic reaction.

Typically, hives look like mosquito bites or welts, but the size may vary from an eighth-inch to as much as several inches across. The color may be white (blanched), pink, or sometimes only pink around the edges, especially in the case of large, irregular hives. Small hives are usually round, though larger ones may coalesce into irregular shapes. Usually hives are fairly symmetric in distribution, occurring equally on both sides of the body, though localized hives may also occur. The welts tend to come on fairly quickly, within a space of minutes to hours, and may seem to move from one site to another.

The causes of hives are myriad. Potential culprits include allergic reactions to foods, plants, or inhaled chemicals, drug reactions (both truly allergic and non-allergic), insect bites or stings, infections (viral, bacterial, worms, sometimes fungal), physical trauma (including cold, heat, sunlight, or water exposure), and emotional stress. Foods likely to induce hives include seafood, berries, and distilled liquids such as wine. Any new food or medicine is a likely suspect, but sometimes the amount of a particular food is the problem – a few berries may not trigger hives, but a whole bowlful may. Likewise, a single bee sting may not induce urticaria, but three or four stings may. It often takes a real detective to determine the etiology, but even then the cause often remains undetermined. If you can't figure out why you or your patient has a case of hives, don't worry – half the time doctors don't know for sure either.

Common sense dictates to avoid any suspected food or chemical. If an infection is the suspected cause, the accompanying hives should resolve in the same time frame as the underlying infection. Fortunately, even if you have no hint as to the cause, hives nearly always resolve on their own, given enough time (hours to weeks).

Aside from figuring out what to avoid, the main problem with hives is the itching – it can drive a person mad! Patients may suffer insomnia, anxiety, or depression in their desperation to escape their own skin.

Most hives respond well to full doses of an antihistamine, including over-the-counter Benadryl (diphenhydramine), Claritin (loratadine), Zyrtec (cetirizine), Allegra (fexofenadine), or chlorpheniramine. Those which cause drowsiness are especially useful at night. The histamine-2 (H-2) blockers used for acid reflux are also effective (Zantac, Axid, Tagamet, Pepcid, and their generics, but note – the stronger anti-acid medications including Prilosec and Prevacid do not relieve hives). Effective prescription options include Clarinex, hydroxyzine, tricyclic antidepressants (Elavil, Sinequan), and prescription strengths of the H-2 blockers listed above.

Corticosteroids are sometimes used for intolerable itching or widespread hives, but keep in mind that hives will go away eventually untreated. Assuming you have a limited supply of steroids on hand, do you want to use a potentially life-saving medicine just to stop itching? I certainly would not treat hives simply for appearance sake.

However, if a case of hives is accompanied by difficulty breathing (wheezing, shortness of breath), steroids are often mandatory. For a patient who's really in trouble (**anaphylaxis**), seek professional help if readily available. Otherwise, administer epinephrine (Primatene Mist or injectable) or albuterol for immediate relief, along with an antihistamine (Benadryl or whichever you have on hand), followed by steroids. For an extreme case of hives, with or without anaphylaxis, 40 to 60 mg of prednisone orally for 5–7 days works wonders. The rash may re-emerge once the steroids are stopped, so tapering the medication over several days is advisable. Decreasing the dose by 10–20 mg every 2–3 days works well.

Generalized rashes

Suppose your child awakens covered head to toe with bright red spots. Would you know what to do? Would you panic?

Rashes which appear all over the body are frightening – especially to an inexperienced parent. Children tend to get generalized rashes more often than adults, though adults may exhibit similar skin diseases from the same causes.

Most American doctors are no longer expert at recognizing the common rashes of yesteryear, especially **measles** and **rubella**. I haven't seen either one myself in decades. The general U.S. population is immunized against these illnesses via the measles-mumps-rubella (MMR) vaccines administered in childhood. Young doctors may never have seen a case. However, these viral illnesses will reappear if society collapses and immunizations are no longer available.

How is this possible if the population is fully immunized? The fact is, the population is *not* fully immunized. Some parents refuse immunization on religious or medical grounds. In other cases, the vaccine does not produce a sufficiently long-lasting immune response.

The primary reason people are little concerned about vaccination is that they simply do not believe these diseases will occur. They are benefitting from what is known as "herd immunity" – when most people are immunized, the relevant diseases are less common in the community.

But like smallpox, have these viruses been completely eliminated from the population, so that no reservoir of the disease survives? Not by a long shot.

Per the CDC there were only 140 new U.S. cases of measles in 2008. However, two decades earlier an outbreak occurred, claiming 123 lives among the 11,000 children hospitalized for measles, with a total of over 55,000 U.S. cases between 1989 and 1991. Yet this is chicken feed compared to what occurs in unimmunized populations. Worldwide funding for combating measles has dropped, prompting the CDC to estimate a "worst case" scenario for 2010–2013, with 500,000 deaths from measles projected to occur worldwide in 2013 alone, assuming vaccination rates remain at the 2008 levels.[20] Clearly, this would not improve in an Armageddon situation.

I start with measles not because it's so common, but because it's so preventable. If you and your family are fully immunized, the risk of acquiring measles is very low – essentially nil – and that's one less rash you'd have to worry about – two actually. Antibiotics are NOT effective for measles or German

---

[20] See http://www.cdc.gov/mmwr/preview/mmwrhtml/mm5847a2.htm

measles (3-day measles, rubella). Children should receive two doses of measles-mumps-rubella (MMR) vaccine (at 12–14 months, and again at 4–6 years old). Adults can be tested for immunity, or simply re-immunized if their status is in doubt (exception: pregnant women and immunosuppressed patients). In short, get the vaccine now, while you can. If society collapses, it will simply be too late.

For those concerned about recognizing measles, which you may encounter even if your family itself is immunized, look for a fever of 103° F or higher, cough, runny nose, and red eyes to start – but at this point there will be no rash. However, checking inside the mouth may reveal what looks like a rash on the inside of the cheeks (Koplik spots). A few days later, a pink, bumpy rash begins on the face and head, moving downward, and lasting 5–6 days. Some patients experience diarrhea or ear pain, but pneumonia is the killer. If the pneumonia is caused by a secondary infection (which you'll have little way of knowing) antibiotics *may* help. If the pneumonia is purely viral, they will not.

Excellent pictures of the rash caused by measles are available online at: http://www.vaccineinformation.org/measles/photos.asp .

Rubella, the three-day measles, is a milder but similar infection, with the biggest risk being birth defects in children of infected pregnant women, including deafness, cataracts, heart defects, and mental retardation. With a 1 in 5 chance of one or more of these birth defects, it behooves young women to assure their immunity *before* they become pregnant, especially in a situation where the disease may become epidemic. Again, there is no effective treatment for three-day measles.

Most of the acute, generalized rashes you are likely to encounter are caused by viruses, with the exception of strep-related rashes and drug reactions. Young children sometimes get a faint, pink, slight bumpy, generalized rash with certain **cold viruses**, which may be difficult to distinguish from a strep rash, but if the child has no sore throat, swollen glands, or fever, it's probably just a virus. Teenagers may develop a similar rash with **mono**. Infants are prone to **roseola**, a rosy rash that appears after a preceding unexplained fever resolves. Both adults and children may contract **Fifth Disease** (erythema infectiousum), a rash caused by human parvovirus B19, and often accompanied by cold symptoms such as a runny nose, sore throat, or headache. In young children the rash often begins with bright red cheeks (the so-called "slapped cheek" appearance), before spreading to the body. Doctors often describe the rash as "lacy" because it forms a lace-like pattern, superimposed on normal-appearing skin. Adults contracting this virus sometimes develop joint pain that may last for weeks or months after the rash has resolved. By the time the typical rash appears, erythema infectiousum is no longer contagious.

Again, for all the viral rashes discussed above, there is no specific treatment. Tylenol may help symptoms of fever or pain, but antibiotics will have no curative effect.

Chicken pox, caused by the varicella virus and discussed above under "Blistering Rashes," is the last of the common viral rashes.

One other fairly common rash that may or may not be caused by a virus is **pityriasis rosea**. This condition is usually most visible on the trunk, more often the back than the chest or abdomen, though it may be generalized. The rash is usually fairly symmetric, with a pattern on the back sometimes resembling a Christmas tree. The red, slightly raised spots seem to form in upward- and inward-slanting bands of lines across each side of the back. This sometimes itchy rash may be diagnosed on the characteristic pattern, but is especially easy to identify when a herald patch is discovered. A herald patch, often mistaken for a spot of ringworm, is a round or oval, dry, sometimes scaly, pink patch, usually on an extremity, that heralds the later onset of the widespread rash. Again, no treatment is necessary, although the itch sometimes drives patients to request relief in the form of an antihistamine or steroid. In times of scarcity, these medicines are best reserved for more serious conditions.

The one childhood rash to be a little more concerned about is **scarlatina**, and other rashes associated with strep throat. For the most part these rashes are only important as clues to streptococcal infection (see **Chapter 9** on **Sore Throat**). Most common is the dry, fine, sandpapery rash that sometimes appears in children, primarily on the torso. Some doctors call this scarlatina, though the term is also used for true **scarlet fever**, which is fairly uncommon. Scarlet fever looks more like a bad sunburn, which will often peel several days later. The specific strep bacterium that we encounter today is probably not the same as that which caused more severe disease a century ago.

Besides infection-associated rashes, drug reactions are the other common type of generalized rash, usually in the form of either hives or a fine, pink, bumpy rash. A drug rash may occur anytime during the administration of a drug, or even weeks afterward. A drug reaction is easiest to diagnose when a patient has recently started a new medication, and when the reaction coincides with the administration of the drug. However, even patients who have been on a particular drug for years can develop sensitivity to a medication. Fortunately, most of these reactions resolve on their own when the medication is discontinued. For a severe allergic reaction, especially one causing shortness of breath, the treatment is the same as for hives with anaphylaxis (as discussed above). Mild drug reactions do not require medication, though antihistamines and/or corticosteroids will relieve symptoms – but again, reserving these medications for serious situations is advisable.

Armed with the preceding approach, you should be able to diagnose and treat the majority of skin problems you encounter. Those I have not addressed are either primarily cosmetic, fairly uncommon, or too difficult to treat without the benefits of modern medicine.

Chapter 13 – Checklist

Items to include in your medical supplies:

- ☐ OTC Nizoral or Selsun Shampoo (or prescription strengths)
- ☐ OTC antifungals: Lotrimin, Lamisil, Tinactin and Vicks VapoRub
- ☐ OTC hydrocortisone cream 1% (or prescription strength)
- ☐ OTC antihistamines for itching: diphenhydramine, cetirizine, chlorpheniramine, loratadine, fexofenadine
- ☐ OTC H-2 antihistamines for hives (and acid reflux): ranitidine, famotidine
- ☐ OTC Primatene Mist for severe hives or shortness of breath, or bee-sting kit
- ☐ OTC benzoyl peroxide acne product
- ☐ Ball-point pen to outline areas of cellulitis or large insect bites
- ☐ OTC bacitracin and prescription Bactroban antibiotic creams
- ☐ Prescription antibiotics, per text
- ☐ Prescription steroid creams (betamethasone or triamcinolone) and steroid pills (prednisone)
- ☐ #11 scalpels for lancing abscesses, along with hemostats and dressings

- ☐ Large supply of dye-free, perfume-free skin moisturizer
- ☐ High quality nail clippers

Actions to take:

- ☐ Make sure all family or group members are immunized against measles, mumps, rubella, and chicken pox (also shingles for those age 50 years and older)
- ☐ Buy a dermatology picture book or make your own by downloading pictures of common diseases from www.dermnet.com or other online dermatology atlas – many are available.
- ☐ Download **Botanicals in Dermatology: An Evidence-based Review** Am J Clin Dermatol. 2010;11(4):247–267, online at: http://www.medscape.com/viewarticle/723144

SECTION FIVE

Pain

Chapter 14

An Approach to Pain

The daily queue of suffering seems endless. Toothache, stomachache, headache, earache, back pain, leg pain, joint pain, neck pain, sore throat, sore feet, sore muscles, sore eyes. People come to you seeking relief – relief from their pain, and relief from fear. Are you up to the task of helping others, or ready to run away? Becoming a healer is not for the faint of heart.

If and when the medical community collapses, those left to carry on will need an armamentarium of tools to deal with pain. Even if it's only your own problems and those of your family that you'll be facing, learning how to relieve pain now, before you're in the midst of crisis, will spare you needless worry. Pain is the #1 symptom that drives patients to physicians today. Pain will remain a fearsome opponent tomorrow, no matter what catastrophe brings the world to its knees.

Pain and fear go hand in hand, two sides of the same coin. Fear is pain's best friend, its evil ally. Relieve one and the other may subside, at least to tolerable levels. I know what it is to fear pain. Every time I visit the dentist my childhood dread of drilling on a nerve rears its ugly head. It's not a rational process. My childhood dentist didn't believe in novocaine. I'll never get over it.

People can often tolerate an amazing degree of pain if given hope that the condition is only temporary. Labor pain is every bit as bad as any other sort of pain, yet how many women suffer through hour after hour of gut-wrenching torture without requesting so much as an aspirin? People will also endure an incredible amount of pain if they believe good will come of it – such as a new baby, or saving another's life.

As a healer, you'll need to dispense more than a dose of narcotics. Having enough medical knowledge to understand a disease process will help you foresee the course of the disease and offer hope of recovery. Even if you cannot relieve the pain, you can relieve fear – both fear of unending pain, and fear of being alone. If you lack the tools to deaden the pain, don't think you're doing no good. Like a child who wants his boo-boo kissed, adults, too, want to know that someone cares.

In this regard, doctors are not necessarily the best healers. Physicians are aloof by training and sometimes by nature. Once you try helping others, you'll learn that part of the patient's suffering becomes your own. Taking on the pain of the world is a crushing burden. Doctors cannot function when they are overwhelmed by too heavy a load, and so often limit their emotional involvement. But emotional involvement is a powerful salve. An infant with an earache may be comforted in its mother's arms. "Hold me" may be a laboring wife's request of her husband, knowing he cannot take the pain away.

I emphasize the non-medicinal treatments of pain because: 1) sooner or later they may be all you have; 2) stretching your supply of pain relievers will help you treat more patients; and 3) many people are intolerant of or allergic to pain medications.

The best way to relieve pain is to eliminate the underlying cause. Deliver the baby, lance the abscess, pass the kidney stone. Pain is your friend when it comes to diagnosis (as discussed throughout this book), but sometimes you'll just have to treat it regardless of cause.

> The English language has many words for various kinds of pain: aching, stabbing, burning, stinging, piercing, numbing, cramping, throbbing, tingling, smarting, lancinating, agonizing, and nagging, to mention the most common. The type of pain will clue you as to both cause and severity. The fluent or bodily-aware patient will be able to describe their discomfort in some detail. Others will simply say they hurt.

Beyond what a patient may say, their body language will alert you to the intensity of their distress. A smiling teenager flirting with her beaux does not need narcotics, even though she says she's dying of pain. A silent man curled up in the fetal position has something serious going on.

The art of medicine includes deciphering both what a patient wants and needs. Some patients request no medicine, if they can only be permitted a day off work. Others prefer to pop a pill and keep going. In America, we overmedicate because we rest too little. Sleep is a powerful analgesic. If pain medication is not available, simply getting a person to rest and/or sleep may be the ticket to relief.

Doctors use many classes of drugs to alleviate or prevent pain: anti-inflammatories, steroids, narcotics, antidepressants, anti-anxiety drugs, anti-seizure drugs, beta-blockers, calcium channel blockers, triptans, muscle relaxers, sedating antihistamines, caffeine, nitroglycerin, antacids, oxygen, anesthetics, and even alcohol. We don't always know how these drugs work. A patient does not have to be depressed for an anti-depressant to relieve pain. Thinking beyond traditional pain medications will broaden your ability to offer relief.

On treating pain

Whereas patients focus on pain abatement, doctors often focus on functional improvement. Generally speaking, physicians do not necessarily aim for complete relief of pain, but rather sufficient improvement to permit adequate functioning. Relieving all pain can actually make a situation worse, allowing the patient to injure himself. A truck driver with chronic back pain may say he's feeling no better, but now is able to unload his cargo. A migraine patient may report her headaches are as bad as usual, but hasn't missed a day of work in a year. It is difficult to measure how much a patient hurts. It's much easier to measure how well a patient functions.

Despite current medical thinking, I'm not much of a believer in patient-reported pain scales, though others find them useful. Among my patients, they seem to make little difference in clinical treatment, at least with chronic pain. Patients have difficulty remembering how much they were hurting last week or last month compared to now.

The one situation where a pain scale may be useful is where short-term observation (hours to days) of a hurting patient is possible. Asking the patient to report pain on a scale of 0 to 10 may yield a measure of improvement, or lack thereof. In the current medical environment, pain scales are often more a matter of documentation than a meaningful addition to medical care. It makes little sense to collect the information if it is not going to be used as a basis for treatment. Patients must understand the scale well to offer significant feedback. Many patients will report their pain as 8 or 9 out of 10 when it is obvious from their behavior that it is not this intense. If you are going to use a pain scale, take the time to explain it thoroughly. It also helps to use words or pictures to demonstrate the degree of pain, as in the table below. Check online if you want an example with pictures.

0	1	2	3	4	5	6	7	8	9	10
No pain		Annoying		Uncomfortable		Dreadful		Horrible		Agonizing

When doctors evaluate pain, one of the immediate goals is to determine if it is life-threatening or not. Is chest pain a heart attack? Is abdominal pain appendicitis? If you think you have an emergency on your hands and have the option of referring to a hospital or physician, please do so. But the goal of this discussion is to focus on what you can offer on your own, without emergency back-up. Here are a few examples to consider.

Say a patient is experiencing excruciating chest pain in association with a likely heart attack. What can you do about it? First, give the patient an aspirin, to thin the blood a little, and perhaps limit further damage. This will not alleviate the pain, but may do some good in the long run. If you have oxygen available, have the patient inhale it at a rate of 2–3 liters per minute (per the machine's gauge). The pain of a heart attack is partly due to inadequate oxygen within the heart muscle, somewhat like leg pain in a runner, and improving oxygenation may lessen the discomfort. Assuming you don't have oxygen available, have the patient lie in the bed with his upper body propped up on several pillows. This decreases the work of breathing compared to lying flat, with less demand on the cardiac muscle. Next, give nitro. Nitroglycerin lessens heart pain by opening up the coronary circulation, thus delivering more oxygen to the heart. Nitroglycerin sublingual (dissolved under the tongue) offers very quick but short-term relief; nitroglycerin paste, patches, or delayed release capsules offer longer-term relief, but are slower to take effect.

Up to this point, we haven't mentioned pain relievers per se. Oxygen, positioning, and nitroglycerin may not only improve the underlying problem, but also relieve the patient's discomfort to a degree. As for direct pain treatment, you probably won't have injectable morphine available, but oral Vicodin, Percocet, or even tramadol may offer some relief. Nausea frequently accompanies severe heart pain, and you may need to treat with OTC meclizine or a prescription anti-emetic (Phenergan, Vistaril, Compazine) to allow the patient to keep narcotics down. Also, if the patient is agitated, calming him may decrease his oxygen consumption, thereby decreasing chest pain. Valium, Xanax, or Ativan (all controlled prescription drugs) may be helpful.

Medically speaking, this is about all you can do – but still it's not *all* you can do. Hold the patient's hand or rub their neck, if this seems to comfort them. Offer a cool washcloth if they are sweating. Allow a calm, supportive family member to assist you. Keep disturbing or anxious relatives out of the room. Offer to pray with the patient, if this seems appropriate. Offer fluids unless the patient is vomiting. Two reasons fluids are withheld in the hospital are that the patient is getting an I.V. anyway, and that a surgical procedure may be around the corner, with associated anesthesia and risk of vomiting. Your post-Armageddon patient is not going to undergo a heart bypass or stenting, and does not need to suffer dehydration on top of a heart attack. Be careful, though, if the patient is short of breath, as excess fluids may worsen a case of congestive heart failure.

Now, whatever you've done with the equipment at hand, don't blame yourself if the patient dies. We are simply not in control of everything. You did not cause the patient's heart attack and you've done what you can to help.

Your next patient is a 45-year-old woman, complaining of chest pain as well, but who doesn't appear ill. Chest pain in a person under about 50 years of age is more likely related to the lungs, ribs, or digestion than to the heart. In an asthma patient, when the lungs are tight and the patient is short of breath or wheezing, opening the airways (with an inhaler or steroids) may do more to relieve pain than any pain reliever. If the patient is breathing normally but complains of pain on inspiration, this is usually pleurisy (inflammation of the lining of the lungs) or rib-cage pain. Either way, anti-inflammatory medicine such as ibuprofen, naproxen, or even aspirin is helpful. (Remember, though, that if you're wrong and the pain is coming from the stomach, these drugs may aggravate the problem.) *In our index case, there is definite tenderness when you palpate along the rib margins.* The heart and lungs cause pain, not tenderness. If rib tenderness is present, you can be fairly confident the problem is musculoskeletal, that is, not serious, and again an anti-inflammatory should help relieve the discomfort. Heat or ice (and not wearing an underwire bra) often help as well.

Next in line is your 30-year-old nephew who works hard and parties harder. His chest is hurting, too, sort of burning, and you can see he's hung-over. Home-brew will be available even in the worst of times. Chest pain due to acid reflux (often aggravated by alcohol or anti-inflammatory medications) requires a different approach altogether. Pain medication is *not* the answer. Decreasing the amount of stomach acid refluxing into the esophagus will alleviate this pain. Baking soda and liquid antacids offer almost immediate relief, which is a diagnostic test in itself. Any of the OTC antacid reducers (Pepcid, Tagamet, Zantac, Axid, Prilosec, Prevacid) will afford longer-term acid suppression. Since these medications will not be available forever, avoiding heartburn triggers is only sensible (NSAIDs, alcohol, tobacco, spicy food, fried or fatty food, citrus fruits, tomato products, chocolate, caffeine – yes, avoid all the good stuff).

At first your 40-year-old cousin thought the pain was in her right lung, but now it seems focused in the upper abdomen, toward the right. She's pretty sure it came on after eating half a jar of peanut butter. The pain is dull to sharp, mostly aching, but with cramps coming in waves, with intermittent nausea. This type of pain is typical of gut pain, probably stemming from gallbladder irritation. With gut pain, narcotics may help, but NSAIDS (anti-inflammatory drugs) should be avoided. Sleep, relaxation, a hot bath, and abstaining from eating also offer partial relief. These same measures help individuals with colitis, kidney stones, kidney infection, diverticulitis, and other intra-abdominal irritations.

Very light massage is a technique that helps gut pain by distracting the mind from the deeper pain. This is part of the basis for the efficacy of effleurage, a TENS unit (transcutaneous electrical nerve stimulation unit), and even a hot shower. Just as an Internet connection can only carry so much information at once, the human nervous system can only process so much neural input at one time. The heat of a hot shower takes at least several minutes to penetrate sore muscles, but partial relief begins the moment the skin is stimulated. Laboring women sometimes massage their own bellies to lessen the deep pain. Anyone can experiment with this superficial massage technique, which works not only for gut pain, but other deep pains as well. Light oil massage works similarly.

Deep massage is best described and taught by a professional masseuse, which I am not. But even an untrained friend can give a good backrub that relieves the tensions of the day. I've had many patients obtain as much relief from a professional massage as from medication or physical therapy. The relief may be short-lived, and the massage may need to be repeated in a day or two, but this natural remedy is used worldwide for pain relief. In fact, in countries where there isn't a drugstore on every corner, touch therapy is the primary mode of pain relief.

Doing anything at all is nearly always better than doing nothing. Placebos, which have no physical basis for helping, still do so about a third of the time. Hope is a natural narcotic, and people will try a multitude of peculiar and likely ineffective therapies on the basis of hope alone. This is also how so many crackpot therapies work their way into the health care field. Anything, even a sugar pill, will help somebody. Part of the benefit is mind over matter; part is giving your body time to heal on its own. Many patients who think an antibiotic cured them overnight were simply going to be better by the next day anyway. Applying cool cabbage leaves to tender, engorged breasts is purported to relieve the discomfort, but perhaps grape leaves, lettuce leaves, or a cool wash cloth would accomplish as much. Still, applying cabbage leaves lies in the realm of "doing no harm," plus it gives the mother something active to do. People prefer to be in charge of their own bodies.

As a physician I struggle with the need to be honest with my patients versus the desire not to deprive them of the placebo effect. Modern medicine prides itself on "truth." But for anyone who believes in a certain therapy, even one proven by medical science to be ineffective, for that individual the relief is real. After an Armageddon event, the placebo effect may be a doctor's strongest ally. A placebo may be a pill, a procedure, an activity, or a dressing. Whatever you do, choose your placebos wisely and first, do no harm.

Natural remedies also include biologically active chemicals such as opium and salicin (from which aspirin is derived). Through the years, the pharmaceutical industry has developed many refinements, but these two are the original basis of all narcotics and anti-inflammatory medications, including codeine, morphine, hydrocodone, oxycodone, ibuprofen, and naproxen. When supplies of pharmaceutical pain relievers run out, healers will need to resort to the original, naturally-available painkillers.

White willow bark contains the natural pain-killer salicin. For a full discussion, see the University of Maryland Medical Center (UMM) Web site, which includes details of dosing, drug interactions, side-effects, and recipes for willow bark preparations made from commercially available supplies.[21] Of course, stockpiles of willow bark will run out as quickly as stockpiles of aspirin, and it makes more sense to learn to recognize the tree, and either locate it within your community or plant your own. Other types of willow may also be effective.

Willow Bark Tea Recipe (from UMM)

Boil 1–2 teaspoons of (commercially-available) dried
white willow bark in 8 ounces of water

Simmer 10–15 minutes and let steep for half an hour.

Drink one cup 3–4 times daily as needed.

[21] University of Maryland Medical Center: http://www.umm.edu/altmed/articles/willow-bark-000281.htm

Narcotics are the strongest pain relievers and will be the hardest for preppers to come by. Doctors are extremely unlikely to prescribe enough to stockpile and so, aside from learning to prepare your own, are there any alternatives?

Tramadol is a prescription painkiller, nearly as strong as codeine or hydrocodone, at least in the narcotic-naïve patient. People who get a "high" on narcotics are not fond of this drug. Whereas a few years ago it was quite expensive, now the cost is on a par with ibuprofen. Because it is not addicting, doctors are happy to use it much more freely for many conditions ranging from headaches and stiff necks to sciatica and broken bones. If you have a good relationship with your doctor, you may be able to obtain a reasonable supply, which you should plan on reserving for serious pain. The normal dose is 50–100 mg every 4 to 6 hours.

Secondly, the combination of Tylenol plus an anti-inflammatory is nearly as strong as the narcotics hydrocodone or codeine, and in many patients, works as well or even better. As long as a patient can tolerate the ingredients separately, they are well-tolerated in combination. With 500-count bottles of Tylenol, ibuprofen, and naproxen sodium readily available over the counter at minimal cost, anyone can lay in a good supply for future use.

Of course, anti-inflammatories (NSAIDs) are not tolerated by every patient. Any NSAID may cause stomach discomfort or even an ulcer with prolonged use. They should always be taken with food to minimize contact with the stomach lining. Some patients are able to tolerate an NSAID if they take an acid-lowering drug (such as Pepcid, Zantac, Prilosec, or Prevacid). Allergies to NSAIDs are not uncommon, and sensitive individuals may develop hives or wheezing.

For musculoskeletal pain (strains, sprains, fractures, injuries), the NSAIDs, narcotics, and Tylenol are useful, but again, don't limit yourself to thinking of pills as the only way to alleviate pain. Rest, ice (or heat), splinting, wrapping, and taping are all measures that decrease pain by lessening the stress on the affected body part.

Again, the main point is to get beyond thinking that pain pills are the answer to pain. Yes, they have their place, when the pain is disabling and nothing else works. But overall, especially with the supply of narcotics severely limited, do what you can to avoid them, and save the "big guns" for situations that truly warrant their use.

Chapter 14 – Checklist

Items to include in your medical supplies:

- ☐ Tylenol and OTC NSAIDs – ibuprofen, naproxen sodium, and aspirin
- ☐ Prescription tramadol, narcotics, muscle relaxers, sleep aids, antidepressants, beta-blockers, calcium channel blockers
- ☐ Oxygen tank or concentrator; extra tubing
- ☐ Hot water bottle or reheatable rice bag
- ☐ Athletic tape; Coban; elastic wraps; ankle, wrist, finger, and hand splints; slings
- ☐ OTC Prilosec, Prevacid, Pepcid, Zantac (or generics); liquid Maalox; baking soda
- ☐ Oil of clove for dental (nerve) pain

Actions to take:

- ☐ Learn about using willow bark at the University of Maryland Medical Center Web site (at http://www.umm.edu/altmed/articles/willow-bark-000281.htm); also, locate a local source of willow bark or plant your own trees.
- ☐ Study up on massage and effleurage techniques
- ☐ Download a pain scale you find useful

SECTION SIX

Acute Injuries

Introduction to Acute Injuries

This section is aimed at injuries that would normally require the attention of a physician, but which could be treated successfully without professional care. These are conditions encountered on a regular basis in family practice, pediatrics, urgent care, and emergency rooms. Common injuries include burns, strains, lacerations, bites, stings, and concussions, among others. Each chapter begins with a snapshot of a situation in which you may one day find yourself, and outlines an approach to diagnosis and treatment.

Severe injuries, such as traumatic amputation, skull fracture, or bullet wounds, are beyond the scope of this book. Anyone interested in treating such serious conditions should invest in medical reference books on surgery and trauma.

Chapter 15

Burns

With the public water supply no longer reliable, you'll likely be boiling water for drinking and cooking purposes. Now suppose, when your daily work is done, you decide to reward your efforts with a cup of hot coffee. As you head to the back porch, you trip over a pile of firewood, spilling the entire cup on your thighs. You cry out in dismay, as you desperately try to loosen your jeans. When you finally wriggle free of them, you realize you've torn open several large blisters. The pain is excruciating. The hospital has been closed for months and you don't know the whereabouts of any doctor. Is there anything you can do on your own?

The above scenario is typical of the most common type of burn that medical practitioners encounter, that is, a second-degree thermal burn. Patients generally seek treatment due to the pain, the appearance, and fear of infection. But with a little knowledge, yes, you can treat yourself effectively.

Before discussing treatment, we should first address diagnosis. Burns are divided into three basic groups. **First-degree burns** cause erythema (redness) of the skin with mild discomfort, but no blistering. A mild to moderate sunburn is the prototype of a first-degree burn. No special care is required beyond keeping the area clean and avoiding further exposure to heat. Such a burn may cause superficial peeling a week or so after the initial injury, but should leave no scar. Most patients do not seek treatment for a first-degree burn. Other types of first-degree burns include brief exposure to hot water, hot cooking dishes or utensils, mechanical devices, and occasionally chemical burns.

The initial treatment of a first-degree thermal burn is cooling the affected area, preferably by immersion in cool water, to prevent further tissue damage. Chemical burns are much less common than those caused by exposure to sunlight or excessive heat. The initial treatment for a chemical burn is likewise to rinse the affected area with water, to prevent further injury. Applying a dressing to a first-degree burn is optional, depending on location, and is primarily aimed at avoiding physical trauma to the area. Because the skin remains intact with such a burn, antibacterial creams are unnecessary.

Skipping over to **third-degree burns** for a moment, these would present a challenge for home treatment. Fortunately, such severe injuries are much less common than first- or second-degree burns. A third-degree burn causes deep tissue damage, penetrating below the skin into the subcutaneous tissues or even muscles, commonly resulting in localized nerve damage. It's a bad sign when a significant burn is not painful, as this generally indicates a deep injury. Nowadays, most patients with third-degree burns are treated at a burn or wound center. In the event of societal collapse and total absence of professional healthcare, treating a third-degree burn as you would a second-degree burn would be the place to start, with extreme attention to cleanliness and preventing infection. Fluid loss also becomes an issue, as does shock and sepsis. A localized third-degree burn may certainly heal (with scarring), but without specialized care, an extensive third-degree burn may well prove fatal. Again, these severe burns are thankfully uncommon.

Back to **second-degree burns**, which will be our focus here. Common causes of second-degree burns include prolonged exposure to bright sunlight, brief or prolonged exposure to hot liquids, inadvertent exposure to steam, or skin contact with mechanical or household devices such as a skillet, soldering iron, etc. A second-degree burn is usually quite painful immediately, with residual discomfort persisting for a few days to a few weeks. Pain medication may be necessary for a large injury.

Initially, the skin may appear quite red in the area of exposure, or demonstrate immediate blistering, or appear as an open wound denuded of skin, or sometimes look white (ash, actually) from brief exposure to a very hot surface. Additional blisters may develop over the next several hours, often with residual redness (first-degree burn) at the periphery.

The rule of nines

To estimate the extent of injury, the following percentages of total body surface area (TBSA) may be used. These numbers include only skin damaged by 2nd-degree or higher burns.

Head/neck	9%
Each arm	9%
Anterior thorax	18 %
Posterior thorax	18 %
Each leg	18 %
Perineum	1%

The palm of the patient's hand is approximately 1% of total body surface area, and may be used to estimate patchy areas. Normally a 2nd-degree burn involved 10% of TBSA or more would be referred to a specialized burn unit.

The percentage of TBSA is included in the Parkland Formula for initial fluid resuscitation (see next page).

There is actually quite a range of severity among second-degree burns. A splash of hot oil might cause a 1-cm area of painful blistering, qualifying the injury as a second-degree burn. However, a severe, total body sunburn, as might occur after a day at the beach without sunscreen, would be of greater medical concern. Thermal injury of a large skin surface may cause nausea, fatigue, fluid loss, dizziness, and a general feeling of unwellness. Most patients actually seek medical treatment for smaller, painful burns which have blistered. Location is also significant. A three-inch burn on the face, hand, or genitalia is of more concern than a similar wound on the leg or torso, due to the risk of infection, scarring, disability, or proximity to vital structures such as the eyes.

A badly burned patient requires intensive care with special attention to excess fluid loss and intake. Care of these patients is beyond the scope of this book and a professional text should be consulted. Initial fluid needs for a critical patient are addressed in the Parkland Formula, below.

Initial fluid resuscitation in the badly burned patient:

The Parkland Formula for Adults

Administer 2–4 ml of Lactated Ringer's I.V. solution* for each kg of patient body weight multiplied by the percent total body surface area involved.

2–4 ml LR x BW in kg x % TBSC

Administer half this amount evenly over the first 8 hours after injury, and the remainder over the next 16 hours.

* In a patient able to take oral fluids, especially when I.V. fluids are unavailable, oral rehydration solution should be substituted.

As with a first-degree burn, cooling the area immediately helps prevent further tissue damage (the cooking of your own tissue). Of course, primary prevention is a better idea. If you must be in the sun, use sunscreen or protect your skin with long sleeves and long pants. Don't forget a hat to protect your face and nape of your neck. If you're working with hot liquids, fire, steam, or hot utensils, make sure to have a supply of clean, cool water available, in case of accidental injury.

The major concern with second-degree burns is potential infection. If the skin is blistered but intact, it should be left intact. Your own skin is the best Band-Aid. Blistered skin rarely becomes infected as long as the blisters haven't opened. Occasionally a blister will enlarge to the point that it threatens to burst. Blisters exhibiting this much pressure can be decompressed by nicking the corner of the blister, using a sterile needle or other sharp, sterile utensil, thus allowing the clear blister fluid to escape. Afterwards the skin should lie flat against the underlying raw tissue, providing a clean, natural dressing. Protecting this fragile skin with a padding of gauze will help prevent further accidental injury. Decompressing a blister also causes less discomfort than removing the loose, blistered tissue. Sometimes the blister fluid will re-accumulate and the process will need to be repeated. Blisters remaining intact should be protected from potential trauma for several days with a soft bulky dressing.

If the blisters have already popped, or if the skin has sloughed off, or if you have decompressed a blister, a non-stick dressing should be applied, such as a Telfa pad coated with an antibacterial cream or ointment. Bacitracin is used by hospitals and physicians, and may be purchased over-the-counter. Because this medicine is both inexpensive and effective at preventing infection, laying in a good supply is an excellent idea. Silver sulfadiazine cream is an elegant antibacterial burn cream often prescribed for a significant injury. If you have a good relationship with your family doctor, he or she might be willing to prescribe a supply for emergency use. Again, the cream is applied to the dressing, which is then applied to the wound. The use of honey in the treatment of burns is addressed in **Chapter 30**.

Change the dressing daily to check for the possibility of infection. The primary wound will already appear red, but an infected burn may develop an expanding area of pinkness around the edges. Although many second-degree burns are surrounded by an area of first-degree burn, after the first 24 hours, this zone of erythema (red or pink skin) should be starting to fade, rather than enlarge. Other signs of infection include foul odor, pus, increased pain, fever, increased warmth, or red streaks extending from the burn upwards, following the venous or lymphatic channels. Cultures from infected burns typically demonstrate skin bacteria, usually staph or strep germs. Occasionally wounds will become colonized or infected with fecal or other organisms, but this is uncommon if both the injured area and caregiver's hands remain clean. A second-degree burn may be gently rinsed daily with warm or cool water (cool is usually more comfortable), with a little soap added if desired.

If the burn exhibits signs of infection, especially if the wound seems to be enlarging, then treating with an oral antibiotic is appropriate. First-line antibiotics for infected burns include cephalexin, Augmentin, (or possibly an erythromycin in a penicillin-allergic patient). If these are not effective, you may be dealing with methicillin-resistant *Staph. aureus*, or other resistant organism such as *Pseudomonas*. A trial of a sulfa drug, doxycycline, ciprofloxacin, or Levaquin would be a good second choice. (Generally speaking, amoxicillin and penicillin do not work well for skin infections.) The length of antibiotic therapy depends on the extent of the infection and the response to treatment. I suggest treating at least two days beyond apparent resolution of the infection. A small area, say an inch or so across, may resolve with as little as three or four days of oral antibiotic therapy. A larger infected burn may require 7 to 10 days of treatment. Using a topical antibacterial preparation (such as bacitracin, Bactroban, silver sulfadiazine, or even honey) in conjunction with an oral antibiotic may help limit length of treatment and conserve your supply of life-saving oral antibiotics.

Depending on the size of the injury and any secondary infection, second-degree burns usually heal within a few weeks, although it may take several weeks to a few months for the appearance to return to normal. Sometimes scarring is permanent.

Chapter 15 – Checklist

Items to include in your medical supplies:

- ☐ Medical grade honey or standard clover honey
- ☐ Non-stick bandages such as Telfa pads; sanitary napkins for large wounds; large Band-Aids
- ☐ Sterile and/or non-sterile gauze rolls for bulky dressings and coverings; medical tape or Coban
- ☐ Sterile needle for puncturing tense blisters
- ☐ Silver sulfadiazine cream (or possibly colloidal silver); bacitracin; Bactroban
- ☐ Oral antibiotics for skin infections (per Chapter 13)
- ☐ Oral pain relievers (acetaminophen, ibuprofen, naproxen sodium, tramadol, narcotics)

Actions to take:

- ☐ Educate yourself about colloidal silver preparations at: http://www.silver-colloids.com/index.html

Chapter 16

Back Strain

(Continued from Chapter 15 . . .) Remember that water you were boiling before you burned yourself? It takes a lot of firewood to keep the stove going. Is all that heavy lifting the reason your back's killing you?

A sprained back is usually caused by lifting too heavy a load, often while twisting or bending, or by repetitive lifting of a lesser load. Perhaps you experienced immediate pain, and were therefore able to identify the cause. Or, just as likely, your backache developed several days after prolonged work, leaving you uncertain as to the etiology. Because the onset of pain is often delayed, make sure to ask patients with back pain about their activities for up to a week prior to the onset of pain. The original injury may not have caused as much discomfort as the swelling that develops a few to several days later. Family physicians see patients with back pain on a daily basis, so count on treating this common malady.

What is a back strain anyway?

Basically a strain or a sprain is a microscopic tear of a muscle, ligament, or tendon. In the case of the back, this is usually one of the large muscles that support the skeleton of the lower back. These injuries do not show on X-ray, except for minor changes in the alignment of the spine caused by tight muscles. The body's response to a strain or sprain is localized swelling with resultant muscle stiffness, pain, and sometimes tenderness. Additionally, pain on movement occurs, alerting the patient to the need for rest to allow the affected area to heal. Frayed muscle fibers can grow back together more quickly if they're not being stretched and pulled repeatedly.

The pain of a **simple back strain** is confined to the muscles of the back, and does not travel down the legs, as a sciatic nerve injury might. Isolated back pain may also be caused by an underlying injury to the **intervertebral discs** or **vertebrae** themselves, which is often difficult to differentiate from a simple strain. A **slipped disc** usually causes pain into the legs, though the discomfort is sometimes isolated to the lower back. Anyone suffering from low back pain that shoots down the back of the leg, especially if it is accompanied by numbness or tingling, is probably suffering from a degree of **nerve impingement** (**sciatica** or **lumbar radiculopathy**). Fortunately, most of these patients benefit from the same therapies that help a muscular back strain. Don't worry too much if you can't pinpoint the diagnosis – doctors frequently are unsure themselves.

In an elderly person, especially a frail woman, a **vertebral compression fracture** of the lumbar spine is a common cause of isolated back pain. Vertebral compression fractures generally occur after a fall, and cause significant back pain (but not leg pain, unless a nerve is also pinched). In an elderly patient with advanced osteoporosis, a compression fracture may occur with normal activities of everyday life, even just sitting. Pain on movement may be extreme. The treatment of such a fracture is rest and pain medication for several weeks. Nearly every other cause of low back pain benefits from low-impact exercise early on, whereas with compression fractures weight-bearing exercise should be delayed a few weeks, then gradually reintroduced. A walker or wheelchair may be necessary if walking is too difficult. Encourage these inactive patients to breathe deeply in spite of the pain, to avoid developing pneumonia.

Acute back pain is best treated with relative rest and pain relievers. Relative rest means to avoid heavy lifting and repetitive bending, especially the activity which brought on the problem to start with, but it does not mean to lie in bed (although a day or two of bed rest may be beneficial). Walking at a slow to moderate pace tends to loosen the muscles of the back. Anyone fortunate enough to have a pool available would benefit from swimming or walking in chest deep water. Sleeping on one's side with a pillow between the knees helps align the back and reduce discomfort. Back massage, along with heat or ice to the affected area, may help as well.

Over-the-counter pain medication affords adequate relief in most patients, in the form of ibuprofen (200–800 mg three times a day) or naproxen sodium (200–400 mg twice daily) (the higher dosages equaling prescription strength). Since any anti-inflammatory medication may cause gastritis (stomach irritation), always administer these drugs with food and observe carefully for stomach upset. Some patients are better able to tolerate them if given simultaneously with a stomach acid-reducing medication, such as Pepcid or Prilosec. In patients who cannot tolerate ibuprofen, naproxen, or aspirin, acetaminophen is an option (500–1000 mg every 4–6 hours). Also, any anti-inflammatory drug may be combined with acetaminophen if necessary for pain relief. Patients unaccustomed to narcotics find this combination quite effective. Narcotics such as Vicodin, Percocet, or Tylenol #3 are effective as well, but should be reserved for serious injuries. It is quite unlikely your doctor will be willing to prescribe a narcotic for stockpiling, so laying in a supply of over-the-counter anti-inflammatories and acetaminophen is your best bet. Other medications sometimes useful are prescription tramadol, muscle relaxers, and sleep aids.

Except in extreme cases, even slipped discs and pinched nerves are treated about the same as simple back strains. Orthopedic surgery is unlikely to be an option after an Armageddon event, and people will have to make-do with what is available. Hands-on medicine, i.e., physical therapy, massage, and chiropractic therapy, is also therapeutic. The bottom line is that most backs heal, given sufficient rest and appropriate exercise, and there is little likelihood you will cause further injury if you discontinue the activity which brought the problem on. By two years post-op, many patients who have undergone surgery for slipped discs are no better off than those who declined surgery.

X-rays or MRI scans will be scarce or non-existent after an Armageddon event. Diagnosis will be made according to history, symptoms, and physical examination, which are the bedrock of medical diagnosis in any event. If a person's back pain is clearly attributable to an injury, other causes of back pain are probably irrelevant. However, for a person with gradual onset of lower back pain with no prior acute or overuse injury, other causes of back pain should be considered, including urinary infection, shingles, intra-abdominal problems, and prostate infection, as discussed previously.

Non-pharmaceutical relief of back pain

Sleep position

Sleep with a pillow between the knees to align the hips and lower spine, and with a neck or head pillow that maintains proper alignment of the head and neck with the body.

First morning exercise

Before arising in the morning, roll over on your stomach and use your arms to help curl your torso backwards, similar to a push-up from the waist. Hold 5 seconds and repeat 10 times.

Daytime activity

Change position frequently, from sitting to standing, every half hour, and walk around for several minutes.

Daily exercise

Walk (or better yet, swim) half an hour daily

Tens Unit

Obtain a prescription for a Transcutaneous Electric Nerve Stimulation Unit, with extra pads, wires, batteries, and electrodes. Experiment to ascertain the best position and settings for optimal relief.

Proper lifting technique

Avoid bending at the waist – better to squat and lift with your legs, not your back. Strengthen your abdominal and leg muscles to take the load off the lumbar spine and supporting tissues.

Lumbar support

Obtain an elastic lumbar support for use during exercise.

Massage

Have a loved one visit a massage therapist with you to learn effective techniques for back muscle relaxation for future use.

Chapter 16 – Checklist

Items to include in your medical supplies:

☐ OTC pain relievers (acetaminophen, ibuprofen, aspirin, naproxen sodium)

☐ Re-usable hot water bottle and ice packs

☐ Prescription tramadol and muscle relaxers (cyclobenzaprine) for pain relief

☐ Wheelchair or transport chair, walker, and crutches

☐ Orthopedic lumbar support

Actions to take:

☐ Watch or download videos for treatment of low back pain at: http://www.spine-health.com/information/back-exercise-videos

Chapter 17

Cuts and Lacerations

(Continued from Chapter 16 . . .) In your surprise at burning yourself, you dropped your china coffee cup to the floor, which has shattered. Your preteen daughter runs into the room barefoot when she hears your cry of pain. Suddenly she shrieks in alarm as she steps on a knifelike shard. Blood gushes from her foot as she hops to safety, fortunately avoiding further injury. For a moment you are distracted from your own misery as you catch sight of a 2-inch dagger of glass protruding from her foot. Where in the world is a doctor when you need one?

Lacerations are among the commonest of injuries. Sooner or later everyone succumbs. More often than not, these are caused by personal carelessness rather than injury inflicted by a second party. In an era when antibiotics may be scarce and infection may be lethal, keeping one's skin intact becomes vital. Wearing well-fitting shoes even indoors is an essential part of foot care when the consequences of injury may be dire. Diabetics and other patients with peripheral (foot) nerve damage are especially at risk, since they may not know if they step on a tack, or if their shoes have rubbed their feet raw. My own father developed large, deep blisters from wearing ill-fitting shoes, which took months to heal even under ideal circumstances.

People often use sharp instruments carelessly, partly because, in the back of their minds, they know medical care is available. But if it is not, what will you do if you slice your finger on a kitchen knife or cut your arm with a chainsaw? Anytime you use a utensil with the potential of tissue damage, think first and take necessary precautions. Not only may a stitch in time save nine, but a little forethought may prevent stitches altogether.

The unfortunate victim of our story is now sitting at the kitchen table holding her foot up, staring at a 1-1/2 inch gash in the sole of her foot, with the 2-inch glass dagger protruding from it. Such an injury is actually worse than most lacerations you may encounter. To start with, let's deal with a simpler situation.

One of the most common injuries is a gash caused by a knife or other clean, sharp instrument. These lacerations are typically straight or curvilinear (curved in an arc, but not jagged). They may pierce part-way through the skin, all the way through the skin, or deeper into the subcutaneous fat and connective tissue. (Rarely do they sever a muscle or tendon, and complex wound repair is beyond the scope of this book.)

The primary goal of wound treatment is to allow the body to repair itself. In order to accomplish this (at least with a good cosmetic result), the edges of the wound must be close together in order for cells to bridge the gap. This is all that stitches really accomplish. Wounds heal best when they are clean, so the first step is to remove any visible contamination, such as skin fragments, gravel, splinters, shards, etc. Even if no contamination is visible, microscopic contamination from the skin surface itself or the sharp implement is likely. An open wound should be rinsed with a clean liquid, either water, saline, or if these are unavailable, possibly hydrogen peroxide or alcohol (both of which will sting considerably). Plain clean water is fine, or mild soap may be added if necessary for adequate cleansing, rinsing with clear water afterwards. Using surgical soap such as Hibiclens is optimal but not mandatory.

If the wound is oozing blood, applying pressure for several minutes will usually stop the flow. There is no hurry here. If it takes 15 or even 30 minutes of pressure to get the bleeding to stop, don't worry. Even a small spurting artery will slow down if pressure is applied long enough. Cleaning a wound may cause it to re-bleed, but once the wound is clean, pressure may be reapplied until the bleeding once again ceases.

With a linear laceration, the next question is how far apart do the edges lie? Patients often seek treatment for lacerations that are not even quite through the skin. These may look somewhat fragile, as if putting traction on the edges might separate the wound completely (which could accidentally happen – no big deal, though. See below for repair of a deeper wound). A laceration only part-way through the skin does not require suturing, but is benefited from some external support to prevent further injury. Steri-Strips or butterfly dressings can be used to pull the edges together a bit and stabilize them. If medical supplies are unavailable, strips of clean electrical tape or duct tape may suffice. Using an antibiotic ointment often loosens adhesive dressings, and is usually unnecessary for this type of laceration. If you do choose to use an antibiotic ointment, make sure the adhesive strips are as secure as possible before applying the ointment. Overall, it's better to clean the wound thoroughly first, tape it, and avoid the antibiotic ointment. Scalp wounds can be closed by braiding the hair across the wound, drawing the edges together.

How long should any sort of adhesive closure be left on? On thin or fine skin which is not under tension, 4–6 days is probably sufficient. On an area that is under tension or subject to movement or friction, 6–10 days is adequate. For patients who must continue using their lacerated hands or other body parts, I often supplement the wound closing with an elastic bandage all the way around the arm, hand, leg, or foot, to lessen the chance that the tapes might loosen.

Next, what about an injury that is all the way through the skin? The fortunate patient will have such a wound aligning with the skin lines or folds. These wounds often lie flat on their own with the edges in good position, at least as long as the injured area is not used. In a patient able and willing to remain with the injured part in a good position with the wound edges well-aligned, these areas may be simply taped, as above. The longest wound I've ever taped shut was a 3-inch laceration straight down a patient's shin. After taping I wrapped her entire lower leg with an elastic bandage for additional support. This patient was happy not to have stitches and was careful to prevent re-injury. She healed wonderfully – as well as, or better than, had she had sutures. Suturing a wound actually introduces the element of a foreign body, and sometimes causes more inflammation than simply taping the wound together.

But what if the wound gapes open? Wounds that go "against the grain" or against the skin lines are often under tension, which causes them to gape open. In general, these wounds do not heal with as nice a scar as those that go "with" the skin lines. One common example is the incision of a cesarean section. Most women prefer the bikini cut, a horizontal incision low across the abdomen, above the pubic hair. These scars do not widen and often are nearly invisible. However a vertical incision, even though it is not under tension (since the abdomen is loose after childbirth), will be significantly wider and sometimes feels a little "lumpy" (with subcutaneous retractions).

A laceration that goes against the skin lines, i.e. one that gapes open, will usually require suturing. Suturing (stitching a wound together) is not rocket science. Installing a zipper in a pair of pants is much more difficult. The important points are to place sutures 1) deeply enough and 2) closely enough, but not too close. For a wound that is barely through the skin, placing the sutures an eighth to a quarter inch apart is about right. Again, the goal is to have the wound edges lie right next to each other. If the stitches are too far apart, the wound will gape or bunch up between sutures.

There is usually no need to shave the area before suturing, unless you cannot see what you are doing, or unless you cannot keep the hair out of the wound edge. Hairs caught within a wound may prevent proper healing or cause an "ingrown" hair or local irritation.

For a gaping wound, it is usually best to start at one end and work towards the other, making sure the edges align properly as you go. (Some doctors prefer to start in the middle and work their way outward, repeatedly bisecting each half of the laceration with a new suture.) The depth of the sutures should be about the same as the width. For a laceration just through the skin, the sutures should be about an eighth to a quarter inch deep and an equal distance across the wound. The depth of the suture should be near or just above the bottom of the wound. If only the surface skin is brought together and not the underlying tissues, fluid may accumulate in the gap, which prevents healing.

Curved medical needles are very convenient for suturing because they allow the operator to suture more deeply than with a straight needle. When using a curved needle, the point of the needle should be directly perpendicular to the skin as the needle is inserted. Following the natural curve straight down into and then out of the opposite side of the wound yields a good result, without the edges of the skin dipping down into the suture line, which you want to avoid. A slightly humped-up appearance, with the upper wound edge *very slightly* open will heal better than one with the edges "bent" into the wound. Really this is only common sense: one intact skin surface does not adhere and grow onto another one. If you are using a straight sewing needle, gently pinching or pulling the wound edges upwards as you insert the needle will allow you to place the suture deeper and will result in a slightly humped-up appearance and improved healing.

For a shallow wound the needle may be inserted in one side and out the other in a single step. For a deeper wound it is best to insert the needle from one edge of the laceration, bringing the needle up in the middle of the wound. The suture may then be completed by repositioning the needle and sewing from the inside of the wound to the opposite outer edge, where a knot may be placed.

Doctors usually place interrupted sutures, that is, one stitch at a time, rather than running sutures (like sewing a seam). These keep the wound better aligned, and if one is accidentally removed, they don't all fall out.

How tight to make the knots is another concern. They should be snug, pulling the edges of the laceration together, yet without excess tension on the wound. Excess tension is apparent when the skin bunches or gapes between sutures, and is common when the sutures have not been placed deeply enough. Also, when the knots are too loose, the sutures will lengthen, allowing the wound edges to gape apart. This is often caused by slippage of the suture material. Nylon or other synthetic suture material is great for suturing skin wounds, because germs adhere less well to the slippery surface. However, for the same reason, knots are more likely to slip. The best way to get around this is to use a "surgeons knot" for the first loop of the knot. This merely amounts to looping around twice instead of once with the first throw of the knot. (Children sometimes use this technique on slippery shoe laces.) Subsequent throws of the knot should all be singletons. Make sure you use square knots, and not Granny knots. The Girl Scouts teach "right over left and under, then left over right and under." A total of four or five throws is sufficient. If you happen to mix in a Granny knot among your chain of square knots, it is rarely necessary to remove the errant knot. Simple add on a few more correct throws.

What sort of suture material should you use? For thin or fine skin, such as a child's skin or that on an adult face, 5-0 nylon or other synthetic is advisable. This thinner suture material is less likely to leave scars where the sutures themselves have been placed. With a thinner suture material, the individual stitches will need to be closer together. Although this may amount to more stitches than with a thicker material, the cosmetic result is usually better. For a standard laceration on an extremity or the torso, 4-0 material is good. For a very deep gash, 3-0 suture is a consideration. Of course, you may not have medical suture materials available. Thick nylon thread or fine fishing line could be substituted. The 5-0 material described above is a little thicker than a human hair; 4-0 is about twice as thick; 3-0 is 2 to 3 times thicker yet.

When suturing a wound, local anesthesia is optional. The pain of each stitch is no worse than getting a small injection without numbing. Some patients find the administration of a local anesthetic more painful than the placement of a few simple stitches or staples. Fear of pain is often a bigger problem than the pain itself. If you do have 1% or 2% lidocaine available, this may be used for numbing the surrounding skin. Infiltrating about 1 mL of lidocaine solution per inch of laceration should be sufficient. Both sides of the wound need to be numbed. I generally inject into the open area of the wound underlying the skin because this is less painful than injecting into intact skin. If you do inject, try to stay superficial enough inside the wound to cause the overlying skin to bulge upward a little. Injecting deep into the wound will not numb the skin. Lidocaine with epinephrine is good for scalp wounds and other areas with significant bleeding. (Epinephrine causes vasoconstriction, that is, narrowing of the blood vessels, which results in less bleeding.) Lidocaine without epinephrine is generally used on fingers and toes, and should probably be used for lacerations in the feet of diabetics and others were compromised circulation. For a patient allergic to lidocaine, injectable Benadryl (diphenhydramine) may be substituted.

Anesthesia without pain

The trick to painless anesthesia is patience. Nowadays doctors are always in a hurry. They inject local anesthetics quickly, knowing the discomfort won't last long. If you've ever had stitches, you know lidocaine stings enough to frighten a child (and some adults). However, it is possible to numb a wound painlessly, though doing so takes longer.

Start by simply dripping lidocaine into the wound, allowing it to absorb a few minutes. Then *very slowly*, from inside the wound, inject a tiny amount of anesthetic under the skin surface and into the edges of the wound, a little at a time with a 25 or smaller gauge needle. Talk reassuringly to the patient as you do this, and avoid drawing attention to the wound. Taking five minutes to complete what is otherwise a 20-second procedure may earn you a cooperative child and thankful parent.

Flap lacerations are also common. These are caused when a sharp object encounters the skin at an angle, nearly slicing off a flap. Sometimes they occur when sudden tension is placed on the skin and a flap of skin is pulled back. (I have a scar from a full-thickness flap laceration on my hand caused by stopping a self-propelled dog toy on it as a child. This one-and-a-half-inch injury was not sutured and healed quite well merely by taping the flap in place.) Flap lacerations may be through the very superficial layers of skin, or all the way through. If you think of the tip of the laceration as the point of the letter "V," this area must be thick enough to suture, otherwise it will tear through. The tip is almost always the thinnest tissue, but if it is thick enough to suture (which is a judgment call), the first suture should anchor the tip in place with good anatomic alignment. Subsequent sutures are then placed one by one from either end. If the tip is too thin to suture, two anchoring sutures may be placed on either side of the flap where adequate tissue thickness allows, and the tip subsequently taped in place. Again, simply taping a flap laceration often works quite well.

Back to our unfortunate victim, who is still dripping blood on the kitchen floor. With a two-inch dagger of glass protruding from her foot, she was unsure what to do regarding applying pressure. If professional care is available, it is best to stabilize the patient, leaving the foreign object in place for later removal by a physician. However, unless an injured victim can be transported for definitive medical care, the foreign body should be removed. (I am not an expert on what to do if a knife is sticking out of your eyeball, but unless a neurosurgeon or ophthalmologist is available, it is best removed.)

In a way you should count yourself lucky: the foreign body is visible. Removing splinters, even large ones, often amounts to what I call a "fishing expedition." You'd think that such foreign bodies are easy to find beneath the skin, but this is often not the case. They may be quite distant from the entry wound, and in the deeper tissues are often difficult to palpate. When covered with blood, splinters are hard to discern from human tissue by sight alone.

Upon removing the glass dagger, you should expect more bleeding. You may as well irrigate the wound now, despite the bleeding, to remove any additional shards that may be lurking. If there is a question of glass splinters deep within the wound, do not use your own finger to explore for them. Instead use a pair of forceps or tweezers, feeling for a hard, glasslike surface. If you've done your best to clean the wound, then it is time to move on. Small foreign bodies that are left behind sometimes work their way out at a later date. Apply pressure to the wound until the bleeding stops.

With the wound clean and dry, the next consideration is whether deep tissue damage has occurred, as in tendon or ligament disruption, or even bony injury. Perhaps a damaged tendon is visible, though this is usually difficult to determine in a bloody environment. Doctors usually ascertain tendon damage by observing whether the patient can move his extremities as he should. For example, an injury to the bottom of the foot might cut the tendons that permit a person to curl their foot or toes downward. An injury to the top of the foot might prevent a patient from pulling his toes backward. If the function of a hand, foot, or other body part is compromised, it would be ideal to have a surgeon or at least a physician of some sort repair the wound. Tendon repair is beyond the scope of this book. Assuming no deep tissue damage has been found, or if it is present, that you have no one to help you, then closing the wound is the next consideration.

Ideally, a half-inch deep gash in the sole of the foot would be repaired in layers, with absorbable sutures placed deep in the wound, to draw the deep tissues together. Afterwards, 4-0 synthetic suture material could be used to close the skin. However, most non-physicians will not feel comfortable doing a multi-layer closure. In this event, it is probably better to use heavier-duty suture material such as 3-0 nylon, placed with a large curved needle. Again it is important to place the suture clear to the bottom of the wound. With deeper sutures, it is easier to place half the suture (from the outside to the inside of the wound), then reposition the needle to place the other half (from the inside to the opposite side), rather than try to bridge the entire wound diameter with one fell swoop.

What if the bleeding resumes every time you release the pressure? If you have the equipment, you could try hyfercating (locally cauterizing) a bleeding blood vessel, or tying off a visible bleeder. (A paper clip heated to glowing could be used as a cautery, preferably after local anesthesia.) But assuming these are not really options, simply sew the wound shut and then if needed, continue applying pressure, even if you have to do so for hours. The bleeding will stop eventually in almost every situation when sufficient pressure is applied for long enough. For an injury on the foot, not walking on the injured limb for several days would help prevent re-bleeding.

Next, for injuries on the foot, prevention of infection is paramount. Again, ideally, a patient would refrain from walking on the injured foot for about a week. But whether or not this occurs, the foot must be protected from contamination with dirt or dust, using a bulky protective dressing.

Any time there is concern for infection, the wound should be examined daily. Look for redness, swelling, pus, increased pain, or heat. If these symptoms occur, they should be treated according to the guidelines for soft tissue infections discussed in **Chapter 13**. This also raises the question of whether prophylactic antibiotics should be given to prevent infection. In the example above, we have a potentially dirty foot but a relatively clean cutting implement. The table below outlines other possibilities and my personal recommendations for using prophylactic antibiotics. If these are employed preventively, three days of therapy should be plenty, using either cephalexin or Augmentin (or possibly erythromycin in a penicillin-allergic patient). Therapy for established infection would, of course, require a longer treatment period, typically 5 to 10 days, according to guidelines discussed earlier for skin infections.

Wound Type and Prophylactic Antibiotics

Body area	Cause of Wound	Circulation	Antibiotics?
Clean	Clean	Good	No
Clean	Clean	Poor	Probably not
Clean	Dirty	Good	Probably yes
Clean	Dirty	Poor	Yes
Dirty	Clean	Good	Maybe
Dirty	Clean	Poor	Yes
Dirty	Dirty	Good	Yes
Dirty	Dirty	Poor	Yes

While the above instructions for laceration repair do not cover every possible scenario, they do offer an approach to addressing the majority of injuries a layman is likely to encounter. Other wound closure options exist. Stapling could be substituted for closure of wounds on the scalp, torso, and fleshy parts of the arms and legs. Staples are not good for the hands, feet, genitalia, or face. The primary advantages of stapling are speed and ease of use. For certain scalp lacerations, the hair could be twisted or braided across a laceration, pulling the skin together as effectively as sutures would. (Most doctors have never actually used this technique, however.) Pincer ants have been used to close lacerations, breaking off the ants' heads after the pincer has been applied. Perhaps your own creativity will lead you to new techniques professionals have not yet considered.

Chapter 17 – Checklist

Items to include in your medical supplies:

- ☐ Sterile water or saline, or the means to sterilize water (iodine, bleach, heat)
- ☐ Autoclave or other sterilization equipment (e.g., Cidex for instruments)
- ☐ Baby hairbrush for cleansing wounds; WaterPik; antibacterial soap (Hibiclens)
- ☐ Sterile drapes, gauze, and dressings
- ☐ Needle holders, hemostats, tweezers/forceps (flat and toothed), suture scissors
- ☐ Suture material (3-0, 4-0, and 5-0) – nylon and absorbable
- ☐ Wound-closure tapes (Steri-Strips or similar); Duct tape for emergency use
- ☐ Local anesthetic: lidocaine (with and without epinephrine)
- ☐ Syringes – most useful are 3-cc syringes with 25-gauge, 1-inch needles attached

Actions to take:

- ☐ Watch instructional videos demonstrating suturing techniques
at: www.armageddonmedicine.net
- ☐ Make sure your family and loved ones have been immunized against tetanus

Chapter 18

Knee Injuries

(Continued from Chapter 17 . . .) Your injured daughter is recovering well, happy to nurse her injured foot, leaving it up to you to gather firewood despite your burns and backache. As you make your way deeper into the forest, you step in a hole and twist your knee hard enough to swear. Limping back with the single log you've found, you wonder if you'll ever walk normally again. Can your family survive if you find yourself crippled?

Knee injuries can be permanently disabling, especially if surgical intervention is unavailable. Fortunate, most are not. The basic rule for knee injuries is: if it hurts, stay off it.

A twisting movement of the knee is probably the most common mechanism of injury. Other potential modes of injury include direct impact, lateral pressure to the knee while the foot is fixed, hyperextension of the knee, and excessive flexion. Twisting injuries may result in a mere sprain, or sometimes damage to the cartilage or ligaments that support and stabilize the knee joint. Knee fractures are fairly uncommon.

If the knee swells and feels mushy (like a water balloon) after an injury, this is most likely due to damage inside the knee joint, i.e., damaged cartilage (meniscus) or ligaments. Although there are ways to differentiate between these problems, without the possibility of surgery the treatment will be much the same. In certain circumstances walking on a hurting knee will cause more trouble than with other injuries, especially in the case of a torn cartilage where the loose piece gets stuck in the knee, much like jamming a pencil in a door hinge. Some patients can tell when their knee "goes out," and occasionally they will feel it slip back into place. Walking on a malpositioned piece of overlapping cartilage will cause considerable pain and further damage.

No matter how an injury of the knee is sustained, getting off it as soon as possible is advisable. If you twist your knee in the woods, make yourself a crutch. If your knee feels more comfortable in a certain position, try to leave it in that position until you can get off your feet. For most injuries this means keeping the knee slightly flexed (bent). When you are able to sit down, apply ice as soon as possible to limit swelling. An elastic bandage or knee brace will help stabilize the joint.

Unlike back strains, where staying mobile helps keep the muscles loose, knee sprains respond best to rest. The period of recovery will be lengthened if you walk on it and cause further damage. An unstable knee is susceptible to repeat injury.

Although doctors sometimes withdraw fluid from the knee to relieve pressure, do not, repeat, *do not* try this yourself. Introducing skin bacteria inside the joint is a recipe for serious, possibly incurable infection. A joint effusion (water on the knee) acts somewhat like a splint, preventing unwanted movement. Wrapping the knee with an Ace wrap will help counterbalance this inner pressure. For adults, a 4–5 inch high quality elastic wrap and a size large Neoprene knee brace with metal side supports are good additions to your medical kit. For children, a 3-inch wrap and size small knee brace are appropriate.

Avoid taking large amounts of pain medicine that permit you to walk comfortably. Masking the pain and walking on a damaged knee will only lead to further damage. Using ibuprofen, aspirin, or acetaminophen for discomfort present at rest is reasonable and unlikely to camouflage a serious injury. Most knee pain is related to weight-bearing. Once you're off your feet, applying ice is often all that's needed. If you must walk, consider crutches or a walker. Continue using the knee brace until all discomfort, swelling, and instability resolve.

A simple knee sprain may recover in minutes to hours. An average knee sprain will take a few days of limited movement before the swelling resolves and you can walk comfortably. A serious knee sprain will take weeks before full recovery, and a badly torn ligament or meniscus may never be the same again, causing recurring pain or a permanent limp. Again, prevention is key. Knowing that surgical treatment is not an option should make a person more careful. Is it reasonable to play tackle football today when you may need to march 20 miles to safety tomorrow?

Chapter 18 – Checklist

Items to include in your medical supplies:

☐ Neoprene knee braces – sizes small, (possibly medium), and large

☐ Hinged knee brace and/or knee immobilizer

☐ Ace wraps – 3″, 4″, and 5″ widths

☐ Crutches and/or walker and wheelchair

☐ OTC NSAIDs – ibuprofen, aspirin, naproxen sodium

☐ Reusable ice bags and/or instant ice bags

Actions to take:

☐ If you currently have a bad knee, consider corrective surgery now.

Chapter 19

Ankle Injuries

(Continued from Chapter 18 . . .) Suppose as you stepped in the hole, you had twisted your ankle instead of your knee. You can't walk on it at all and drop your firewood to the ground, searching for a stick to use as a crutch. You manage to hop back inside your (soon to be cold) house. What should you do now?

Ankle injuries are almost always caused by an inversion injury: the outer ankle is forced downward is the foot rolls inward, stretching the outside of the ankle joint. This tears the fibers of the ligaments that support the outer ankle, sometimes breaking off the tip of the fibula (lateral leg/ankle bone). Walking home from high school many years ago, I did this myself. Edging my way around a mud puddle (so as not to splash my sister's coat that I had secretly borrowed), I suddenly slipped, crashing to the ground and breaking my ankle (and ruining the coat).

Ankle sprains are classified as first, second, and third degree. Most patients don't seek treatment for a first-degree sprain – these resolve within minutes to hours, causing some pain but little difficulty walking. With a third-degree sprain, the ligament has been torn in half. These may swell, but often don't hurt as much as a second-degree sprain, since the ligament is no longer under tension. However, with a third-degree sprain, the joint will be unstable. These sprains require prolonged immobilization or surgery. Since we are assuming surgery will be unavailable, treating a third-degree sprain like a severe second-degree sprain is reasonable.

Most ankle sprain patients – probably over 95% – seek medical care for second-degree injury, which still covers a wide spectrum of damage. With a second-degree sprain the ligament has been partially torn. This could mean a few fibers or many fibers. Picture the ligament as a thick elastic band. The more fibers that are torn, the more tension on the uninjured fibers. A big problem with injured ligaments is the poor blood supply, which is the primary reason ankle sprains heal more slowly than a person would expect.

The most common symptoms of a second-degree ankle sprain are pain and swelling of the outer ankle, usually with bruising and tenderness. If relatively few fibers have been torn, there will be little difficulty walking. With many torn fibers, it may be impossible to take even a step. If you have a nasty looking ankle with significant swelling and bruising, and are unable to walk, this raises the question of a small fracture. Sometimes the tip of the bone (fibula) is weaker than the ligament, and thus breaks off if the ligament is stretched too far, too fast. Usually the broken bone is not separated from the main bone by more than an eighth to a quarter inch. The body is able to bridge this gap with new calcium formation if the ankle is sufficiently immobilized. That's all a cast does – immobilize the ankle to allow healing and prevent further injury. Again, this is not rocket science.

A mild second-degree ankle sprain will require immobilization for a few days in the form of an Ace wrap, a gel cast, a splint, or other immobilizing device. For a person who is able to stay off his or her feet, keeping the injured limb elevated for a few days with ice applied may be all that is required. A moderate injury will require immobilization for a few weeks and probably the use of crutches. A severe injury will necessitate prolonged immobilization, from approximately 4 to 8 weeks, along with crutches for most this time.

How soon to begin walking? Let joint pain and stability be your guide. When weight-bearing is well-tolerated *without* pain medication, the ankle should be sufficiently healed to allow gradual resumption of exercise. Walking too soon may cause additional injury. For mild to moderate sprains, the discoloration may lag behind ability to ambulate. Anyone who has suffered a moderate to severe ankle sprain should continue to wear an elastic bandage or gel cast when walking for at least a few weeks after the ankle seems better, to prevent re-injury. A mild ankle sprain might convert to a severe ankle sprain if re-injured during the recovery period.

An avulsion fracture of the fibula (where the tip of the bone has broken off) heals about as quickly as a severe second-degree sprain (6–8 weeks). Without an X-ray, you will not know if you have a small break. Unless the ankle appears deformed (aside from the swelling discussed above), it won't matter much if you have a small, undiagnosed avulsion fracture. Both require prolonged immobilization and rest.

As part of your medical kit purchase at least two 3-inch and two 4-inch high-quality elastic wraps. (The cheap ones don't provide sufficient support for more than a few days.) Although an ankle could be immobilized with cardboard, a broom handle, a piece of plastic, etc., you may want to purchase an appropriately-sized gel cast, air cast, or nylon/Velcro splint for emergency use.

Chapter 19 – Checklist

Items to include in your medical supplies:

- ☐ Ankle braces of various types and sizes: Velcro, air cast, gel cast, inversion-prevention (sizes S, M, L, XL – most adults use large or extra-large)
- ☐ Ace wraps – 3″ and 4″ widths
- ☐ Reusable and/or instant ice packs
- ☐ Crutches and/or walker; wheelchair

Chapter 20

Insect Bites and Stings

(Continued from Chapter 19 . . .) You made it through spring. Your ankle has healed and your daughter's foot is as good as new. (Though the weather is warm, she now wears her shoes 24/7.) You decide to spend the day outside, but as you gather a pile of brush, you inadvertently disturb a hornet's nest. Though you both sprint inside, you and your daughter each suffer a dozen stings. As you catch your breath, you notice your daughter is more short of breath than you are. Is she just out of shape from the long winter? Could she be at risk of dying from an anaphylactic reaction?

Having acquired this book before TEOTWAWKI, you should have on hand:

- A bee-sting kit (epinephrine injection) and/or Primatene Mist (epinephrine) inhaler
- An antihistamine, preferably diphenhydramine, cetirizine, or chlorpheniramine

Give both immediately. Even without a true stinging insect allergy, a large number of stings may have the same effect. My own neighbor, who was not allergic to bee stings, died after being stung half a dozen times. Better safe than sorry. Expect your daughter to feel a little jittery from the epinephrine, which may also increase her heart rate. Her breathing should slow within several minutes. The antihistamine will take longer to kick in, but should take care of any hives that may develop. If symptoms recur hours later, the dose of one or both medications (epinephrine and/or the antihistamine) may need to be repeated, although this is uncommon.

Fortunately, most people only suffer one or two stings at a time. If these lesions are itchy or a little painful, giving an antihistamine orally should help. Swelling at the site of the sting is considered a local reaction, but if hives develop elsewhere on the body, or if wheezing, nausea, or shortness of breath occur, this would be considered a true allergy. The epinephrine relieves all allergy symptoms quickly, but doesn't last long. The antihistamine is to prevent additional symptoms later.

If you don't have epinephrine on hand, an albuterol inhaler should be effective for rapid relief of bronchial constriction, in combination with an antihistamine for hives and other symptoms. Other probably less-effective substitutes for epinephrine include pseudoephedrine and/or caffeine, in combination with an antihistamine. The controller-inhalers Symbicort and Advair may be useful if albuterol is unavailable, but these have a slower onset of action. Steroids may help, but usually take hours to begin working (prednisone 40–60 mg or methylprednisolone 12–24 mg daily, for 1–3 days).

Primatene Mist is available OTC without a prescription, at least until 12/31/2011. An epinephrine bee-sting kit may only be purchased with a prescription. Will your doctor prescribe one – especially with no history of bee sting allergy? Maybe. I would prescribe one to a bee-keeper, even if the bee-keeper had no history of bee-sting allergy. (If he were allergic, I'd suggest a change in vocation.)

Some people develop large, local reactions, up to several inches across. How can you tell the difference between a large local reaction and an infected sting? Local reactions occur sooner, usually within minutes to hours of a sting, though in a few patients the area might enlarge for up to about 24 hours. Infections usually don't begin until 24–48 hours after a sting. (Of course, a local reaction could become infected, and the symptoms merge from one to the other, making it difficult to discern.) Local reactions tend to be itchy, whereas infections tend to be tender, but there is considerable overlap. Either way, the overlying skin appears slightly raised and pink. With soft tissue infection (cellulitis) the color tends to be somewhat redder, though this would be difficult for the layman to discriminate. Also, a simple local reaction should be quite symmetric, with the edges tending to be more distinct than those of an infection. These differences are more difficult to appreciate in darker-skinned individuals

What if you can't tell the difference? Waiting a day or two often reveals the clinical course of the problem. A local reaction should be fading by then, especially if the patient has taken antihistamines on a regular basis. Outlining the affected area with a ballpoint pen will help to distinguish whether improvement or worsening has occurred. If the area of redness and swelling is enlarging after 24–48 hours, infection requiring antibiotics is more likely.

Infections of insect bites or stings are generally caused by the common skin germs *Staph* or *Strep*, which have penetrated the skin via the puncture. Cephalexin and Augmentin are among the best choices (erythromycin may be considered in a penicillin-allergic patient), unless resistant staph is suspected, in which case trimethoprim-sulfamethoxazole or doxycycline should be substituted (or added). You can't know which germ is present without a culture, which is unlikely in an Armageddon scenario. Take your best guess (like Dr. House) and then observe what happens. If there is no improvement by 2–3 days, a change of antibiotics is a consideration. Other antibiotics that may work include clarithromycin, azithromycin, and Levaquin. The following are unlikely to be effective: penicillin, amoxicillin, ampicillin, nitrofurantoin, ciprofloxacin, and metronidazole.

What about spiders? A spider bite is not a spider bite unless you've actually seen the spider bite you – which is rarely the case. People simply assume a small, raised red mark, possibly with a central puncture, has been caused by a spider. At least in America, what people attribute to a spider bite is more commonly a MRSA infection (MRSA = methicillin-resistant *Staph aureus*, pronounced "mersa"). If such a spot enlarges, antibiotics may be needed. Penicillin-type antibiotics will not work. Effective drugs include trimethoprim-sulfamethoxazole, doxycycline, or sometimes the macrolides or quinolones.

Mosquito bites usually don't become infected but do carry the risk of transmitting other diseases including West Nile Virus and malaria (not to mention Yellow Fever and various encephalitis viruses). With current mosquito control techniques, these have not been a major issue in America, but could be if the status quo changes.

Chapter 20 – Checklist

Items to include in your medical supplies:

- ☐ Bee sting kits
  (Prefilled syringes or vials of (1:1000) epinephrine 0.3mg/0.3ml plus diphenhydramine 25-mg capsules)

- ☐ Fast-acting inhalers: Primatene Mist (available OTC at least until 12/31/11) and/or prescription albuterol inhaler

- ☐ Antibiotics for skin infections, per text

- ☐ Antihistamines: diphenhydramine, cetirizine, and/or chlorpheniramine

- ☐ Prescription steroids (prednisone and/or methylprednisolone)

- ☐ Insect repellant with 10–30% DEET

- ☐ Full-coverage clothing for everyone

- ☐ Insect repellant clothing (sold at L. L. Bean and elsewhere)

Chapter 21

Concussion

(Continued from Chapter 20 . . .) Your daughter did well with the epinephrine and diphenhydramine, but is afraid to go back outside. Unfortunately, she trips over the shovel you dropped in the hallway, hitting her head on the wall as she drops to the floor, unconscious but breathing. A few minutes later she awakens, slightly dazed. How will you know if she has brain damage without a CAT scan?

At a minimum, she's suffered a concussion, that is, a mild traumatic brain injury associated with rapid onset of short-lived neurologic impairment. A person needn't be knocked out, though this is typically the case. "Knocked silly" is sufficient to diagnose a concussion. Symptoms may include confusion, headache, amnesia, dizziness, nausea or vomiting, visual disturbances, slurred speech, drowsiness, irritability, disorientation, staring, trouble focusing or answering, or simply not thinking straight.

Nowadays most people who suffer a concussion undergo a head CT or MRI scan. But these scans are not looking for a concussion – rather, they are looking for additional problems, such as skull fractures, bleeding within the brain, strokes, neck injuries, or brain swelling. There is no X-ray or laboratory test that confirms the diagnosis of concussion, other than to say nothing else is wrong. Skull X-rays are not useful unless a skull fracture is suspected, and unless you have a surgeon on hand, the information gained from a radiologic exam will be of little help.

In a person who has experienced a concussion but who feels, looks, and acts fine, or in a person with minimal symptoms, a brain scan would probably be normal anyway. Most patients who suffer a concussion have normal CT scans and enjoy a full recovery.

That is, unless – and this is a big one – the patient suffers a second head injury before fully recovered from the first. The so-called "second impact syndrome" can be devastating, resulting in massive brain swelling, leading to death or severe, permanent disability. If a second concussion (or even lesser head injury) occurs within minutes, days, or even weeks after the first concussion, what could have been a mild injury may be devastating. Clearly, the lesson to be learned is: avoid a repeat head injury at all costs. That said, most doctors have never seen a "second impact syndrome." Few patients actually experience two head injuries within a short period of time. Athletes, who are most at risk, are usually sidelined until their symptoms resolve.

Without a neurosurgeon and hospital care, treatment of brain injury will be extremely limited, making prevention the only reasonable strategy. If a patient's condition seems to be worsening over the course of minutes, hours, or days, this may be a sign of bleeding within or around the brain, which may require emergency surgery. Professional care should be sought if at all possible.

Possible Symptoms of Concussion

Most common	Headache, amnesia, confusion
Other early signs	Fatigue, slurred speech, ringing in the ears, dizziness, nausea or vomiting, slurred speech
Symptoms which may occur either immediately or up to days after injury	Impairment of memory or concentration Disorders of sleep, taste, or smell Irritability, depression, personality changes Sensitivity to light (photophobia) or noise
Symptoms in young children	Difficulty walking or loss of balance Sleeping more or less, or tiring easily Change in eating Loss of interest in normal activities or toys Irritability or crying
Worrisome signs	Prolonged unconsciousness, seizures, uneven pupils, a change in breathing, blood or fluid from the nose or ears, repeated vomiting **Any symptoms that are growing worse**

A simple concussion will resolve within 7–10 days. Obviously, you cannot know this at the outset. Concussion grading scales are being abandoned because their correlation with severity of injury is unclear. The degree of injury is best assessed in retrospect, after the patient has returned to normal.

A complex concussion is one in which initial loss of consciousness persisted for over one minute, or one in which seizures have occurred, or when concussion symptoms have continued beyond 10 days. Such an injury would normally be handled by a neurologic specialist.

Without a CAT scan or MRI scan it may be difficult to differentiate a minor intracranial bleed from a concussion. When blood accumulates within the skull, the pressure may produce stroke-like symptoms or cause the brain stem to herniate, resulting in death. However, a minor bleed may produce few symptoms, and the leaked blood may reabsorb with minimal residual effect.

No matter what, the take-home lesson is prevention. Would you allow your son to play football if you knew no ambulance would come – ever?

Chapter 21 – Checklist

Items to include in your medical supplies:

☐ Bicycle, football, or motorcycle helmet

☐ Several ounces of prevention

Chapter 22

Fractures

(Continued from Chapter 21 . . .) What if, in your rush to help your daughter, you had tripped, falling forward to the floor, catching yourself on your hands? Your wrist looks a little funny, perhaps slightly deformed. Though you ice it and apply an elastic bandage, the pain mounts, making you wish you had a narcotic available. Could it be broken? Will it heal without an X-ray?

I pose this last question because I've heard it so often: will a broken bone heal without an X-ray? X-rays have nothing to do with bone healing, only with imaging the bone, to check for fractures, displacement, and alignment. X-rays do help doctors know if they've realigned a bone correctly during surgery or casting, but unless a bone is markedly deformed, it's probably best NOT to attempt realignment on your own. For bones protruding through the skin, seek orthopedic care if at all possible.

For the purposes of this discussion, we will cover only those fractures which a layman could treat with readily available over-the-counter supplies. I'd say not to bother stocking fiberglass casting material, which holds up better than plaster, but is more difficult to remove. If you apply plaster and don't have a cast-saw, the cast can still be removed by wetting it down or chipping it off, or using garden snips, etc. Just don't hurt yourself. Even plaster is overrated. The purpose of a plaster or fiberglass cast is twofold: 1) immobilizing the extremity to keep the bone well-positioned for healing; and 2) prevention of re-injury. These goals could be accomplished with a variety of alternative materials.

Starting with the simplest of fractures, we'll begin with the toes. **Toe fractures** are exceedingly common. They usually occur in one of two ways: dropping a heavy item on the toe or slamming the foot into a bedpost or other immovable object. Small toes are by far the most likely victims, especially the littlest toe. A broken toe may appear swollen, reddened, or black and blue, and hurts quite badly for a few hours to a few days. Without an X-ray you won't know if your toe is broken, but this rarely matters. Most broken toes remain well-aligned or are only slightly askew. If the toe feels more comfortable buddy-taped to the adjacent one, then by all means do so. Elevating the foot and applying ice usually offers sufficient pain relief, with or without over-the-counter pain medication. Wearing a flat-soled shoe for a few weeks to limit movement of the toes is not mandatory, but may make walking more comfortable. Walking on a broken toe is permitted as tolerated. Most people voluntarily limit their activity for several days.

One concern with a fractured toe is any overlying laceration, which might allow bacteria to enter the wound, causing infection of the soft tissues and possibly the bone. An infected bone may require weeks to months of antibiotics to heal, and may lead to chronic pain, eventual amputation, or even death. All cuts on the feet should be kept clean and closely monitored. It is acceptable to suture a laceration overlying a broken toe only if done so within the first 24 hours. If additional redness, swelling, heat, or pus develops, antibiotics should be started right away (cephalexin, amoxicillin-clavulanate, and levofloxacin are good choices, and perhaps erythromycin in penicillin-allergic children).

Another exception is a **broken big toe**. Unlike the smaller toes, the large toe is used for balance and is essential for normal gait. Fortunately, the bones of the big toe are much sturdier and therefore less likely to break. It would be nice to have an X-ray of an injured big toe, but lacking this, you'll have to make do. If a big toe injury is suspicious for a fracture, treat it as though it has been broken. Ordinarily, this would involve internal fixation (surgery with pinning). The best you can accomplish will be external immobilization. If the toe looks crooked, do your best to straighten it by applying traction (which will likely hurt). When the toe is as straight as you can get it, splint it straight and/or buddy-tape it to the second toe. Since additional swelling may occur, apply a dressing such as Coban, a material that looks like a thin elastic wrap, but which adheres to itself and may be easily loosened and reapplied.

Big toe fractures frequently involve the joint surface and/or growth plate, and therefore may lead to permanent arthritis and/or deformity at any age. Currently doctors rarely get the opportunity to observe how these fractures heal without intervention, since referral to an orthopedist is the rule. Unlike the smaller toes, walking on an injured big toe before it is healed may damage the joint further, so if at all possible, avoid weight-bearing for at least a few weeks, possibly longer. (That said, in a crisis situation, the need to escape may outweigh the threat of future arthritis.)

Moving upward, **fractured metatarsals** (long bones in the feet) are common now and will become more so if sedentary people begin walking long distances of necessity. The so-called "march fracture" occurs when the foot bone is overstressed by prolonged marching (or walking, running, or jogging). The mid-foot (between the toes and ankle or heel) becomes increasingly painful and swollen, with tenderness over the weakened area, but generally without bruising or redness. The bone does not break in half, but rather undergoes micro-fractures, with the bone structure weakening a little at a time. Weight-bearing becomes intolerable. With a mild case, merely decreasing activity may suffice. Wearing a flat or stiff-bottom shoe will decrease the rocking motion of the foot. Padded insoles, ice, or heat may help as well. Crutches and/or an air cast may be necessary for a more severe injury, but full casting is rarely needed. Minimizing activity that causes foot pain will allow the foot to heal, generally within a few weeks. Unless your life depends on remaining mobile, taking strong pain medication to mask the pain is a bad idea and will only result in further injury.

A second common metatarsal fracture is a break through the fifth (outward-most) metatarsal. This injury is caused by forceful kicking (accidental or purposeful) or sometimes with twisting or rolling the foot inward, and occasionally by direct impact. Pain, tenderness, swelling, and sometimes discoloration or visible deformity occurs over the outer-most foot bone. Such a fracture may be treated as a march fracture (see above). A mild break may allow limited weight-bearing, but a complete fracture may require staying off the affected foot altogether for 2 to 6 weeks.

Heel fractures (calcaneal stress fractures) are seen primarily in runners, as the posterior heel weakens from repeated impact. Suspect a heel fracture in active athletes with heel pain, or in anyone who has been on their feet much more than usual. (Do not confuse this with pain and tenderness a little toward the arch of the mid-foot, which is likely to be plantar fasciitis.) As with any injury caused by overuse, relative rest is the only answer. Weight-bearing exercise must be decreased or temporarily eliminated to allow the bone to heal. No casting or other specific immobilization is required. This is another situation where you do not want to mask the pain with narcotics or other pain-relievers, unless the situation mandates mobility.

The importance of good shoes

Surely the above discussions have convinced you that sturdy, well-supported, good-fitting shoes are as vital to your health as any medication. If your feet hurt and prevent fleeing from danger, bad shoes may kill you. If they rub a deep blister in your foot, infection may kill you. If you can't secure sufficient food, starvation may kill you – and your children.

Leg bone fractures are caused by sudden strong impact, the sort of trauma where additional injuries should be considered. The major exception to this is the fractured distal fibula, just at or above the outer ankle bone, which is actually the most common leg fracture seen in a primary care setting. A small fracture of the distal fibula is caused by the same mechanism that causes a lateral (outside) ankle sprain, i.e., rolling the ankle inward as the outer ankle collapses downward (see **Chapter 19**). A fractured fibula may be difficult to distinguish from a bad ankle sprain, and the initial treatment is much the same: Rest, Ice, Compression, Elevation (mnemonic RICE). Early measures are aimed at preventing further internal bleeding, swelling, and dislocation. Swelling is gravity-dependent, so keeping the injured limb elevated limits the potential for fluid accumulation. Swelling is also pressure-dependent, so applying an elastic wrap firmly (but not so tight as to form a tourniquet) will both prevent and treat swelling.

Even if the ankle (fibula) is broken, there is no rush to apply a plaster cast. In fact, you DO NOT want to apply an encircling cast until the swelling has stabilized. A rigid cast applied to a still-swelling extremity may act as a tourniquet or cause frictional soft tissue damage. Both you and your patient will be permanently scarred if premature casting of a simple fracture leads to unnecessary tissue death and amputation. The goal of casting is immobilization, which may be accomplished using an air cast, a gel cast, a stiff magazine or cardboard, or anything you may have on hand that will support the injured bone without unduly compressing it or compromising the circulation. Narcotics may be necessary to relieve pain, but the goal is to allow rest, not activity.

How will you know if or when the bone is healed (or if it's even broken, for that matter)? Without X-rays, you won't, and so you'll need to rely on symptoms. If the leg/ankle is too weak to walk, a serious injury has occurred. If resting and splinting the injured limb for a few days does not allow weight-bearing, then continuous immobilization and crutches should be continued a few weeks, at which time the injury can be reassessed. At this point, if the patient feels as good as new, and there is no residual swelling or discoloration, a second-degree ankle sprain is likely to have occurred, and gradual resumption of activity may be permitted. Otherwise, continued immobilization for a total of 4 to 8 weeks is indicated. Children will heal more quickly than adults, and of course, minor breaks may knit more readily than major injuries.

More serious leg fractures are beyond the scope of this book, but the same general principles apply. Over the years I have observed even serious fractures heal without casting or pinning. All is not lost if you happen to break a bone.

Although bleeding to death internally (from a punctured blood vessel) is theoretically possible, this is rare. Compound fractures, where the bone is sticking through the skin, may cause a fatal infection, but these are rare as well, aside from war, car wrecks, and contact sports. Injuries from motor vehicle accidents will naturally decrease when we run out of fuel. Sports injuries should decrease if we all become farmers. Hopefully people will become more careful in preventing injuries once they realize orthopedists are not available to put them back together again.

In the elderly, **compression fractures of the spine** are common. If your granny falls out of bed or trips on the way to the bathroom, an age-weakened vertebra may collapse like a piece of Styrofoam. In a patient with full-blown osteoporosis, simply rolling over in bed may crush a weakened bone. Typically a compression fracture causes severe back pain and difficulty moving. Walking or even sitting up may be impossible. The patient may have trouble localizing the pain and should be evaluated for other injuries. Because compression fractures occur in weak bones, they take a long time to heal, typically several months. Narcotics may be needed for weeks (which may lead to obstructing constipation if stool softeners are not also administered). Although bed rest should be limited to 3–5 days to prevent blood clots and deconditioning, this requires liberal use of pain medication and hands-on help with many activities of daily living. Including a walker among your medical supplies is a good idea for anyone with family members in their sixties or beyond.

A vertebral compression fracture may put a formerly active patient out of commission long-term. The pain and disability, along with medication-induced mental changes may require one-on-one assistance for weeks. Diminished breathing (due to pain) may lead to pneumonia. What is currently considered a routine fracture may end up consuming vast amounts of medical resources, thus threatening your entire group. Will you need to ration medication? This will be difficult when your own mother is moaning in pain. If narcotics are unavailable, sedation may be the answer to severe pain. If an alcoholic beverage (or perhaps Nyquil) allows an injured person to rest, this may conserve your limited supply of pain medication.

Rib fractures occur in both the young and old due to falls or blunt trauma. Although the risk exists for a broken rib to puncture the lung, this is uncommon. Unless a patient is quite short of breath, odds are the underlying lung has not been damaged. (Explaining how to recognize and treat a pneumothorax is beyond the scope of this book.) Typically a patient can point to the exact location of the pain. Sometimes a broken rib has a little "give" to it, but most patients won't allow the examiner to press hard enough to determine this. Occasionally an overlying bruise or abrasion will signal the presence of a fractured rib.

Anyone who's ever broken a rib knows it feels better to avoid taking a deep breath. Patients spontaneously splint a broken rib, either by shallow breathing or by applying external pressure to the general area. Years ago doctors would recommend a rib binder, but this leads to inadequate lung expansion, and often subsequent pneumonia, especially in the elderly. For a younger person who has no choice but to remain active, wearing a binder for a few hours a day to permit necessary activity may be helpful, but when the binder is removed, which should be done hourly, the patient must force himself to breathe deeply in order to expand the lungs fully.

Broken ribs are acutely painful for a week or two, with gradual resolution over 4 to 8 weeks. Narcotics and anti-inflammatory drugs are useful but not mandatory. Patients may experience relief from holding a pillow against their chest when coughing, or the topical application of heat, ice, Aspercreme, Lidoderm, capsaicin, or a TENS unit. No specific therapy is required to enable broken ribs to heal. What is needed is special attention to preventing pneumonia by keeping the lungs expanded.

A **collar bone fracture** is usually an injury of the young. This superficial bone has little fatty or muscular protection from direct trauma. Your son or daughter may snap the bone simply by falling and landing on the adjacent shoulder, or even on an outstretched hand. Given a history of falling, a tender bump along the mid-clavicle (collar bone) is likely a fracture. Wearing a figure-of-eight strap positions the shoulders back a bit, offering partial pain relief and correct position for healing. The figure-of-eight splint is available without a prescription for under $20. If such a splint is not included in your supplies, simply immobilizing the affected arm in a sling may suffice. Pain-free movement of the shoulder is usually possible by 3–4 weeks in children, or 4–6 weeks in adults.

Fractures of the upper arm (the humerus, or bone between the elbow and shoulder) are more common in older patients. Imagine how bad you'll feel if your granny trips over your shoes, lands on her shoulder, and shatters her humerus. No one will be laughing. A younger person who sustains high-energy trauma, such as being thrown from a horse or motorcycle, may experience similar injury, with pain, tenderness, and swelling, located a few inches below the shoulder.

Fortunately, in a typical fractured humerus (as is the case approximately 85% of the time), the bony fragments are little displaced and therefore neither surgery nor casting is required. (Again, this book is directed toward common presentations of typical injuries. You can't become an orthopedic surgeon after reading a single chapter.) Supporting the arm with a sling swathed against the body for three weeks allows initial bone healing to occur. (Alternatively, have the patient fold their arm against their chest, then pull the lower half of their shirt up over the arm, pinning the hem near the collar, thus creating a sling.) In this position, wrist and hand exercises should be started immediately. Within two to three weeks, depending on pain, pendulum exercises should begin: with the arm free, the patient leans forward and allows the arm to swing gently in a pendulum, but without active movement of the arm muscles, for about 5 minutes, four times a day. A week or so later, the shoulder may be gently moved while the arm is supported by an assistant. By 6–8 weeks, full range of motion should begin, with complete healing requiring up to 12 weeks.

Wrist fractures can be tricky. Is it the wrist bones, the forearm, or the joint? Orthopedic doctors won't treat injured wrists without knowing what's going on inside the joint. A layman could hardly be expected to guess at the proper treatment. Because diagnosis and treatment cannot be reviewed in a few short paragraphs, I'm leaving this topic to the orthopedic textbooks. In the meantime, elevate the injured limb, apply ice, and splint the wrist in the most comfortable position, securing it with an Ace wrap. Ideally this would be with the wrist extended (bent backward) a little and the fingers free, similar to the position of the hand when typing. (If this is the only reference book you have, maintain immobilization in this position for 2–8 weeks, or until the pain diminishes, meanwhile encouraging movement of the fingers. If the fingers are not permitted to move during this period, they may become permanently restricted.)

Lastly, **finger fractures** are common, often resulting from direct trauma and crush injuries. Well-aligned breaks that occur *between* joints will heal well simply by buddy-taping them to the adjacent finger for a few weeks. Fractures that occur *at or near* joints may cause permanent disability and are best left to an expert. If there is no expert around, hopefully you have an orthopedic book to consult. If not, align the finger as best you can, immobilize it with a splint or by buddy-taping, and protect it from further injury. Even now doctors don't have the answer to every injury. My own daughter had a fracture through a finger joint that will never be quite right, despite two surgeries.

Like everything else in America, we tend to think our bodies are replaceable. But at TEOTWAWKI, you may not have a second chance. Thankfully, as I've shown, many fractures will heal with minimal intervention. For those that will not, permanent disability and/or deformity may result. So take good care of the one body God has granted you.

Chapter 22 – Checklist

Items to include in your medical supplies:

☐ Mobility aids: crutches, walker, wheelchair, flat-soled shoes (post-op shoes)

☐ Medical tape; sports tape; Coban

☐ Finger splints; wrist splints (Velcro, cock-up, carpal-tunnel); ankle splints

☐ Plaster casting/splinting supplies (and possibly a cast saw)

☐ Figure-of-eight splint; slings

☐ Rib belt (only for short-term, emergency use)

☐ OTC NSAIDs, acetaminophen, Aspercreme, tramadol, narcotics

☐ Calcium foods and/or supplements to maintain strong bones; Vitamin D

Actions to take:

☐ Acquire a used orthopedic textbook

☐ Make sure everyone in your family has properly fitting well-supported shoes

SECTION SEVEN

Selected Conditions

Chapter 23

Selected Conditions

Introduction

This section includes information on common problems likely to be encountered at TEOTWAWKI that a person could usually manage on one's own with a little know-how. The text should not be considered all-inclusive, and medical textbooks should be consulted for additional detailed information. Consider the following a starting place for typical presentations of common conditions.

Anemia

Is anemia always due to low iron? Most people think so. However, although iron-deficiency anemia is most common, other causes exist and present according to age-related patterns.

If your bouncing baby boy grows increasingly tired, pale, underweight, or listless, this may be due to **inadequate dietary iron**. Although I do advocate breast-feeding, iron-rich supplementary formula or iron-containing vitamins may be required to prevent anemia. For preppers with infants, stocking a supply of one or both is advisable.

For toddlers and school-aged children, anemia is rare. One exception is again dietary – for **vegetarians**, be cautious with children who shun iron-rich green leafy vegetables. Kids like carbs, which won't supply sufficient iron.

Once your precious little girl becomes a young lady, **menstrual blood loss** is the most common culprit for iron-deficiency anemia, especially in girls who don't replace the iron loss with iron-rich foods. Be sure to include high-iron foods such as raisins, canned greens, and red meat among your food stores. Iron pills are cheap and also worth stockpiling. Ibuprofen or naproxen will slow menstrual blood flow in some girls who bleed heavily. Birth control pills to regulate menstrual flow are another option, though require a prescription and may be a challenge to stockpile. As for boys, anemia is quite rare.

Once the child-bearing years are behind you, new woes arise. Occult (invisible) **gastrointestinal blood loss** becomes the leading cause for anemia, due to **medications** (primarily NSAIDs such as aspirin or ibuprofen), **colitis**, **polyps**, **diverticulitis**, or **cancer**. If visible blood is present in the stool, it's there – no need for a test. (Rarely red foods such as beets may mimic the appearance of blood.) If anemia is suspected in a pale, tired, easily-winded middle-aged or older adult, it is prudent and simple to check for blood in the stool using a hemoccult test, which you can currently purchase online or at your pharmacy.

Not sure if you're anemic or just feeling old? Performing a hematocrit (blood count) is simple if you have the proper equipment to measure the fraction of blood composed of cells, an experiment easily performed in high school science class. The cells will sink to the bottom of a column of blood via gravity (or centrifugation). In women, cells should comprise at least 35% of the blood, and in men about 40%. (Note – babies run much higher. Consult a pediatric text for specifics.) People don't usually feel especially bad until the count drops below 30%; blood transfusions are reserved for symptomatic patients with counts below about 26%. For the technically-minded, you may want to obtain finger lancets and appropriate capillary tubes to practice on your family and friends.

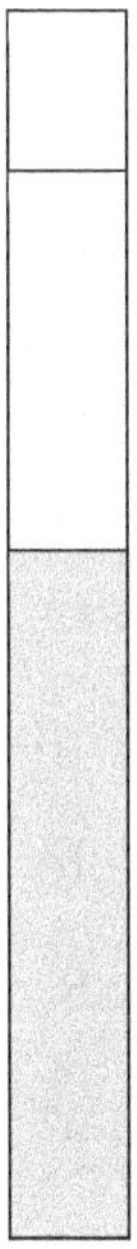

Measuring a hematocrit

In a column of blood, the cells (dark gray) will sink to the bottom,
leaving yellow-tinged serum (light gray) at the top.

Measure the height of the cells (dark gray),
and divide this by the total height of the fluid column
(both light and dark gray, but not the white (air) at the top).

In the illustration to the left,
the hematocrit would be approximately 2/3 or 33%.

Treatment of anemia due to GI bleeding is aimed at preventing further loss. In a patient taking warfarin (Coumadin), Plavix, or an NSAID (aspirin, ibuprofen, naproxen, and prescription NSAIDs), these should be discontinued immediately. If your upper abdomen hurts or burns, you may have a bleeding ulcer, which should be promptly treated with acid-reducing agents (see entry on heartburn and ulcers). Colitis, causing abdominal pain and blood-tinged rectal mucus, could be treated with oral steroids if X-rays, colonoscopies, and gastroenterologists are unavailable (prednisone, 10–40 mg daily, aiming for the lowest dose which works, for as short a time as possible – but best to consult a medical textbook for this). If diverticulitis is suspected (maroon stools, lower abdominal pain, diarrhea), antibiotics may be curative (see *Diverticulitis*). At TEOTWAWKI cancer will be treated primarily with prayer and compassion.

What about Grandma and Grandpa? In the older patient, the above reasons for blood loss are common, as are dire causes of intestinal bleeding, such as ischemic colitis. An elderly person who appears severely ill and has rectal bleeding may not survive. You may want to try treating for diverticulitis, but surgical causes of acute intestinal bleeding will be fatal without the appropriate care. Narcotics may ease severe intestinal pain in a person expected to die.

Fortunately, chronic anemia is often well-tolerated in the elderly. Anemia of chronic disease (as is found with chronic kidney failure or inflammatory conditions such as rheumatoid arthritis, and which is unrelated to iron intake or blood loss) rarely drops the hematocrit below about 27%. Since the decline in blood count occurs over a prolonged period of time, the body is gradually able to accommodate the decrease. No special treatment is needed for most individuals. Fatigue and shortness of breath occur primarily in patients with underlying heart disease or COPD.

If anemia is also accompanied by mental changes or tingling of the toes or fingertips, vitamin B_{12} or folate deficiency should be considered. Since it's unlikely you'll be able to assess serum levels of these nutrients, a therapeutic trial of both B_{12} and folate should be given (though better to prevent the problem with adequate nutrition). Some older adults are unable to absorb B_{12} from the diet efficiently. Although these patients are usually treated with injections, high dose oral B_{12} is often effective.

The above is only a primer on anemia, but covers the majority of situations commonly encountered in modern medicine. Radiation exposure, hemorrhagic viruses, worms, chemical poisonings, bone marrow disease, and a host of other conditions may cause anemia as well, but you'll need a medical textbook to deal with these.

As you prepare, don't forget to include:

Iron rich foods, iron supplements, iron-rich formula for babies

Liquid vitamins with Vitamin K (for babies)

Multi-vitamins including B_{12} and folate (for all, especially the elderly)

Capillary tubes and lancets for hematocrit determination

Ibuprofen and/or birth control pills to slow menstrual bleeding

Arthritis

Are your knees killing you? Do your knobby fingers remind you of the Wicked Witch of the West? Is a trip upstairs torture on your hips?

Arthritis is very common from middle-age onward. I probably have some myself. Osteoarthritis, also known as degenerative arthritis, or old-age arthritis, is the most common form of degenerative joint disease. Joints hurt, enlarge, and sometimes become hot, red, or swollen.

Younger individuals may also suffer from arthritis, although this is more likely to be of an inflammatory nature, such as lupus. Nowadays fancy drugs such as methotrexate, Plaquenil, Humira, and Embrel are sometimes used to treat rheumatoid and other inflammatory arthritis. In post-modern medicine, options will be severely limited. Inflammatory arthritis will be treated much the same as osteoarthritis, as it once was, with the exception of perhaps using steroids more liberally for rheumatoid arthritis, lupus, and similar entities.

Treatment is aimed at decreasing pain and inflammation. Although resting a hurting joint short-term is helpful, lack of exercise can cause increased stiffness. Patients need to find the right balance of exercise and rest for optimal functioning. With the decreased caloric intake that may face us if society collapses, obesity will decrease, thus lessening the impact of foot, knee, hip, and back problems (if we don't do ourselves in with all the increased walking). Ice tends to improve acutely arthritic joints, whereas heat is helpful for chronic arthritis. Tylenol, tramadol, and occasionally narcotics are usually prescribed to lessen the pain of arthritis.

As for inflammation, a host of non-steroidal anti-inflammatory medications (NSAIDs) exist for treating arthritis. Most of these are prescription medications, but aspirin, ibuprofen, and naproxen are available over the counter. As cheap as these are, laying in a deep supply of thousands of pills seems prudent, especially since they have multiple other uses for acute problems such as headaches, menstrual cramps, low back pain, acute strains, pleurisy, phlebitis, gout, and fever. Keep in mind that even these OTC drugs are not free of side-effects, especially stomach irritation or even bleeding.

Once our stockpiles of medicine are used up, we'll have to revert to herbal anti-inflammatory medicine. Willow bark is the prototype salicylate-containing remedy, and can be chewed or made into tea. Commercially-available willow bark preparations are unlikely to have a shelf-life exceeding that of pills, so it makes more sense to plant your own willow tree, or locate one in your area.

The wonder drug for arthritis is corticosteroids, either injected directly into the joint or taken orally. Patients with lupus or rheumatoid arthritis would love to take prednisone every day if not for the side-effects of weight gain, swelling, insomnia, abdominal discomfort, bone calcium loss, and diabetes. Having a reserve of steroids on hand is reasonable if combined with a large supply of restraint in using them. Two to ten days of prednisone 20–60 mg daily can work miracles, but should be reserved for rare, intolerable, or emergency occasions.

As you prepare, consider including:

- OTC NSAIDS (ibuprofen, naproxen, aspirin)
- Possibly prescription NSAIDs or Celebrex
- OTC acid-reducers, if NSAIDs bother the stomach
  (generics of Pepcid, Zantac, Prevacid, or Prilosec)
- Prescription corticosteroids (prednisone, methylprednisolone)
- Calcium supplements to counter calcium loss due to steroids
- Pain killers (Tylenol, prescription tramadol, possibly narcotics)
- Topical preparations (Aspercreme, Icy Hot, heat, ice)
- Supportive wraps and braces
- Willow bark or source thereof
- OTC glucosamine supplements, possibly chondroitin
- Ambulatory aids such as a cane, walker, or wheelchair
- Paraffin bath (hot wax treatment) for hand arthritis

Asthma and COPD

It's the middle of the night. You can't breathe. You reach for your last rescue inhaler, hoping it contains one final dose. Fortunately, it does. But what will you do tomorrow . . . and the rest of your life?

I posed this question to my asthmatic nephew. If things go bad, this law-abiding citizen plans to raid every pharmacy he can find. The competition may be fierce.

Not so long ago severe asthma attacks were a common occurrence, often necessitating hospital admission. In the past decade, since controller medications became a mainstay of therapy, the incidence of severe illness has markedly decreased (in medication-compliant individuals), although deaths from asthma still occur. With so many options now available, it is nearly always possible to keep an asthmatic patient healthy and out of the hospital.

But what will you do if the drug supply chain is interrupted? Will you be able to breathe freely? If an evacuation is ordered, will your lungs allow you to keep up?

Asthma does not behave the same in every patient. Many cases are so mild that the affected individual is unaware of the diagnosis. In other patients the disease is life-threatening. But in every situation there are steps you can take to limit the impact of the disease.

COPD, or chronic obstructive pulmonary disease, behaves much like asthma, but is caused by smoking tobacco. Many of the same medications are effective. The first-line treatment, however, is to **<u>STOP SMOKING</u>**!!! Can I emphasize this any stronger?

Probably the most common type of asthma is the mild, intermittent form. These patients usually have no symptoms, though they may develop a cough, wheeze, or shortness of breath on occasion, usually in response to a trigger. Common triggers include respiratory infections, allergies, dust or chemical exposure, changes in temperature, or vigorous exercise. People who are subject to chest colds may well have low-grade asthma (or COPD, in the case of smokers).

These patients require either no asthma medication or only occasional use of an inhaler or oral steroids. Avoiding triggers is the best way to prevent an asthma flare: limit exposure to respiratory infections, get an annual flu shot, and stay away from pets or anything else to which you are allergic. Although the printed directions for many antihistamines say to avoid their use in asthmatic patients, for allergic asthma, over-the-counter antihistamines may actually be helpful (Benadryl, Claritin, Zyrtec, Allegra, and chlorpheniramine). Pseudoephedrine, the best decongestant for upper respiratory tract congestion, is also often effective for lower respiratory congestion, and may improve mild bronchial swelling. Singulair, a prescription asthma medication, is more likely to be effective in allergic than non-allergic patients, and is intended for chronic daily use.

Albuterol (Ventolin, Proventil, ProAir) is the most widely prescribed rescue inhaler for acute symptoms. Anyone who uses such an inhaler even on an occasional basis should talk to their physician about obtaining additional supplies for future needs. Promise your doctor that you will still follow up with him or her on a regular basis as long for as the medical establishment is not disrupted; otherwise it is unlikely you'll be prescribed extra to stockpile. Why? Doctors are actually encouraged by asthma experts to prescribe no more than one albuterol inhaler at a time because patients needing them on a regular basis should also be on a controller drug, and may ignore this advice if given unlimited access to albuterol. For COPD patients, ipratropium inhaler may work better than albuterol, and some patients do better using both (as in Combivent inhaler). If you cannot obtain a stockpile of one of the above, at least procure a supply of Primatene Mist (see below).

For patients with mild, intermittent symptoms, although albuterol works quickly and reliably, it is not the only option. Caffeine opens the airways much like aminophylline, the mainstay of asthma therapy twenty years ago. Regarding side-effects, essentially any medication that has the benefit of opening the airways by dilating the bronchial tubes has the potential of caffeine-like side-effects, including jitteriness, insomnia, and sometimes elevated blood pressure or increased heart rate.

How does mild asthma compare with a severe case? Patients with severe asthma or COPD never breathe normally. They may think they do so because they've become accustomed to the situation over the years, but on pulmonary function tests doctors find their breathing capacity is decreased, particularly the ability to exhale. Fortunately, the human body has a significant degree of reserve capacity. People can live long-term with only one lung or the equivalent.

With multiple medications, severely affected patients can live normal lives. Generally this involves taking an inhaled steroid (Flovent, Pulmicort, Asmanex), perhaps along with another controller drug such as Singulair or a long-acting bronchodilator (as in the combination inhalers Advair and Symbicort, containing both steroids and bronchodilators). Many patients still require albuterol and/or ipratropium inhalers on a daily basis, and would be expected to need oral steroids when a flare occurs (40–60 mg prednisone for 3 to

10 days, or a Medrol Dosepak). Some require daily or intermittent oxygen. For severely affected patients, avoiding triggers is even more important.

People with moderate asthma lie somewhere along the spectrum between mild and severe, and may have spells when the disease is better or worse.

If you or your child suffers from asthma, what can you do besides stockpiling medicine to prepare for the day when drugs and doctors become unavailable? Quite a bit, actually. There's no need to feel helpless, expecting to watch your youngster suffocate.

To start with, asthma and COPD patients should do all they can to remain healthy. Maintain a healthy body weight, don't smoke, exercise regularly, and eat well.

Next, become an expert at avoiding triggers. Stay away from dust, fumes, chemicals, and pollen. Wearing a mask or face-protector is a consideration. Limit exposure to animals, especially mammals and birds (also feather pillows, wool, rabbit fur, and the like). Many patients believe their own pet is not causing a problem, but while an asthmatic may not suffer an acute attack when holding his own pooch, chronic exposure may cause on-going low-level symptoms, difficult to attribute time-wise to animal allergy.

Anyone with a question of true allergic asthma should have allergy testing done, both for the information this provides regarding avoiding triggers, but also in case allergy-desensitization shots might help. I've seen patients suffer asthma for years whose symptoms abated after several months of weekly injections. It's the closest thing to a cure for asthma (aside from a child eventually outgrowing it.) Your family doctor may offer this service, but more likely you'll need to see an allergist.

Patients who have exercise-induced asthma may spontaneously avoid the level of exertion that brings on symptoms. On the other hand, many of these patients may find they can actually exercise longer if they first induce asthmatic symptoms with a short bout of exercise, followed by a recovery period of 10 to 30 minutes. When breathing has returned to normal and exercise is then again attempted, the airways frequently exhibit less of a tendency to constrict.

All patients with asthma or COPD should own *and use* a peak flow meter. Repeat, *get a peak flow meter*. This handy little device, costing under $30 (and often covered by insurance) will help you assess your breathing even before you experience symptoms. Knowing your peak flow rate when you are well as compared to sick helps determine treatment. Physically, you may not notice a 10% reduction in your breathing, but it may be a signal to you that a flare is about to occur. Forewarned, you can act proactively to ramp up your medicine or adjust your behavior if needed. You must get to know your body, your triggers, and your response to therapy.

Peak flow rates depend not only on degree of airway constriction, but also somewhat on body size as well as age. Large, healthy men may have a rate as high as 800 L/min, whereas for tiny octogenarians 300 L/min may be entirely normal. More typically, healthy women run about 400–500, and men 500–700. People with chronic asthma or COPD often have peak flow rates 200 points lower even when they think they're doing fine, and may drop another 200 when a flare occurs. Knowing your baseline is essential in evaluating the severity of both chronic and acute symptoms.

Medication remains the mainstay of asthma treatment. Naturally you should stockpile both the rescue and controller medications you normally require. Beyond this, though, are there any over-the-counter remedies that actually work, something easy to stockpile without a doctor's permission? Fortunately, yes. The following are currently sold in the United States and elsewhere, although see below regarding future availability.

- **Caffeine** is the most universally-available chemical to open the airways. A review of the medical literature by the Cochrane collaboration concluded that the ingestion of caffeine offers modest improvement in lung function for 2 to 4 hours after consumption (a 12–18% increase in FEV1, which is similar to a peak flow measurement, as discussed above). Doses as low as 5 mg/kg body weight were shown to have an effect. For a 70-kg (154 pound) man, that's 350 mg of caffeine, or about 2 cups of strong coffee or black tea. Caffeine is also available as 200 mg tablets, generally sold to promote wakefulness. Your peak flow meter will help you assess your improvement.
- It's amazing that **Primatene Mist** (epinephrine) is available over-the-counter. Epinephrine used to be a mainstay of asthma treatment. It is certainly effective, but quite likely to cause rapid heart rate, increased blood pressure, nervousness, and jitteriness. It is the same as adrenaline, which causes the rush that you feel when someone jumps out of a dark corner and scares you. Doctors advise patients against the use of this medication, not so much because it is ineffective, but because of side-effect concerns. Another drawback is the short-acting nature of the drug, lasting at best a few hours. Primatene Mist is currently scheduled to be withdrawn from the market as of December 31, 2011, although the manufacturer hopes to have a replacement available using a different FDA-approved propellant.

- **Primatene Tablets** containing ephedrine are currently available over the counter. Related to pseudoephedrine, ephedrine behaves similarly, with a somewhat greater risk of the same side-effects (see below).
- **Pseudoephedrine** is one of my favorite medications. It decongests the airways from top to bottom, alleviating symptoms of sinus pressure, ear pressure, nasal congestion, and lung congestion. Although patients now have to sign for the medication (thanks to the methamphetamine labs), it is an excellent drug to stock up on. Common side-effects include insomnia, anxiety, rapid heart rate or palpitations, and sometimes increased blood pressure. Some patients find pseudoephedrine too drying, although this effect is dose-related. A few patients have the paradoxical side-effect of drowsiness.
- **Antihistamines** help dry up secretions and minimize the body's reaction to substances to which a person may be allergic. If you suffer from mucus accumulation (phlegm) as part of your obstructive lung disease, you may find an antihistamine helpful. (Note: some patients have the opposite reaction, and find the thicker, drier mucus more difficult to expel. These patients may do well with an **expectorant** (guaifenesin or SSKI)). Patients with allergic asthma do particularly well with antihistamines. The over-the-counter products are as good as prescription medications (and once were). Benadryl (diphenhydramine), Claritin (loratadine), Zyrtec (cetirizine), Allegra (fexofenadine), and chlorpheniramine are all available OTC in inexpensive generic form. Claritin, Allegra, and Zyrtec are less sedating than Benadryl or chlorpheniramine. Some patients have the opposite effect and feel wired when using an antihistamine.

- **NasalCrom** is a nasal inhaler for nasal allergies. It contains cromolyn sodium, one type of controller medication also useful in alleviating chronic asthma. When originally released, all forms of cromolyn sodium were available only by prescription. (The lung inhaler and eye drop remain prescription drugs.) Although NasalCrom is intended for nasal allergies and is inhaled through the nose, some of the medication reaches the lungs. Used on a daily basis, and inhaling deeply as the mist is sprayed, NasalCrom may decrease the overall severity of chronic asthma symptoms. Other advantages are the cost (less than $20 for a bottle containing 200 sprays) and excellent safety profile, even at the high end of dosing. This medication will not cause jitteriness, rapid heart rate, drowsiness, nor insomnia.
- **Antibiotics.** I add these here merely as a reminder that patients with lung disease should take antibiotics sooner rather than later during a respiratory infection. Fish antibiotics are the only U.S. source of OTC antibiotics, intended for aquarium use for fish diseases.

As you prepare, consider including:

Prescription inhalers, decongestants, steroids, antibiotics, per text

OTC Primatene Mist/Tablets; NasalCrom; pseudoephedrine

Caffeine pills and/or *caffeinated* coffee, tea, chocolate

Peak flow meter

Oxygen concentrator and power source

Nebulizer; tubing; medication chambers; power source

Nebulizer medications: albuterol, ipratropium; corticosteroids

Blood Clots and Pulmonary Embolism

Although blood clots may occur anywhere in the body, they typically occur where blood stagnates or moves slowly, usually in the veins of the legs. The greatest concern is when a large clot breaks off and is carried upward through the heart to the lungs, which may cause chest pain, shortness of breath, or occasionally death. Fortunately, most blood clots do not dislodge.

The tip-off to a blood clot (deep venous thrombosis, or DVT) is swelling in one leg only, sometimes with posterior thigh tenderness, or localized warmth or redness. Without ultrasound or X-ray equipment to confirm, you'll need to rely on symptoms. DVTs are more common in people who already have bad veins and swollen legs, so in these individuals look for asymmetric swelling – i.e., more than the patient's usual on a single side. Clots below the knee generally produce little swelling and are too small to cause much damage, even if they migrate. Clots forming in the deep veins of the thigh produce swelling from the knee down, and if disrupted, may be large enough to lodge in the heart or main pulmonary artery, fatally obstructing the flow of blood.

Currently treatment of blood clots is primarily aimed at preventing enlargement (as opposed to dissolution) of the clot. Although warfarin is presently the treatment of choice, this medication requires regular blood monitoring and is likely too difficult to manage in an extreme situation. (The rare patient who desires to continue warfarin should invest in a home prothrombin time monitor, available for about $700.) The alternative is aspirin – that's real aspirin, not Tylenol – one 325-mg tablet daily for at least three months, best taken with food. Keeping the effected limb elevated when possible, applying heat, and wrapping the limb with an elastic compression bandage will help limit swelling and discomfort. (Although not currently approved for treatment of blood clots, the new prescription drug Pradaxa is another possibility to thin the blood, as discussed under atrial fibrillation and heart disease, below.)

If the clot moves to the lungs, you now have a **pulmonary embolism**. Typical symptoms include sudden onset of (usually) one-sided chest pain, shortness of breath, and sometimes cough or wheeze – symptoms often confused with pneumonia, asthma, bronchitis, or inhaled foreign body. Make sure to assess the legs for blood clots in any adult presenting with these symptoms.

In modern times, intravenous clot-busting drugs are used in intensive care settings to dissolve large or dangerous clots. This option will be unavailable at TEOTWAWKI. Continuing the aspirin therapy and offering supportive care will be all you can provide. Oxygen, bronchodilator inhalers, and pain medication may be useful, along with a healthy dose of prayer.

As you prepare, don't forget to include:

Aspirin 325 mg and 80 or 81 mg tablets

Willow bark or better yet, a willow tree

Elastic bandages such as Ace wraps

Botulism

A strange illness has struck your small community. Over the winter, three mothers have died of a paralyzing illness. Oddly, no one else has been sick. Should the other mothers be worried? What is the common factor?

By now everyone's heard of Botox (botulinum toxin). What once was considered a deadly poison is now a popular cosmetic injection. Paralyze the muscles of the forehead and *voilà*, your wrinkles disappear. Miniscule doses of the purified toxin are also useful in the treatment of true medical problems, from migraines to muscle spasms.

However, botulinum is considered one of nature's deadliest nerve toxins. Produced by the bacterium *Clostridium botulinum*, the pre-formed toxin usually enters the body through the ingestion of contaminated food. The toxin is disseminated via the bloodstream to every nerve in the body. The muscles of the eyes become paralyzed, causing double vision and drooping eyelids. Chewing, swallowing, and talking grow difficult as the muscles of the mouth and throat weaken. Next, the shoulders are effected, with paralysis progressing downwards to the forearms, hands, thighs, calves, and feet.

Worst of all, the muscles of breathing are attacked, causing shortness of breath, respiratory failure, coma, and death. Untreated, the fatality rate may reach 70%, depending on dosage of the toxin.

Clostridium botulinum is not your ordinary oxygen-loving bacterium, such as those that cause pneumonia and bronchitis. Though *C. botulinum* organisms may be found in low levels throughout the natural world, where they really thrive is in oxygen-free, non-acidic, low salt environments, such as those found in canned food. In a severe case, the gas produced by the organism can produce sufficient pressure to cause bulging of food-containing cans. However, more commonly neither the container nor the contents shows obvious contamination.

With its ubiquitous distribution in soil, consider it a given that a few live botulinum spores will be in every can or jar of food, at least initially. They must be killed to prevent multiplication and subsequent production of the nerve toxin.

The commercial food industry accomplishes this via a "botulinum cook," heating canned foods to 121 °C (250 °F) for 3 minutes. Home canning methods are less standardized and simple boiling at 212 °F for a few minutes may be insufficient to kill every spore.

For safe home canning techniques, download the free *Complete Guide to Home Canning* referenced in the box at the end of this section.

Currently, botulism affects about 1 in 10,000,000 Americans annually. Once identified, these individuals are treated with botulinum antitoxin, which prevents further progression of paralysis, but does not reverse established symptoms. Even with the antitoxin, patients may require weeks to months on a ventilator. With intensive treatment, the death rate has dropped to as low as 2%.

Contrast this with a post-Armageddon scenario, where home-canned goods will be consumed much more commonly. If ingestion of such goods increases a thousand-fold, it is likely the incidence of botulism will increase a thousand-fold as well, to perhaps as high as 1 in 10,000 people annually. But post-Armageddon, there will be no antitoxin, no intensive care unit, no respirators, and no effective treatment. The only answer will be prevention.

What about the mothers who died in our hypothetical community? Many people incorrectly assume that contaminated food will smell or taste bad. The person most at risk is the cook, who may be tempted to sample a product prior to cooking, to judge if it is contaminated. A single bite of food containing botulinum toxin may be lethal. However, the toxin is deactivated by heat. The CDC recommends boiling home-canned foods 10 minutes (plus 1 minute per 1000 feet above sea-level) prior to serving. In our scenario, these mothers had sampled uncooked food before heating them for the rest of the family.

Does this mean it is safe to eat food from a bulging or rusted can, once it's been thoroughly heated? Not unless the alternative is certain death. Even if the toxin has been deactivated by boiling, the spores of *Clostridium* may not be killed. This can lead to a second type of botulism, wherein the bacteria survive within the body, in this case the gut (or in other circumstances, a contaminated wound) and produce the neurotoxin, which remains capable of producing paralysis, although symptoms *may* be less severe. For safe disposal of suspect food, boil for 30 minutes, then carefully dispose of somewhere inaccessible to children, pets, and domestic animals.

Infant botulism is the prototype of disease due to intestinal colonization, and is sometimes caused by ingesting spore-containing honey. Although the adult immune system can destroy the few botulinum spores that may be present in honey, the infantile immune system is incapable of doing so. For this reason, children less than 12 months old should never be fed honey. Constipation (due to paralysis of the intestinal tract muscles) is usually the first symptom of infant botulism, followed by weakness, trouble feeding, an altered cry, lethargy, and possibly the descending paralysis typical of foodborne botulism.

Since the disease is caused by bacteria, why aren't antibiotics the answer? Again, in most cases it is the toxin, not the bacteria, that poses the problem. In a wound contaminated with *Clostridium botulinum*, surgery to remove the infected tissue is the most expedient remedy (although rarely doctors may employ antibiotics as well).

One final comment – those of us residing in the lower forty-eight rarely think about eating a beached whale, but fermented meats and fish, such as those included in the Native Alaskan diet, have also been implicated in botulism, including blubber, beaver tail, salmon, and seal flipper. Other fermented meats may also pose a danger, and in fact the term botulism is derived from the Latin word for sausage (botulus), the first tainted food recognized as causing the disease.

As you prepare, don't forget to:

Include all supplies you will need for safe home canning.

Download the free *USDA Complete Guide to Home Canning, 2009 Revision* online at:

http://www.uga.edu/nchfp/publications/publications_usda.html

Constipation

Most constipation is diet-related, which is why I include it here. If your end-of-civilization diet is lacking in sufficient fiber, you *will* become constipated – count on it. Make sure to include high-fiber foods in your prepper pantry, as discussed in **Chapter 2**.

Patients most at risk for constipation are the elderly and anyone taking drying medications (in particular antidepressants). If you suffer a tendency toward constipation that cannot be resolved with diet alone, you should include a laxative among your medical supplies. If fiber foods are ineffective, fiber laxatives will not work either. MiraLax, Dulcolax, Lactulose (prescription), Ex-Lax, or similar medication may become your best friend. If things really get stuck, then a suppository, enema, or manual disimpaction may be required. If this possibility sounds uninviting, remember, an ounce of prevention is worth a pound of cure.

Diabetes

Basically there are two kinds of diabetes: the kind that can kill you quickly and the kind that won't. Most people in the first category have Type I, insulin-dependent diabetes mellitus. A few have advanced Type II, insulin-dependent diabetes. Without medication, these patients will experience extremely elevated blood sugar levels, leading to coma and death.

Fortunately, most diabetic patients are in the second group. Without medication their blood sugar levels may increase to 200, 300, or even 600 mg/dL, but they won't soar to 1,000 and become rapidly fatal.

At the end of the world as we know it, the outlook for truly insulin-dependent diabetics is fairly grim. Although insulin may be potent a year, possibly a few years, beyond the printed expiration date under recommended storage conditions, a new source of insulin must be established by the time these supplies run out. Currently all insulin in the United States used on human patients is genetically-engineered human insulin. Until the 1990s, insulin derived from animal sources (cows or pigs) was prescribed for both humans and pets. Nowadays human insulin is the mainstay of diabetic treatment for cats and dogs as well as human beings, although one manufacturer is currently producing bovine insulin for use in cats. This is good news – the art is not lost, although neither your doctor nor pharmacist is the least bit likely to be ready to duplicate the process. In an Armageddon event, insulin production would likely revert to manufacturing the drug from animal sources until genetically-engineered insulin is again available. One veterinary pharmacist apparently figured how out to compound bovine insulin on her own by studying old patents.

On another bright note, certain older types of insulin are available over-the-counter, without a prescription in most states, specifically the NPH, Regular, and 70/30 versions of human insulin. Needles and testing supplies are available as well without a prescription, though pharmacists may use their discretion when selling needles to suspicious customers. If you purchase insulin over the counter, insurance and government programs are unlikely to cover the cost. The least expensive supplies I have found are sold through Wal-Mart. Keep in mind the different kinds of insulin are not interchangeable, primarily due to varying onset and duration of action. Discussing this with your physician now is a good idea, as is learning to regulate your glucose and insulin. Most insurance programs pay for diabetic teaching classes at your local hospital. Even if you've had the disease for years, you'll likely learn more than you would expect.

The use of the oral drug metformin in the treatment of Type I diabetes is under investigation. Clearly it cannot control Type 1 diabetes when used alone, however it does yield modest improvement, at least in certain patients. Many of my own questions will never be researched, however. For example, could metformin delay the development of diabetic coma for a few days in an insulin-dependent patient, if insulin supplies run low? This might allow time to find a new source of medication.

Another stop-gap measure to delay coma and death if a re-supply of insulin is likely within a day or two might be exchange transfusion. Successful blood transfusions were performed 200 years ago, without the aid of modern medicine. If my child was dying of diabetes and my blood type was compatible, I would certainly be willing to exchange my blood with my child. I realize this is an extreme solution, but at TEOTWAWKI we'll all need to think outside the box. Cord blood transfusions are also under investigation for treating Type 1 diabetes, and have decreased the need for insulin in some patients. This sounds high-tech, but collecting cord blood is not especially difficult. I mention these potential treatments for Type I diabetes to offer hope. The current medical establishment is constrained from departing too far from accepted thinking. However, novel therapies may be found when there is no choice but to do so.

For Type II diabetics the situation is much less critical than for insulin-dependent diabetics. However, some Type II diabetics do end up on insulin as the pancreas loses its ability to manufacture insulin. Most Type II diabetics actually make more insulin than non-diabetics produce, due to insulin resistance, requiring higher levels of insulin to regulate elevated blood glucose. In the long run, this stresses the pancreas, essentially causing it to wear out.

Fortunately some diabetics can reverse this process via significant weight loss and careful dietary monitoring. For the typical overweight Type II diabetic whose pancreas is still functioning to some extent, caloric restriction (whether now or in times of scarcity) may result in an improvement (or even resolution) of the diabetic condition. In short, if you're overweight and diabetic, lose weight now and preserve your pancreas. Otherwise you may find yourself in the same boat as Type I insulin-dependent diabetics.

In the past few decades the goal of diabetic treatment has changed, focusing on tighter blood sugar control to prevent long-term complications. With this in mind, the definition of diabetes is currently a fasting blood glucose level of 126 mg/dL or higher. However, years ago the cut-off was 140 mg/dL, and any practicing physician can tell you that many patients experience no apparent short-term symptoms even at blood sugars of 300.

In a scenario where blood glucose levels cannot be easily monitored, reverting to older treatment goals and regimens is likely. Of course, you should stock up now on blood glucose testing supplies: monitors, lancets, batteries, and test strips. In times of scarcity you'll want to minimize your testing regimen to preserve your cache. Patients on metformin or acarbose alone run very little risk of low blood sugar levels, and blood glucose testing done only monthly or quarterly may suffice. Patients on sulfonylurea drugs and other medications that can cause hypoglycemia may require closer monitoring (daily to quarterly).

But the question remains, what will you do when you run out of testing supplies?

One of the oldest methods of monitoring diabetes is via frequency of urination. *Diabetes mellitus* actually means *run-through honey*, that is, what a person eats seems to run right through them, coming out in the form of sweet urine, which may be sticky or even taste like honey. Normally the kidneys will reabsorb all the glucose from the blood as it is filtered of impurities. However, at high sugar levels (above 200–300 mg/dL) the kidneys are unable to absorb all the sugar; hence some is excreted in the urine. Glucose (sugar) in the urine acts as a diuretic (water pill), causing increased urinary volume and frequency. Patients often pee more, eat more, and drink more, with or without a change in weight.

Because patients with high blood sugars and resultant excess urination lose calories (as sugar runs-through the body), weight loss occurs (unless you live in America where the calories can be easily replaced). Except where food is unlimited, for many overweight Type II diabetics this can act as a stabilizing mechanism: caloric loss leads to weight loss, which leads to lower body mass index, which may lead to decreased blood glucose levels and a decreased insulin requirement. (Beware: this mechanism does not function in Type I or insulin-dependent Type II diabetics, whose blood sugar will rapidly increase to dangerous levels.)

I know of no doctor who has actually tasted a patient's urine (I certainly haven't), but doing so is one possible test for diabetic control. A motivated prepper might want to determine at what blood sugar level his kidneys tend to spill glucose into the urine. This experiment is fairly easy to do, but I suggest you discuss the plan with your doctor before attempting the procedure. One simply allows one's blood sugar to increase (usually by withholding medication temporarily), meanwhile monitoring blood sugar levels and urinary glucose levels. For example, at a blood sugar of 150 mg/dL you're unlikely to find any glucose in the urine on dipstick testing with OTC urine test strips. However, by the time your blood glucose level reaches 300, you probably will. Tasting the urine at these various levels may also give a clue as to whether the kidneys are leaking sugar.

The whole concept of tasting one's urine probably motivates the reader to stock up on home blood sugar testing supplies. Currently test strips out-date within a short period, at most a few years. However, if stored as directed, in the original unopened packaging, they may well be stable significantly longer. Few strips still have a visual color-code to allow you to manually estimate your blood sugar level if your meter is not working. However, Quikchek Glucose Reagent Strips, intended for veterinary blood glucose monitoring, feature this option

Monitoring frequency and volume of urination is also useful. Elevated urinary sugar levels cause increased frequency due to increased urine volume. In contrast, urinary infections cause increased frequency, usually of small volumes, due to irritability of the urinary tract. A person who finds himself getting up at night with a full bladder, or urinating large amounts several times a day, may well have uncontrolled diabetes. Weighing yourself periodically is another method of determining your fluid loss. A pint of water weighs a pound, and increased urinary losses will soon show up on a scale. Make sure you have the old type of scale on hand, one that requires no battery. A good balance scale should last a lifetime.

Regarding oral medication, for the most part the fancy newer diabetic drugs, those costing $100–200/month, would be difficult and excessively expensive to stockpile, and therefore less suitable for life after TEOTWAWKI. Two inexpensive classes of oral medications would form the mainstay of diabetic treatment: metformin and sulfonylureas. Even if they do not reduce one's blood glucose to normal levels, they should lower it by 50 to 200 mg/dL for most patients. Many patients would be expected to lose a significant amount of weight due to scarcity of food. Both the decreased calories and decreased body mass would tend to lower blood glucose as well. Living with a blood sugar of 300 mg/dL may cause damage to the eyes, kidneys, and heart in the long run, but presumably your immediate concern will be for survival.

If all this is worrying you, do what you can now to get your diabetes under control. Eat well, aim for a healthy body weight, discuss your medications with your physician, stock up on testing supplies, learn how to check your urine, and have your eyes, kidneys, and heart tested.

Next, what about herbal medicine?

Chromium picolinate is known to lower blood glucose levels in both humans and animals, probably by lowering insulin resistance. The medical literature reports improvements in long-term blood sugar control in patients taking 100 to 500 micrograms twice daily. There have been a few reports of renal failure with high dosages. Although additional studies are needed to confirm and quantify the effect, laying in a store of chromium picolinate might be considered.

It has been proposed that garlic may lower blood sugar levels in humans, since it is effective in alloxan-diabetic rats. How garlic may do so remains under investigation, and it is not recommended for treatment of diabetes in humans at this time. However, with the ready availability of garlic, you may want to study your own response.

Alpha lipoic acid (found in meat, broccoli, and potatoes) may help treat nerve damage due to diabetes, but does not lower blood sugar levels. The dosage noted to be effective is 600 to 1200 mg per day.

Ginseng and psyllium may also lower blood sugar a little, but again, this effect cannot be guaranteed. However if no medication is available, Panax ginseng (100–200 mg per day) may be somewhat effective . . . if you can find it.

Cinnamon is a more recent entry into the race to find an herbal preparation to help control blood sugar. A review article in the journal *Pharmacotherapy*[22] concludes that cinnamon has "a possible modest effect in lowering plasma glucose levels in patients with poorly controlled type 2 diabetes." The various trials used different dosages (1 gm to 3 gm of cinnamon per day), and demonstrated no harmful effects. However, they were each done in select populations and were continued for only a few months, making it difficult to extrapolate to long-term treatment in the general population.

Among my patients, I've had some who have tried these herbal preparations for their diabetes, but none who experienced a reversal of the disease. If an herb can lower your blood sugar 10–50 points, that's great, but also much less effective than medication. Still, it's better than nothing, and when combined with calorie restriction and weight loss, herbal preparations are certainly a consideration when or if medication is unavailable. Of course, most of

[22] *Pharmacotherapy*. 2007;27(4)

us are not growing ginseng in our backyards, and assuring an on-going supply would be a challenge for herbs as well as drugs.

For a good review of the literature regarding herbal treatment of diabetes, see *The American Family Physician*, September 2000, available online at http://www.aafp.org/afp/20000901/1051.html.

For information regarding use of ginseng see *The American Family Physician*, October 2003, also available online at http://www.aafp.org/afp/2003/1015/p1539.html.

For a review of studies examining the role of cinnamon in the treatment of diabetes, see *Pharmacotherapy*. 2007;27(4):595–599, also available online at: http://www.medscape.com/viewarticle/555433.

As you prepare, consider:

Stockpiling insulin and oral diabetic medications

Stockpiling blood sugar testing strips, monitor, batteries, and lancets

Stockpiling test strips for urinary ketones and glucose

Stockpiling veterinary Quikchek blood glucose test strips

Stockpiling cinnamon, chromium picolinate, garlic, alpha lipoic acid

Losing weight and stabilizing your blood sugar now

Discussing alternative/inexpensive medication options with your doctor

Investigating at what blood sugar level your kidneys spill glucose

Diarrhea

Nowadays people get upset if diarrhea continues beyond a day or two – three at the most. If that's all you have to worry about, skip this chapter.

But what if it goes on and on, day after day after day? Or what if you begin bleeding, or have cramping, or prolonged vomiting? Is your whole family at risk? Will you become dehydrated? Could it be food poisoning, or a parasite, or perhaps an unknown toxin?

The infectious causes of diarrhea are covered in detail in **Chapter 11** under *Gastrointestinal Infections*. Here I'll cover a few general principles in the diagnosis and treatment of diarrhea.

What is meant by diarrhea should first be specified. An occasional loose stool does not qualify. Most people understand diarrhea to mean increased frequency of bowel movements or decreased consistency. Medically speaking, diarrhea denotes higher volume (weight) of daily stool, due to higher water content. For practical purposes, we'll call diarrhea a condition that persists at least 24 hours, featuring runny bowel movements occurring in greater number than is usual for a given patient. It may or may not be accompanied by other symptoms, such as nausea, vomiting, gas, fever, or fatigue.

The evaluation of diarrhea centers on likely causes, as well as the overall condition of the patient, which is by far the most important consideration. A person who feels generally well, is able to eat, and is not losing weight has little to fear from most causes of diarrhea, including food poisoning. The default diagnosis for simple diarrhea is viral gastroenteritis (a stomach or intestinal flu), which usually lasts a few days, or occasionally as long as a few weeks. Common non-infectious causes include food intolerance or allergy, chemical poisoning or intolerance, medication side-effects, hyperthyroidism, anxiety, and colitis. Often, by eliminating a suspect food or chemical, the problem can be identified and avoided.

As mentioned, most cases of diarrhea are caused by intestinal viruses. Medication does not remedy the cause, but it may improve symptoms. Medical treatment is aimed at slowing the transit time through the gut (as with Imodium) or absorbing extra intestinal fluid by adding fiber (as in Metamucil). However, medication is rarely needed for typical short-term diarrhea.

When diarrhea continues beyond a few weeks, or if the patient appears significantly ill, a thorough investigation should be considered, beginning with infectious causes. In the meantime, treatment is aimed at preventing dehydration and electrolyte imbalances. Assuring sufficient oral fluid intake to balance the loss (using oral rehydration therapy, as per recipe in **Chapter 2**) is much more important than slowing down the diarrhea. If vomiting is also present, I.V. fluids may be helpful, but lacking this option, administering an anti-nausea medication may be required to keep fluids down (oral OTC meclizine, or prescription Phenergan or Compazine, by mouth, injection, or suppository).

As you prepare, consider including:

Imodium AD or generic loperamide; Pepto-Bismol

Fiber anti-diarrheals (Metamucil, Citrucel)

I.V. fluids (Ringer's Lactate) and I.V. administration supplies

OTC anti-vomiting drugs (meclizine, Bonine, Dramamine)

Emetrol for mild nausea (canned peach syrup also works)

Oral or rectal prescription for nausea (Phenergan or Compazine)

Gout

Has your toe ever hurt so badly that you couldn't stand even a bed sheet to touch it? Unless you injured yourself, this is likely gout. Living through an attack without medication could be a nightmare. Let's hope you won't need to walk anywhere.

Gout is a recurring form of arthritis that for some patients is a black or white issue: either they feel fine – or terrible. Typically gout occurs in the toe or foot, though other joints may be affected, particularly knees, hands, and elbows. Gout is caused by an inflammatory response to uric acid that crystallizes within the joint. The affected joint is swollen, warm, often red, and, boy, does it hurt.

For other patients gout assumes a more chronic form. The joints (usually of the foot) are sore to a varying degree, but not exquisitely so. Sometimes chronic gout leads to a degenerative type of arthritis, or coexists with osteoarthritis. Unlucky patients suffer both the acute and chronic varieties of gout, with kidney stones thrown in for good measure.

The serum uric acid is a reflection of what the joint uric acid level may be. The best test to diagnose gout is to withdraw some synovial fluid from a swollen joint and look for crystals under a polarizing microscope. Such a test could be done even after global catastrophe, but the truth is, the test is usually omitted even today. Patients don't like having needles inserted into painful joints, and often the diagnosis can be made by eyeballing the problem, especially for someone who's experienced gout before.

Some patients suffer from gout on a hereditary basis; for others it is diet-related. Gout was once called the "rich man's disease" – only the rich could afford a diet high in animal protein. Still other patients experience high uric acid levels as a result of medications they are taking, particularly diuretics. Anyone prone to gout is more likely to suffer the problem in the winter months, when the lower temperature allows the crystals to precipitate out of the synovial fluid.

Gout can be confused with other types of arthritis or bony problems, including osteoarthritis, rheumatoid arthritis, sprains, fractures, joint infection, and trauma, so knowing a patient's history is always important.

But assuming the diagnosis is correct, what can be done when no doctor is around?

For gout sufferers it should come as a relief to learn that over-the-counter medication can help (and sometimes works wonders). Although traditionally prescription drugs such as colchicine and indomethacin are used to treat an *acute* case, OTC anti-inflammatory medications (NSAIDs) are equally effective in full dose. Ibuprofen, naproxen, and aspirin all work quite well (and all have the potential side-effect of heartburn or stomach upset, so be sure to take them with food. Some patients may require an acid-lowering medication such as omeprazole as well, to protect the stomach). Short-term steroids (5–10 days of prednisone or Medrol) are occasionally required, but are only available by prescription. Anti-inflammatory drugs are also effective for *chronic* gout. For acute gout, doctors recommend higher doses of NSAIDs than is typically advised for over-the-counter use, e.g. 800 mg of ibuprofen three times daily, or 500 mg of naproxen twice daily. Higher doses of aspirin may cause hearing damage or ringing in the ears and should be avoided. Tylenol (acetaminophen) does not have anti-inflammatory properties, and so does not work well for gout, but it can be used in addition to the NSAIDs for additional pain relief, if needed. Rest is a better answer than narcotics when the pain is severe.

Colchicine is not an NSAID, but does work great for gout. As of spring 2011 generic colchicine is currently difficult to obtain, however brand-name Colcrys is available by prescription. Although the drug is derived from the roots of the flowering herb *Colchicum autumnale*, ingestion of the plant can be fatal and has no antidote. Even at therapeutic doses of colchicine, most patients experience some nausea, vomiting, or diarrhea. I would leave the use of this drug to a trained professional.

Gout is not a type of arthritis where ice will help; it should, in fact, be avoided. Gentle soaking in warm water may provide some relief, or a heating pad if the patient can tolerate the foot being touched.

Don't be tempted to take a drink of alcohol to decrease the pain of gout. Alcohol tends to slow the elimination of uric acid from the body, and may instead prolong an attack.

The most important aspects of a gout-prevention diet are: 1) to drink plenty of fluids to dilute and remove uric acid from the body; 2) to avoid animal proteins (particularly organ meats, red meat, fatty fish, and seafood); and 3) to avoid alcohol, especially beer. Some gout sufferers may find their symptoms improve with the significant change in diet likely to accompany the end of civilization as we know it.

Currently patients with recurrent gout attacks are commonly treated with allopurinol on a daily basis, to decrease the serum uric acid level (and hence, the joint uric acid level). There is no OTC equivalent of allopurinol, so if you have a heavy duty case of chronic gout, you may want to stock up. There are a few newer medications, especially useful for patients who have decreased kidney function (elevated BUN and creatinine), but these are quite expensive. Decreased kidney function is not the same as trouble urinating, and is determined by blood testing. You're unlikely to know how well your kidneys are functioning unless a doctor informs you. For the majority of patients, this will not be a concern (especially if civilization is falling apart around us).

Most physicians have not used herbal preparations in the treatment of gout, but the inclusion of caffeine and dark-colored fruits such as cherries, dark berries, and purple grapes in the diet has been shown to lower serum uric acid levels.

How likely are you to suffer a case of gout? The incidence of gout in the general population is quoted as being under 1%, but in my own patient population of middle-aged and older adults, I'd put it at a few per cent. If you yourself don't have gout, odds are quite high that you know someone who does, most likely an older man, although women may develop gout as well. Someday sharing your stockpile of inexpensive anti-inflammatory drugs may win you a friend for life.

If you or a family member has gout, don't forget to stock:

OTC NSAIDs (ibuprofen, naproxen, aspirin)

OTC Pepcid, Zantac, Prilosec, or Prevacid to protect the stomach

Prescription Celebrex if intolerant of NSAIDs

Allopurinol (generic) or Uloric (expensive) to prevent chronic gout

Prescription steroids (prednisone or methylprednisolone)

Herbal therapies: caffeine and dark-colored fruits

Headache and Migraine

Suppose your nephew complains his head is killing him. When is it serious? Can you help him? When should you worry?

Nowadays any ER patient with a terrible headache will get a CAT scan – not an option at TEOTWAWKI. Fortunately, most patients do not have brain tumors, aneurysms, or intracranial bleeding (and what could you do about it if they did?) Without a neurosurgeon, serious causes of headache will need to be treated symptomatically.

The most serious headaches are those that occur with additional symptoms, such as slurred speech, one-sided muscle weakness, blurred vision, or facial droop. If professional referral is an option, these patients should be referred. Thankfully such headaches are rare in younger patients, though definitely a concern in the elderly.

In middle-aged and younger patients, **migraines** are typically the most painful headaches. These are usually one-sided, and often accompanied by nausea and intolerance of light and/or noise. Sometimes the headache is preceded by an aura (such as seeing flashing lights) 10–30 minutes before the onset of the headache. **Tension headaches** occur in the back of the neck, or the forehead, or at the temples, or the entire head. **Sinus headaches** are usually in the forehead, face, or top of the head (or occasionally cause referred pain in the back of the head), and are usually accompanied by allergy or cold symptoms.

There are entire textbooks devoted to the treatment of headache. Assuming you are working with extremely limited resources, here are the main points to be aware of:

1. Most headaches, even severe headaches, are not life-threatening or serious.
2. Underlying causes of headaches should always be considered and treated accordingly, including infection, high blood pressure, dental problems, trauma, and neck problems.

3. Reassurance is as important as pain relief. If you find no underlying cause or additional problems, the great majority of the time you will be correct if you reassure the patient that nothing serious is wrong.
4. Elderly patients with persistent headache (especially around the temples), and without other neurologic symptoms, may have temporal arteritis or polymyalgia rheumatica, which responds to steroids (10–20 mg prednisone daily for several weeks, then slowly tapered).
5. The elegant treatments currently available for migraine are unlikely to be an option if civilization collapses; if you suffer from migraines, stockpile whatever medication is working well for you (e.g. triptans).
6. The majority of patients will need to be treated according to symptoms, using pain relievers, anti-inflammatory drugs, muscle-relaxers, nausea meds, and sleep aids. Read **Section Five** on Pain.
7. Unless you're a neurosurgeon, you won't be able to do much more for someone with an intracranial problem such as an aneurysm.

Hearing loss

Does your granny use a hearing aid? Has she procured a lifetime supply of batteries? If the technology is lost, what will you do yourself when you get old, should you survive so long?

Before discussing treatment, let me say a word about prevention. Avoid loud noises, probably the most preventable causes of hearing loss. If you can't hear someone sitting next to you unless they raise their voice, the music is too loud. If you're young enough to snigger at this advice, beware: your turn will come.

Hearing loss is divided into two basic kinds: conductive hearing loss and nerve damage. Conductive loss is caused by damage to or scarring of the ear drums, often from recurrent infections. It also includes transient, correctable loss of hearing from eustachian tube dysfunction, as well as excess earwax accumulation (cerumen impaction). With conductive loss, the sound waves are not transmitted through the ear efficiently, which may be reversible (see chapters on ear pain and respiratory infections). With nerve hearing loss, the damage is permanent, and sound cannot be transmitted to the brain effectively.

Most types of deafness are treated with hearing aids. For certain types of nerve deafness, fancy treatments such as cochlear implants are currently employed. Either way, if technology is lost, electronic devices will be of no use.

What do you do then? Learn sign language? Sign language is only a reasonable alternative if those around you know the language as well.

Without technology, treatment of hearing loss will be set back nearly a century. Before digital equipment, before transistors, before vacuum tubes, before carbon amplifiers, there were ear trumpets. I still remember a medical school professor saying if a mechanical amplification device didn't help a patient hear better, then an electrical one would not either. These acoustic models amplify sound through the use of a cone-shaped device and are effective for mild hearing loss. For a look at the past, visit the Hearing Aid Museum at www.hearingaidmuseum.com. Online auctions feature various historical models for purchase; current manufacturers have proven difficult to locate. Even a paper cone helps better than nothing. If you or a loved one suffers hearing loss, best to explore your options now.

Heart disease

A volume such as this can scarcely serve as a treatise on heart disease, but a few common problems will be briefly addressed.

For the most part, heart problems fall into three categories: **conduction disturbances** (rate and/or rhythm), **angina** (chest pain due to clogged arteries), and **congestive heart failure**. The first includes fast, slow, and irregular heart rates. The latter two are related to inadequate functional capacity of the heart.

When dealing with heart rate problems, an underlying cause should always be sought. The normal heart rate is about 60–100 beats per minute, although athletes and certain other healthy individuals may have a resting heart rate as low as the mid-40s. When symptoms of a **slow heart rate** (bradycardia) occur, they are due to inadequate blood flow to the brain or body as a whole, producing light-headedness, dizziness, easy fatigability, or tiredness. Several medications slow the heart rate, including beta-blockers, calcium channel blockers, digoxin, and amiodarone. These may need to be tapered or discontinued in a symptomatic patient. Hypothyroidism should be considered, and would probably produce other symptoms if the heart rate is affected (see entry on **Thyroid Disease**). Intrinsic heart disease may cause a slow heart rate, and is typically treated with a pacemaker. Medications that increase the heart rate (as a side-effect) may be a somewhat effective treatment (caffeine, pseudoephedrine, mild amphetamines). If the medical establishment collapses, treatment options for symptomatic bradycardia will be quite limited.

Rapid heart rate (tachycardia) is more common than slow heart rate, and may be constant or intermittent. Fortunately, it's also easier to treat. For a persistently elevated heart rate, underlying causes should be considered, including hyperthyroidism, stimulant medications, prolonged fever, dehydration, and of course, heart disease. If an underlying (non-cardiac) cause cannot be found, the possible need for slowing the heart rate arises. Some patients always run a resting heart rate of 110–115 without other symptoms, and may require no treatment. Potentially disturbing symptoms that often accompany a rapid heart rate include the sensation of palpitations, anxiety, and light-headedness. At a prolonged rate above about 115–120, patients often begin experiencing symptoms of heart failure (shortness of breath, fatigue, dizziness, leg swelling), especially older patients (see below). Slowing the heart rate reduces these symptoms, and may be accomplished with beta-blockers or calcium channel blockers (and rarely both together).

Rhythm problems include occasional erratic beats, runs of rapid heart rate, and persistent irregular rhythms. Of these, *asymptomatic* irregularities don't require treatment, with the exception of atrial fibrillation and ventricular tachycardia. Again, beta-blockers (metoprolol, atenolol, propranolol) and calcium channel blockers such as verapamil and diltiazem may be used in *symptomatic* patients.

Atrial fibrillation produces a persistent, irregularly irregular heart rhythm, which is often diagnosable on physical exam, although it's preferable to confirm with an EKG. With this problem, the rhythm-generating upper chambers of the heart (atria) are quivering at a heart rate of about 300 beats/min. Fortunately, most of the electrical signal is blocked at the level of the major pumping chambers of the heart (ventricles), yielding a heart rate of 150 or less. Still, rates above about 110 beats per minute may make a person uncomfortable, anxious, dizzy, tired, or short of breath.

Ideally treatment of atrial fibrillation would restore the heart to normal rhythm; this is sometimes achieved with medication, but often requires cardioversion (shocking the heart) or radioablation (destroying the heart tissue responsible for triggering the problem). Without modern medical back-up, the goal of treatment will revert to rate control (which is often the case nowadays anyway). Again, beta-blockers, calcium channel blockers, or digoxin may be used to lower the heart rate. Remember that beta-blockers may worsen breathing in an asthma or COPD patient. Digoxin (or the herb foxglove) must be used with caution, since monitoring of a patient's digoxin level will likely be impossible. The most common symptoms of too high a dose are nausea, vomiting, and excessively slow heart rate . . . which may be lethal.

The other concern with atrial fibrillation is stagnation of the blood flow through the heart, which may allow clots to form, sometimes leading to a stroke. For this reason, atrial fibrillation patients are administered blood thinners, most commonly warfarin, which requires regular blood monitoring. Without this capability, the safer approach is to use aspirin, 80–325 mg a day. Pradaxa, a new blood thinner, is a third possibility. Drawbacks of Pradaxa include cost ($100–$200/month) and lack of an antidote.

Persistent **ventricular fibrillation** (v. fib.) is much more serious than atrial fibrillation, and without cardioversion (shocking the heart), usually leads to death within minutes. Implanted ventricular defibrillators are the most effective treatment for patients who live through an episode of ventricular fibrillation, but without our modern medical establishment, many of these patients will die. Beta-blockers and/or amiodarone may slow the heart rate or help prevent recurrent episodes of ventricular fibrillation.

Most patients who have an intermittent rapid heart rate have SVT (supra-ventricular tachycardia), which is much less serious than ventricular fibrillation, and may be treated with the drugs outlined under rapid heart rate, above.

Angina, or chest pain caused by too little oxygen to the heart, may be treated with rest, beta-blockers, calcium channel blockers, nitroglycerin, other nitrates, oxygen, or heart surgery (stents or by-pass). The arteries are typically narrowed by build-up of cholesterol-containing plaque (arteriosclerosis), which sometimes obstructs blood flow completely. This starves the heart of oxygen, sometimes killing the affected myocardium (heart muscle), causing a heart attack (myocardial infarction). When this process disrupts the rhythm of the heart, patients often die. Otherwise, if enough functioning heart muscle remains, patients often survive, though may never recover their full strength.

Patients with **high cholesterol** are at higher risk for arteriosclerotic heart disease. Statin drugs are the most effective medications to lower serum cholesterol and decrease risk of heart attack, especially in men. If you are taking a statin drug, you may want to stockpile several years' worth, although blood testing to detect liver or muscle damage is unlikely to be available after an Armageddon scenario. Ideally, a patient with high cholesterol would make dietary and lifestyle changes now, to optimize his or her lipid status prior to societal collapse, rather than waiting for food shortages and forced exercise to improve cardiovascular health. Likewise, if you're planning to rely on herbal treatment of high cholesterol, you may want to investigate now whether such treatment is effective for you, since there may be little opportunity to find out later.

Congestive heart failure occurs when the pumping action of the heart cannot keep up with the body's demands, causing shortness of breath, fatigue, and/or leg swelling. The lungs become congested with backed-up blood or fluid, hence the name. Heart failure usually occurs in the elderly and is typically caused by arteriosclerosis or atrial fibrillation (or other arrhythmia).

The most reliably-effective treatment of congestive heart failure is a strong diuretic to eliminate extra fluid from the body. Furosemide has been used for decades in doses of 10–160 mg per day (20–40 mg is typical). Dangers of furosemide and similar diuretics are dehydration and low potassium. Doctors normally monitor serum potassium levels closely; if this is impossible, giving 10–40 mEq of KCl (potassium chloride) as a supplement is advisable, or at least increasing dietary potassium intake in the form of bananas, citrus, or tomatoes. Potassium has its own dangers in heart failure patients who may have poor kidney function, which you'll have little way of identifying.

Other drugs that may help heart failure include digoxin, beta-blockers, and ACE-inhibitors, but none of these works as quickly or as powerfully as a strong diuretic. Many patients require a combination of two or more drugs.

If you or a family member has heart disease, consider:

Learning all you can now about your specific problem

Seeking a permanent solution to atrial fibrillation (radioablation)

An implanted pacemaker-defibrillator for low heart rate or v. fib.

Definitive cardiac surgery for blocked arteries (stent or by-pass)

Making lifestyle changes (weight loss, smoking cessation, exercise)

Stockpiling aspirin, a beta-blocker, and a calcium channel blocker

Dietary control of high cholesterol and/or stocking statins

Possibly stocking digoxin, lisinopril, furosemide, and potassium

Stocking multiple small bottles of sublingual nitroglycerin

Obtaining an oxygen concentrator and power supply

Heartburn

Do you wake up at night with your chest burning? Does spicy food give you indigestion? Do you experience chest pain whenever you take an aspirin?

Heartburn is a layman's term denoting a burning sensation in the upper abdomen or chest, which is usually due to acid refluxing into the esophagus, or due to excess acid within the stomach itself. The most common symptom of acid reflux is heartburn. However, some patients experience chest pain, nausea, dry heaves, regurgitation or vomiting, either alone or in addition to the burning sensation. *Always* keep in mind that true heart disease may cause many of these symptoms and mimic gastroesophageal reflux, or GERD (see **Angina**, above).

Any acid can burn the GI tract: hydrochloric acid (stomach acid), citric acid (from citrus fruits), acetylsalicylic acid (aspirin). Other chemicals and foods can irritate the stomach as well, including alcohol, tobacco, onions, fatty foods, spicy foods, chocolate, and coffee. Too many of these can overwhelm the body's natural defenses. Although the stomach is coated to prevent acid from burning its lining, this defense is not 100% effective; and although a valve-like sphincter prevents most stomach acid from refluxing up into the esophagus, higher intra-abdominal pressure or a recumbent position can force the valve open, allowing acid to leak upwards.

When the stomach or esophagus is irritated by medications or food, an ulcer may form. Think of an ulcer as a raw spot, similar to what would occur if you scratch a mosquito bite until it bleeds. Naturally an open sore will be more susceptible to further damage from acid. Some duodenal ulcers are due to infection with *Helicobacter pylori*.

Without X-ray or endoscopic examination, it will be very difficult to know if you have an inflammation (gastritis, esophagitis, duodenitis) or a true ulcer. Fortunately, except in the case of *Helicobacter*-related ulcers, the treatment is much the same.

Without a drugstore to run to, treatment of heartburn will focus on prevention. Without a pill for every problem, patients will become more cautious about eating foods they know will cause discomfort. End-of-world events will likely take care of much acid-related distress. We'll run out of cigarettes and beer. Our bellies will shrink, and overeating will become a thing of the past. Starbucks will go out of business and chocolate will become a true luxury. Without alcohol, tobacco, coffee, and overeating, most people will find their symptoms resolve. Other non-pharmaceutical treatments include not eating late at night, avoiding lying down after eating, eating several small meals instead of fewer larger ones, and elevating the head of the bed.

For those planning ahead, stock up now on OTC acid-lowering medications. It's amazing what strong drugs are currently available without a prescription, and some for an amazingly low price. For under a hundred bucks you can buy enough generic Pepcid to last a decade. Generics for Tagamet and Zantac are equally cheap. These were miracle drugs when first released two decades ago – and still would be if Americans were willing to make lifestyle changes. If you rely on a proton pump inhibitor such as Nexium (the "purple pill"), stock up on over-the-counter versions of Prevacid or Prilosec. These do cost more than Pepcid or Zantac, so keep your eye open for discounts. Stock inexpensive OTC antacids as well, for mild or breakthrough symptoms.

For a patient with persistent abdominal burning, it may be reasonable to treat for *Helicobacter* infection. This requires combination treatment with an acid-lowering medication twice daily (see above) plus two antibiotics, all three medicines for 7–10 days. Antibiotic choices are: 1) amoxicillin (1,000 mg twice daily) *plus* clarithromycin (500 mg twice daily) *or* metronidazole (400–500 mg 3–4 times daily); or 2) metronidazole *plus* tetracycline (500 mg twice daily) *or* clarithromycin (500 mg twice daily). If this hasn't helped by 10 days, further treatment probably isn't going to either. In a middle-aged or older individual, persistent symptoms may be due to a stomach cancer, which will be difficult to diagnose without an X-ray or endoscopy.

Hernia

A hernia occurs when the tissues that normally confine the internal organs allow them to bulge through an area that has weakened or that was formed improperly at birth, primarily in the groin or abdomen. Babies born with hernias usually have them corrected in infancy. Adults often develop hernias in mid-life, as a result of straining, weight gain, pregnancy, or surgery.

Hernias into the groin are the most common, especially in men. A bulge may occur in the lower abdomen or into the scrotum. The two other common hernias are umbilical and post-surgical abdominal hernias.

The primary concern with hernias is possible strangulation of intestines that become caught within the hernia sac. Normally a hernia can be reduced, that is, gently pushed back in (temporarily). This often happens spontaneously when a patient lies on his back, the position in which the abdominal muscles are most relaxed. When reduction becomes impossible, the blood supply to the entrapped intestines may be cut off, causing death of the intestines, and without surgery, death of the patient. Fortunately, this rarely happens, especially not in large hernias – I can't remember the last time I've encountered a strangulated hernia. Other concerns include local discomfort and appearance. Some patients worry that a hernia will burst through the skin, but this does not occur.

Surgery is the definitive treatment for hernias, although since surgery is also a potential cause, a hernia may recur. Anyone with a current hernia should consider surgical correction while this option is available, especially anyone with significant discomfort. However, even today many patients choose to forego surgery, and thus I've had the opportunity to observe hundreds of patients who live for decades symptom-free without surgical intervention. A few wear abdominal binders to help keep their hernias from bulging out. Although I cannot find specific statistics, based on my experience the majority of patients, perhaps 90% or more, never suffer a significant problem from an uncorrected hernia.

If medical care is unavailable and you happen to encounter a hernia that seems to be trapped, the best you can do is to try to reduce it. Have the patient relax flat on his back. For a groin hernia, also elevate the foot of the bed a little (20°) to allow gravity to assist. Apply ice or cool compresses to the affected area to decrease swelling. Wait several minutes to a half hour to see if the hernia will spontaneously reduce. If it has not, apply steady, *gentle* pressure to the bulge, guiding it back through the opening. If this is impossible, try to get the patient to relax further (or even fall asleep), and repeat the above steps.

Someone other than a surgeon may be able to help – a family doctor might attempt surgery if the patient's life is at stake, as may a veterinarian, surgical tech, O.R. nurse, or physician's assistant. If the hernia defect cannot be surgically corrected, enlarging it may prevent further trapping of intestinal contents.

Worst case scenario: the hernia will not reduce, the blood supply will be cut off, the tissue will become gangrenous, the pain will be excruciating, the intestines will rupture, and the patient will die. This is a case where morphine would be a blessing – *BUT* I seriously doubt if anyone reading this book will ever be confronted with this situation.

Have a hernia now?

Ask your doctor if you should undergo surgery

Inquire whether your particular hernia is likely to strangulate

For an abdominal hernia, consider an abdominal binder

Lose weight, to prevent excess pressure on a current or repaired hernia

High blood pressure

Treating high blood pressure isn't sexy.

It might be if doctors were rescuing their patients from certain death – or perhaps turning their lives around – or at least making them feel better.

But for the most part, high blood pressure doesn't make people feel especially bad. They wouldn't even know they were hypertensive if they didn't have their blood pressure measured. Of course, there are a few patients who do suffer headaches when their pressure mounts, and a few who would soon suffer organ damage from extremely elevated levels, but for the most part, treating high blood pressure is treating a *risk factor*, not an actual disease, much like lowering cholesterol, losing weight, or cutting back on cigarettes. All of these are risk factors for cardiovascular disease – heart attacks, strokes, and arteriosclerosis – problems which occur down the road, usually after many years.

I've treated many patients for hypertension for two decades already and they haven't had a stroke or heart attack. *How do I know if I've done any good? What if the problem wouldn't have occurred anyway?* Not everyone with high blood pressure dies at an early age.

Statisticians have addressed the question of how many patients must be treated in order to benefit one, that is, to prevent one heart attack, one stroke, or one death. Most patients fall into the mild hypertensive range, with an untreated diastolic blood pressure between 90 and 109 mm Hg (normal being less than140/90). In this group, 141 patients must be treated for five years to prevent one bad outcome.[23] So if I treat about 300 hypertensive patients a year, in the two decades I've been at my office I must have helped prevent about 8–9 cardiovascular events – but there's no way of knowing which were the lucky patients who would have succumbed, but didn't. *And what about the other 292 patients? Have we done any good at all?* Again, hard to say. For patients with severe hypertension (diastolic blood pressure between 115 and 129) the effort seems more worthwhile: only three patients must be treated in order to help one.

I would guesstimate that if all my hypertensive patients would quit smoking, eat healthy, exercise, and maintain a desirable weight at least half of them would see their blood pressure problem resolve. This is the best solution both now and after the end of the world as we know it.

Is elevated blood pressure worth worrying about in times of scarcity? Will there be adequate medication to treat 141 patients for the sake of one? Although this is difficult to answer from a physician's point of view, the individual patient will approach the question from a personal level. Without professional care,

[23] Treating Newly Diagnosed Asymptomatic Hypertension. *Am Fam Physician.* 2002 Oct 15;66(8):1547–1548.

hypertensive patients will need to monitor their own blood pressure. Investing in a professional grade mercury blood pressure monitor, cuff, tubing, and stethoscope is the first step. Relying on battery-powered units is inadvisable. Directions for measuring blood pressure accurately are outlined in **Chapters 33** and **34** on performing a history and physical examination.

Beyond lifestyle modification, the mainstay of first-line treatment of high blood pressure is long-acting diuretics (water pills, such as hydrochlorothiazide) and beta-blockers, both inexpensive time-proven remedies. Diuretics may also be used for treating swelling or heart failure, but may deplete the body of potassium. Beta-blockers are prescribed for a variety of other indications, including migraine prophylaxis, angina, and rapid heart rhythms, but may cause wheezing in asthmatics. Multi-use medicines such as these are highly advisable for stockpiling. A 5-year supply of either would cost only $200, if your doctor is willing to cooperate. Likewise inexpensive are the ACE inhibitors, such as lisinopril (also useful for heart failure) and the alpha-blockers, such as doxazosin (also useful for urinary symptoms associated with an enlarged prostate). Additionally, calcium channel blockers are multi-use drugs: verapamil and diltiazem not only lower blood pressure, but are also useful at slowing rapid heart rates and for migraine prevention. Amlodipine probably yields the biggest bang for your buck, decreasing blood pressure by a greater amount than most other preparations, with leg swelling as the most common side-effect.

For patients on 3 or 4 different medications, simplifying your drug regimen is a strong consideration, as discussed in detail in **Section Eight**. Beyond the second anti-hypertensive drug, there is diminishing effect for each additional medication. It may be better to have sufficient medicine on hand to lower blood pressure to near normal for ten years, rather than to normal levels for only five.

Treating hypertension at TEOTWAWI:

Purchase a professional-grade mercury sphygmomanometer

Obtain several stethoscopes (which are easily lost or misplaced)

Check your own BP readings against those obtained by your doctor

Optimize your health otherwise: quit smoking, lose weight, exercise

Simplify your medication regimen (preferably only 1–2 drugs)

Stockpile several years worth of inexpensive generic medication

If need be, consider alternatives to prescription medications:

OTC Panabrom (Aqua-Ban) or dandelion for diuretic effect

If taking a diuretic, try to stabilize your potassium level by diet alone

Kidney stones

How can something the size of a sesame seed bring a grown man to his knees?

Passing a kidney stone may feel like the end of the world (but it probably isn't). You may think you are dying. You may feel like you're having a baby. But odds are, you'll live through it and emerge on the other side, safe and sound.

Most kidney stones pass without surgical intervention – at least 95% of them – probably more like 99% if you're willing to wait it out. In the era of modern medicine we have an answer for those that don't pass unaided: lithotripsy, surgery, basket retrieval – there's an option for everyone. But in post-modern medicine, what will people do?

Taking a step back, how will people even know what's wrong with them? Naturally anyone who's experienced one kidney stone may recognize another, but a large number of stones occur in patients who've never had one before.

The most common symptom of a kidney stone is one-sided abdominal, flank, or back pain, often associated with abnormal urination. The pain from a kidney stone is related to obstruction of a hollow viscus. In plain English, that means that a tube-like structure in the body, one which normally allows passage of a fluid (or feces), is obstructed by a stone (or a baby, or a plug of feces). In an effort to expel the obstruction, the muscular lining of the tube contracts, much like labor contractions. However, just as not every woman has severe labor pains, not every person with a kidney stone suffers extreme pains. This is partly related to the size of the stone, but probably also related to a person's internal neurologic wiring and whether the stone is jagged or smooth. In general, kidney stone pain is little-relieved by change in position, although patients appear restless and often prefer to move around. The onset is often sudden, as a stone tumbles out of the kidney and lodges in the narrow ureter. The pain may come in waves or be fairly constant.

Kidney stones may also produce bleeding as the stone scrapes along the ureter (the tube between the kidneys and bladder). Once it reaches the bladder, the pressure is relieved and the pain usually lets up, though both bleeding and pain may recur as the stone passes from the bladder through the urethra, and out of the body.

Other symptoms of kidney stones include any or all of the following: strong urge to urinate, frequent urination, inability to urinate, burning on urination, nausea, and vomiting.

At TEOTWAWKI having a skilled health professional to diagnose the condition would be ideal. Visible blood in the urine supports the diagnosis, though infection may cause this as well. Usually symptoms of urinary infection have a more gradual onset than those of a kidney stone.

Patients with mild to moderate pain due to a kidney stone require no or minimal medication. Tylenol or ibuprofen may suffice. Drinking extra water helps push the stone through the ureter (which may hurt); sometimes diuretics (water pills) are employed to increase urine production and help move the stone along. In a person with a prior history of infection or a significant amount of bleeding, taking an oral antibiotic for at least 1–3 days may be advisable to prevent infection (trimethoprim-sulfa DS twice daily, ciprofloxacin 250–500 mg twice daily, nitrofurantoin 50–100 mg twice daily, possibly amoxicillin 250–500 mg three times daily, although this is less effective).

In a person with severe pain, some sort of pain relief is required. Narcotics help most people, but a supply may not be available. Tramadol (a prescription) may be sufficient in many cases (50–100 mg every 3 to 6 hours), as may OTC ibuprofen (600–800 mg every 4–6 hours). Either of these may be combined with acetaminophen (Tylenol, 500–1000 mg every 4–8 hours). If you're not sure of the diagnosis, don't use ibuprofen, naproxen, or aspirin, as these may make stomach problems worse.

A hot bath may relieve the discomfort to some degree. OTC anti-emetic meds (Dramamine, Bonine, meclizine – 25 mg every 6–12 hours) can alleviate nausea and vomiting. If the pain isn't too bad and you're hoping to sleep it off, diphenhydramine (Benadryl, 25–50 mg orally) may help you rest, as may a glass of wine. However, alcohol can irritate the stomach, and if the diagnosis is unclear, it should be used with caution.

Straining the urine through a fine strainer, a coffee filter, or even a T-shirt may help you recover a kidney stone and confirm the diagnosis.

These days, if you think you have a kidney stone or are experiencing similar symptoms, I advise seeking professional help. But in the aftermath of global crisis, you may be on your own. For most people, if the stone doesn't pass in a day, it will within a few days of taking increased fluids. For the few percent that don't obtain relief, let's hope a surgeon is still available. An obstructing stone that does not pass will eventually cause sufficient back-pressure to damage or destroy the affected kidney, and if accompanied by infection, may lead to sepsis and death.

Finally, if you've had one stone, you don't want to suffer another. Kidney stones form in concentrated urine. To prevent stone formation, consistently drink enough fluids to keep your urine nearly clear . . . and continue this practice for the rest of your life.

Low back pain

If your friend (or your spouse or your parent) complained to you of low back pain, would you know how to help them? Where would you begin in deciphering what was wrong?

"Did you lift something heavy?" – you might ask, having strained your back under similar circumstances in the past. Your natural instincts have led you to a good starting place: the patient history.

Seasoned doctors have a good idea what's wrong with a patient before they lay a hand on him or her. The history explains the problem a good 90% of the time – *if* you know the right questions to ask, that is. Questions are directed at categorizing a rather general symptom, such as back pain, into a more specific subcategory: acute versus chronic, musculoskeletal versus internal, injury versus disease.

A person who's only experienced the typical back pain of overwork may not think to ask questions related to other conditions. But muscular strain is not the only cause. Just this week I've encountered patients suffering from gallstones, kidney stones, pleurisy, constipation, bladder infection, menstrual cramps, aortic aneurysm, pinched nerves, compression fractures, shingles, and stomach ulcers, all of whom exhibited back pain as their primary complaint. Two required emergency surgery. Another two were hospitalized for further evaluation. How's a layperson, alone in the wilderness (or anywhere), supposed to figure it all out?

The following strategy helps stratify the patient with back pain into serious concerns and those most likely to resolve on their own. If hospitals and/or surgeons are unavailable, the rare patient with a leaking aortic aneurysm or a perforating ulcer will simply not survive. Fortunately, the other 99% of people won't die from an untreatable disease.

In American medical school doctors are taught, *if you hear hoof beats, think horses, not zebras*, meaning common things occur commonly. (Kenyan doctors might reverse the order.) Rupturing aortic aneurysms are zebras. Back strains from heavy lifting are horses. An addendum to the above rule is that uncommon presentations of common diseases occur more frequently than oddball conditions.

The most frequent causes of low back pain are injury, degenerative problems such as arthritis, and urinary problems. Think of these things first, but don't forget the others.

In taking a patient history, asking the person to describe the problem in their own words is the best place to start. Sometimes it explains the entire situation. "*I got thrown off a horse,*" or "*It burns when I pee,*" are simple examples of what a patient might say to guide further questioning. An older patient who states nothing beyond, "My back hurts," would require significant probing, with detailed inquiry into the various body parts and systems that might be causing the problem.

When I see a patient with back pain I first try to categorize it as musculoskeletal or internal. Musculoskeletal problems involve the bones, spine, muscles, and nerves. Internal problems include the urinary system, digestive system, reproductive system, lungs, heart, and circulation. I include lungs and heart here because some patients are very vague in their descriptions. What they describe as low back pain may actually turn out to be mid-back pain. Requesting a patient to point to or touch the body part that hurts is quite useful. In general, internal problems are of much greater concern and carry a greater risk of death if unrecognized and untreated. I often breathe an internal sigh of relief when I've ruled out internal problems, even though musculoskeletal conditions may take longer to resolve.

Musculoskeletal problems are divided into acute injuries, chronic injuries, and degenerative conditions. In a young person the former is most common; in an elderly person, the latter.

In the young adult (age 16–35), low back pain is commonly caused by an acute or sub-acute strain – either from lifting too much or working too long or too hard. Mothers may suffer from carrying their babies or toddlers, or working in the garden, or playing softball, or carrying the laundry. Weekend warriors and physical laborers may overdo it on an occasional or daily basis. The pain is generally due to strained muscles, that is, muscles which have microscopic tears from overuse. The damage leads to swelling, which worsens the pain, and may stiffen the muscle as a result, thus protecting it. Sometimes the inter-vertebral discs are slightly damaged, and the muscles tighten up to limit further injury.

Questions to help delineate the specific cause of back pain

Was there an acute injury? A fall, a blow, a strain, a twisting? If so, how long ago? Some injuries take a day or two, or even longer, for swelling to occur and cause pain.

Could there be a chronic injury? Even if someone is accustomed to lifting a hundred pounds dozens of times a day, over time it may produce injury.

Where does it hurt? Most musculoskeletal pain is below the level of the waist. Back pain at the level of the ribs or above may be due to the stomach, heart, lungs, pleura, or kidneys.

How much does it hurt? Usually a doctor can tell by looking at a person's face. A patient who is smiling and talking on their cell phone is much less likely to have a serious problem than someone lying on the floor and moaning. Can the person walk? Did they go to work? Often a patient's ability to function is more revealing than their claim of severity.

How long has it hurt? If the problem's been there for months or years, but has only worsened, this is generally a reassuring sign that nothing new or serious is happening.

Has the person had the problem before? Again, a yes answer is reassuring, but still requires re-evaluation. Knowing when and how often the pain occurs is vital.

What makes the pain worse? What makes it better? This is very useful in deciding if something is internal or external. Musculoskeletal problems almost always improve or worsen with a change in position, whereas internal problems are less likely to do so. Does it hurt to bend forward, or backward, or twist to the right or left, or lean in either direction? Is the patient better sitting or standing? Is the pain worse with urinating? Better perhaps? How about eating? Ingesting fatty foods may make gallbladder pain worse. A deep breath often brings on the pain of pleurisy.

Has the patient taken any medication? Did it help? Ibuprofen or aspirin lessen many kinds of pain, but could certainly make an ulcer worse.

Does the pain seem to radiate elsewhere? Intra-abdominal causes of back pain, such as gallstones, ulcers, constipation, menstrual problems, and kidney stones often hurt into the abdomen as well. Pinched nerves, as in sciatica, a lumbar radiculopathy, or spinal stenosis often cause pain into the legs, sometimes along with numbness or weakness.

A typical back strain produces aching or soreness, often with stiffness or difficulty bending forward or in another direction. Unless a nerve is pinched, the pain is limited to the back, and does not travel down the legs nor into the abdomen. Lying down almost always decreases the pain, especially lying on one's side. Anything that decreases the effect of gravity is helpful, such as floating in deep water. Massage, ice, or heat usually decreases the symptoms for at least a short time. Over-the-counter NSAIDs such as ibuprofen, naproxen, and aspirin are effective for pain relief, either alone or in combination with acetaminophen (Tylenol). (A word to the wise – don't combine alcohol with high doses of Tylenol, which can cause liver damage.) Relative rest (that is, avoiding heavy work including the activity which brought on the problem) usually helps and allows the body to improve within several days.

Young women are also prone to urinary infections, menstrual disorders, and problems with pregnancy (see **Chapter 24** regarding female health). Bladder infections may cause low back pain usually associated with lower abdominal discomfort, whereas kidney infections usually cause pain just below the ribs. Either type of urinary infection typically has other symptoms as well: frequent or nighttime urination, pain or burning on urination, nausea, fever, dribbling, bad odor, or cloudy urine (see **Chapter 12** on urinary infections). Over-the-counter urine test strips (Azo Test Strips and others) are available without prescription to check for blood, nitrites, and white blood cells in the urine, any of which may indicate a urinary infection.

Men of reproductive age who have back pain and urinary symptoms may well have a sexually-transmitted disease or prostatitis, although occasionally they will contract a simple bladder infection (see **Chapter 12**).

Young adults may also have conditions discussed below under middle-age. For our purposes I will call the years 35 to 65 middle-aged, although there is certainly a spectrum of illness across this age group, with a tendency to more problems with increasing age.

Middle-aged adults suffer from all the problems of young adulthood – only more so, and worse. Mechanical back pain from injuries tends to last longer and to occur more frequently. The muscles of the back are weaker and cannot take the abuse of younger years. Degenerated discs may cause daily or intermittent discomfort. When the discs or other tissues bulge against the spinal cord or nerves, the pain may travel from the back clear down to the feet. Many adults find they must limit their activity to prevent the pain from occurring. Sleeping on one's side with a pillow between the knees is often helpful. Gentle stretching exercises, walking, swimming, and local application of heat (or possibly ice) help alleviate the pain, as do NSAIDs and Tylenol.

By middle-age most adults are used to a little back pain. More often it's the sciatica (or other pinched nerve) that drives them to the doctor. Nerve pain in the legs, coming from the back, is hard to describe until you've had it. It causes restlessness and a desire to escape. Fortunately, a change of position usually helps. In fact, adults with this type of pain almost always say they need to keep moving. Sitting or standing too long worsens the pain. Conversely, sometimes lying down brings it on. An unpleasant tingly-numb sensation may accompany the pain. Often the patient can't quite say where the pain is, or describes it as moving around. Weakness in the muscles of the calf (or sometimes the thigh) may also occur.

Most people with a pinched nerve do not require surgery. Even with surgery, by two years post-op, there is little difference among patients who have had surgery and those who have not. The interested reader may want to investigate: "Acute Lumbar Disk Pain: Navigating Evaluation and Treatment Choices" in *Am Fam Physician.* 2008 Oct 1;78(7):835-842, available free online at http://www.aafp.org/afp/2008/1001/p835.html.

Treatment for a pinched nerve or sciatica is similar to that for low back pain: relative rest (avoiding heavy lifting and movements or positions that worsen the pain), anti-inflammatory medications, Tylenol, muscle relaxers, and occasionally tramadol or narcotics. Although the afflicted patient experiences pain in the leg, since it is originating from the back, applying heat or ice to the leg is rarely useful. And although the article cited above states that "systemic corticosteroids are no better than placebo for lumbar disk herniation pain," I've seen many patients who seem to benefit tremendously from 3–10 days of prednisone (40–60 mg/day), or an injection of corticosteroids. I've also seen patients who exhibit dramatic improvement after taking sufficient pain medication (short-term) to allow them to relax and "re-boot."

Twenty-five years ago we advised prolonged bed rest for patients with a slipped disk or severe lumbar strain, but now staying active is considered more effective, plus it prevents the muscle atrophy (shrinkage) that weeks of inactivity may produce. Some patients do well with exercises that extend the back backwards, which, in some cases, seems to open up the cramped space where the nerve is being pinched. I often advise my patients to lie on their bed or the floor and curl their upper back backwards while pushing up with their arms (like a push-up from the waist, the goal being to curve the back, not keep it stiff). Repeating this exercise 5–10 times, two or three times a day can loosen the back significantly and decrease leg pain.

The Mayo Clinic offers a list of exercises that help prevent and treat back pain online at: http://www.mayoclinic.com/health/back-pain/LB00001_D .

For patients who have lingering but livable symptoms, a variety of medications can be used to lessen the nerve pain, including Elavil (amitriptyline) and other antidepressants, gabapentin, Lyrica, and other anti-seizure medications. These are taken on a daily basis to gradually relieve the pain. A person should not expect to notice a difference until at least a few days, and often not before a few weeks.

Middle-aged women may also experience urinary infections, as discussed above. Since many women in this age group experience a degree of daily back pain, similar pain from a urinary infection is often overlooked.

Middle-aged and older men with back pain and urinary symptoms (frequent urination, difficulty starting to urinate, dribbling, or pain) may have a chronic form of prostatitis rather than a bladder or kidney infection. This usually requires a longer round of antibiotics (see **Chapter 12**).

Beyond age 65 additional factors come into play. Weakened bones often lead to compression fractures of the spine (primarily in women) that occur with minimal or no trauma. These cannot really be diagnosed without X-rays, but can be suspected in an older woman who has a sudden onset of localized back pain. In a patient with osteoporosis, such a fracture may occur simply by turning over in bed. These patients must limit weight-bearing activity until the bone begins to heal. Usually they require daily pain medications.

Older patients may also have a urinary infection that causes back pain but no other noticeable change in urination. Again, urinary symptoms may be overlooked or ascribed to a dropped bladder or "just getting old." Shingles may cause low back pain that is difficult to diagnose until the typical chicken pox-like blisters erupt, usually in a band-like pattern around half the torso. Aortic aneurysms, heart attacks, and cancer become more common as we age, and may cause back pain, but in an Armageddon scenario without hospital support, nothing beyond supportive care (pain meds) is likely to be available.

Back pain in children is uncommon. In the absence of trauma or injury, a urine infection should be considered, or possibly pneumonia. Kids are not always good at localizing pain, and a complete physical may reveal abdominal pain as well, or wheezing and rattling in the lungs.

As a young doctor, I worried more about my adult patients with back pain. Now that I've joined the middle-age crowd, it seems everybody has it. Most people get better, and most back pain is not cause for alarm.

Sleep apnea

> *Do you awaken frequently gasping for breath? Does your wife sleep in the other room due to your snoring? Are you always tired, despite eight hours in bed?*

It doesn't take a medical degree to question whether you have sleep apnea. When the airways collapse during sleep, restricting the flow of air through the trachea and bronchial tubes, the body becomes highly distressed, triggering the person to wake up enough to breathe deeply. These repeated partial-awakenings take a toll, and deep sleep is never achieved, resulting in chronic fatigue.

The majority (but not all) cases of sleep apnea are related to overweight conditions. Presumably these will resolve when food supplies are limited.

I view sleep apnea as one of America's "pop" diseases. In my medical career, first it was mitral valve prolapse, then came fibromyalgia, now it's sleep apnea. The medical profession discovers a way to easily diagnose a problem that heretofore garnered little attention, and suddenly everyone has it. Doctors' index of suspicion is raised, and the diagnosis is made more frequently, including borderline cases that previously went untreated. This is not to say these conditions don't exist, but that previously people somehow survived without treatment.

Of course, over the past few decades Americans have grown heavier, truly making sleep apnea more prevalent. However, among my patients who have undergone sleep studies and C-PAP titration, even optimum doses of C-PAP seem to make a significant difference only about half the time. When C-PAP does help, patients feel better rested, with more energy for life.

Simple measures which improve breathing should not be overlooked. The lungs fill more easily when the head of the bed is elevated. The airways are less prone to collapse when a person sleeps on his side rather than his back or stomach. Losing weight in the belly and upper body puts less pressure on the bronchial tubes, and thinner people require less air for metabolism. Decongestants or bronchodilator medications may help open the airways, and even Breathe-Right strips may open the nasal passages enough to make a noticeable difference for some. Keeping fit strengthens not only the arms and legs, but also the muscles of breathing.

For those who are truly C-PAP reliant, assuring a reliable power supply, a high-quality machine, and plenty of replacement tubing, filters, and masks is advisable.

Swelling

Edema, or swelling of the legs, is a common problem among the middle-aged and elderly, primarily due to poor circulation plus obesity, but sometimes related to heart failure, diet, excessive standing, medication, or kidney failure. The great majority of the time, edema is gravity-dependent pitting edema, starting in the ankles or feet, and moving up the legs as the fluid accumulates. If you press on the swollen area, especially overlying the shin, it leaves a temporary indent, or pit.

The evaluation of edema begins by discovering the underlying cause. Eliminate the cause, and the swelling may disappear. Medications that frequently cause leg swelling include: 1) amlodipine (and other calcium channel blockers to a lesser degree); 2) ibuprofen, naproxen, Celebrex, or any other NSAID; 3) the diabetic medications Avandia and Actos. Excess salt ingestion may cause swelling in a sodium-sensitive individual; ham seems to be the worst culprit. Anyone with swelling would benefit from salt avoidance beyond the amount of iodized salt needed to prevent a goiter (1/2 tsp daily, see **Thyroid Disease**, below). Being on one's feet too long can cause swelling, as may sleeping in a chair with your legs down, or moving to a higher altitude where air pressure is too low to balance fluid pressure within the body.

Poor circulation in women is often related to prior pregnancies, which have caused damage to the leg veins years earlier. A similar situation can exist in anyone who carries excess weight in the abdomen, whether male or female. This puts pressure on the large veins, much like cutting off the flow of water through a hose, resulting in sluggish blood flow. The resultant higher pressure allows some fluid to leak through the veins and accumulate in the legs.

If the cause of the edema cannot be identified and easily remedied, then treating with a diuretic (water pill) may be necessary. Hydrochlorothiazide (12.5–50 mg daily) causes increased urine production throughout the day and also lowers blood pressure, whereas furosemide (10–40 mg daily) works "fast and furious," with a large amount of urine produced in the six hours following administration. Both of these may cause potassium loss, so it is important to increase dietary potassium intake (e.g., bananas, oranges, tomatoes). The potassium-sparing diuretic triamterene, usually prescribed in combination with hydrochlorothiazide, decreases the need for potassium supplements. Any diuretic may cause dehydration, especially when a person cuts back on fluid intake but continues taking the diuretic. Some people experience muscle cramps or light-headedness. Remember, every drug is a potential poison.

When is leg swelling dangerous? Most commonly this would be due to heart failure, when a patient would also likely experience shortness of breath. Every patient with leg swelling should have his or her heart and lungs evaluated. Irregular heart rhythms, particularly atrial fibrillation, can cause weakened heart function, with resultant swelling and breathing difficulties. Kidney failure is a less common concern, except in the case of dehydration. Heart failure usually improves with a strong diuretic such as furosemide (10–80 mg daily), whereas kidney failure probably won't. Swelling in a single leg suggests the possibility of a blood clot, as discussed earlier (see entry on Blood Clots).

Lymphedema is a much rarer form of swelling. It does not cause pitting when compressed, but rather caused the skin texture to resemble that of an orange peel. It is caused by poor function of the lymphatic system, and is little helped by water pills. The primary treatment is elastic compression stockings or Ace wraps.

Thyroid disease – Hypothyroidism (Low thyroid)

Has your thyroid been irradiated or removed? Were you born without a functioning gland? Have you experienced the sluggishness and fatigue of hypothyroidism? Without Synthroid, are you doomed?

The question of treatment for low thyroid is a great concern among survivalists and preppers. Without traditional medication will you die? The short answer is: likely not – but read on.

Hypothyroidism (low thyroid, or thyroid insufficiency) encompasses a wide spectrum of problems, from asymptomatic (subclinical) hypothyroidism to severe disease including coma. Only once in my 30-year medical career have I seen a patient obtunded from hypothyroidism; current treatment prevents the development of the severe state. Also, like many doctors, I've never seen a patient with an iodine-deficiency goiter, though that disease may resurface after global catastrophe, once iodide stores run low, particularly iodized salt.

For simplicity sake, I'll divide low-thyroid disease into two main classes: those with an absolute deficiency of thyroid hormones and those with a partial deficiency. People with no thyroid hormone whatsoever must receive replacement therapy or they will gradually succumb to severe thyroid deficiency (fatigue, low heart rate, slowed thinking, swollen legs, dry skin, hair loss, and possible coma and death). People with a partial deficiency may live for years or even decades with minimal or even no symptoms.

The real question is: *which sort of patient are you?*

Most people won't know the answer to this question. You can, however, find out, with a little investigation.

Absolute thyroid deficiency is mainly caused by two conditions: 1) severe, intrinsic thyroid disease; or 2) as a result of treatment for hyperactive thyroid (high thyroid, Grave's disease). A few patients are born with congenital hypothyroidism, a subset of the first category, which, left untreated, leads to a whole host of problems, including low I.Q. Patients who have undergone total thyroidectomy or total thyroid ablation via radiation for a hyperactive thyroid should, theoretically, have no remaining functional thyroid tissue. This is not always the case, since some doctors treat hyperthyroid disease with a sub-total thyroidectomy or incomplete irradiation, aiming to leave sufficient thyroid tissue to avoid the need for replacement therapy.

Much more common is partial thyroid deficiency. Decreased production of thyroid hormone may be due to intrinsic thyroid disease, medications (lithium, amiodarone), or surgery. To determine adequacy of thyroid hormone production, what doctors actually measure is the serum TSH level (thyroid stimulating hormone). TSH is produced by the pituitary, and as the name implies, TSH stimulates the thyroid to make thyroid hormone via a fine-tuned feedback system. If your serum thyroid hormones, T3 and T4, drop a bit low, the pituitary responds by producing more thyroid stimulating hormone, which in turn causes the thyroid gland to increase output of thyroid hormone (assuming there is thyroid tissue to stimulate). The opposite is also true: if your serum thyroid hormone level increases, TSH levels drop. Remember: high TSH=low thyroid; low TSH=high thyroid.

Nowadays most patients with hypothyroidism are diagnosed by an elevated TSH level rather than by symptoms. Sometimes a complaint (such as fatigue) triggers the ordering of a test, but mildly abnormal thyroid function does not guarantee that hypothyroidism is responsible for the symptoms. (Who isn't tired, anyway?) I've seen many patients with a mildly elevated TSH level who feel absolutely no different after starting Synthroid. A serum TSH level is a common screening blood test for asymptomatic middle-aged and older people undergoing a routine exam. Therefore, mild hypothyroidism is often identified in patients who have no clue anything is wrong. Another name for this problem is subclinical hypothyroidism, that is, too mild a case to produce symptoms. If you actually felt normal when your doctor diagnosed hypothyroidism, you probably have subclinical hypothyroidism, and could likely live many years without medication. The pituitary is working harder by secreting more TSH, which actually results in normal levels of circulating thyroid hormones, with or without the presence of a goiter.

The normal range for TSH varies from lab to lab, but is approximately 0.3 to 5.0 mIU/L. Patients are commonly placed on thyroid replacement therapy when their TSH is elevated a few points, even if they have no symptoms. However, this practice is controversial. Per a review article in *The American Family Physician*,[24] "In current randomized controlled trials, levothyroxine replacement therapy for subclinical hypothyroidism did not result in improved survival or decreased cardiovascular morbidity. Data on health-related quality of life and symptoms did not demonstrate significant differences among intervention groups. Some evidence indicates that levothyroxine replacement improves some parameters of lipid profiles and left ventricular function." My own experience confirms this data.

So if you are diagnosed with subclinical hypothyroidism, and if treatment won't make you won't feel better or live longer, a reasonable approach is to reserve medical treatment for when (and if) hypothyroid symptoms develop.

---

[24] *Am Fam Physician.* 2008 Apr 1;77(7):953–955, online at: http://www.aafp.org/afp/2008/0401/p953.html

However, there are patients whose TSH levels are elevated by 20, 30, or even 100 points. These individuals are likely to exhibit at least some symptoms and to show decreased levels of serum thyroid hormones. Common symptoms of hypothyroidism include: weakness, dry or coarse skin or hair, fatigue or lethargy, swollen eyelids or face, feeling cold, slowed speech or thinking, and constipation. Of course, many patients have one or more of these symptoms and do not have any thyroid disease. Only in patients with decreased thyroid hormone production will such symptoms improve in response to thyroid supplementation.

Current treatment of hypothyroidism centers on adjusting the dosage of hormone replacement to maintain a serum TSH in the normal range. This is finer-tuning than is probably necessary to keep a patient asymptomatic regarding hypo- or hyperthyroidism. However, whereas subclinical hypothyroidism may not affect health long-term, subclinical hyperthyroidism may deplete calcium from the bones and is associated with a higher likelihood of atrial fibrillation (irregular heart rate). Hyperthyroid patients are often unaware of mild symptoms, such as the ability to eat more without gaining weight, or the need for less sleep.

The mainstay of thyroid replacement therapy is levothyroxine (Synthroid, Levothroid), the same hormone the human body manufactures (T4). It is the form of treatment preferred by most American physicians. The dose can be precisely adjusted (at least using brand-name medication), which allows close monitoring of blood levels. Of course, many patients are on generic medication, which has a +/- 20% bioavailability range (as discussed in **Section Eight, Medication Concerns**). For some patients, this does not matter. Other patients require the exact dosing only available with name-brand medication to maintain a consistently normal TSH level. Generic medication costs as little as $4/month, but even brand-name Synthroid is available for $25/month or less.

Before discussing other treatments, let's again ask the question, are you the sort of patient who must receive thyroid replacement therapy to function?

If, at the time of diagnosis, you were experiencing symptoms of hypothyroidism, and were found to have an extremely elevated TSH, you already have your answer. (You need it.) If you had 100% of your thyroid surgically removed, you're in the same boat.

But most patients that I treat actually have subclinical hypothyroidism, that is, their TSH runs a bit high (say 2 to 10 mIU/L above normal), but they exhibit no symptoms directly linked to thyroid dysfunction. Some of these patients I've observed over several years and have seen their TSH levels fluctuate a little, up or down, with or without treatment. This makes sense, when you consider the underlying problem is usually an autoimmune disorder (Hashimoto's thyroiditis). Other autoimmune diseases, such as arthritis, vary regarding severity of symptoms. If the thyroid is inflamed to a variable degree over time, then the T3 and T4 output would naturally fluctuate. In response, the pituitary compensates by adjusting the output of thyroid stimulating hormone. All this is to say that many of these patients do not require medication. Compare this to the patient with mild diabetes who requires little or no medication, and likely will never become insulin-dependent.

To know if you are this type of patient, consider discussing the following experiment with your doctor. A patient's dose of levothyroxine may be tapered or discontinued and the TSH monitored closely, perhaps once every month or two for a period of time. If lowering or decreasing the dose is going to cause a problem, an elevated TSH would likely show up before a patient experiences symptoms, thus allowing re-initiation of treatment. This depends, of course, on the patient. For a patient in whom I suspect a total lack of thyroid production, I would taper the dose more slowly and/or monitor the TSH every few weeks early on. For a patient whom I diagnosed myself (or have documentation of a minimally elevated TSH level prior to therapy), simply stopping medication and monitoring the result is an option.

Of course, patients do this all the time – they just don't monitor their blood tests. They run out of medicine for a week or a month or longer and often feel no different. Rarely do they become fully symptomatic. (It is possible to monitor your TSH level yourself, by collecting your blood and sending it to an accredited lab. Check online for available services.)

All this is fine and dandy if medication and blood testing are available. (And of course, stockpiling thyroid medication is a good idea for those who need it.) But if civilization collapses, TSH measurements are as unlikely to be available as medication to treat the problem.

However, doctors my age and older remember thyroid treatment before the days of readily available thyroid stimulating hormone determination. Back then, T3 and T4 thyroid levels were assayed in the blood. Although this was (and continues to be) somewhat useful, it does not permit as precise regulation of thyroid function as monitoring TSH allows. Even longer ago patients were diagnosed and treated according to symptoms alone, and many were placed on thyroid medication who probably did not need it. I still have a few patients diagnosed with hypothyroidism 30, 40, or even 50 years ago, who may not require treatment, but who are unwilling to taper their dose to find out. (When a person who does not require thyroid replacement is started on thyroid hormone, the thyroid gland shuts down but the TSH may remain normal; however, if the thyroid medication dose is too high, the TSH level will fall below normal.) Basing diagnosis and treatment on symptom monitoring alone is likely to recur after the end of the world as we know it.

Once stockpiles of levothyroxine run out, and if the manufacturing process has not been re-established, animal sources will once again be used. Even now animal thyroid continues to be available (Armour thyroid), compounded from desiccated porcine thyroid tissue, and is still prescribed by some physicians. For most patients, 60–120 mg of Armour thyroid daily is an adequate dose. Thyroid hormone is absorbed better on an empty stomach, and so should be taken before eating, not only to maximize therapy when supplies are limited, but to obtain the most consistent treatment result.

Until I wrote this book I was unaware that nutraceutical-grade thyroid compounds were available without a prescription. These are desiccated (freeze-dried) whole thyroid tissue from cows or pigs. The sources I found stated the cows were pasture-fed, thus reducing the concern for contamination with Mad Cow disease in animals fed rendered cow parts. I have not found OTC nutraceutical thyroid preparations in local pharmacies, but I do see them online. I'm sure no one in the medical establishment would recommend these, and I don't know if they are honestly prepared, but at TEOTWAWKI, they are a consideration. My main point in mentioning these is that you can stockpile them without a prescription. If you choose to do so, I recommend having a private lab assay the product for the thyroid hormones T3 and T4 so you'll have some idea of your correct dose. Hopefully they are on a par with Armour thyroid.

What about ingesting human thyroid tissue? This certainly smacks of cannibalism, but on the other hand, we harvest blood products from other people, along with hearts, kidneys, faces, livers, etc. Where does one draw the line? Theoretically, human sources from (healthy) cadavers would serve the purpose of thyroid replacement therapy, but somehow taking another person's thyroid, freeze-drying it, then ingesting a little at a time seems barbaric. Aside from cannibalism, however, eating human parts is not unheard of, as in placentophagia (eating of the placenta after childbirth). If I were dying and someone could benefit from my thyroid gland, I'd be as happy to donate that organ as any other. (Perhaps my objection to the whole idea is little different than my abhorrence of eating brains or kidneys – I can't decide.)

According to the product insert for Armour thyroid, the normal human thyroid gland contains about 200 mcg of levothyroxine (T4) and 15 mcg of liothyronine (T3) per gram of gland. Thyroid dosing is usually determined in terms of T4. T3 is the stronger of the two hormones, about 4 times more potent than T4, some of which is converted into T3 in the body. 100 mcg of levothyroxine daily is a typical replacement dose, which would be about 0.5 gram (500 mg) of <u>non</u>-desiccated human thyroid tissue, or about 125 mg of desiccated product. For comparison sake, a baby aspirin weights about 80 mg.

If we revert to monitoring symptoms to determine dosage, what will we look for? An overall feeling of well-being would be the first, although some patients prefer the side-effects of mild hyperthyroidism, which an excessive dose can cause (extra energy, weight loss, or the ability to eat more without gaining weight, along with a decreased need for sleep). As mentioned before, this is dangerous due to the risk of heart rhythm problems and bone weakening (see entry on **Hyperthyroidism**, below). Next, aim for a stable weight, assuming appropriate caloric intake. Weight gain and fatigue may indicate the need for a higher dose, whereas weight loss and hyperactivity may indicate a lower dose is needed. Thirdly, a heart rate between 60 and 100 beats per minute is desirable. A consistently rapid heart rate would suggest too high a dose (in the absence of other causes), whereas a low heart rate suggests the opposite. Keep in mind that certain drugs lower the heart rate (beta-blockers and calcium channel-blockers). Athletic training and other forms of aerobic exercise also tend to lower the resting heart rate, often to about 50 beats per minute. Other symptoms of hypothyroidism such as dry skin, depression, and hair loss would be more difficult to assess, as other causes are quite common. Be careful to guard against the tendency to blame every symptom on an unbalanced thyroid.

Finally, what is the role of herbal medicine in the treatment of hypothyroid disease? In searching the traditional medical literature I could find no studies that substantiate herbal therapy. It is unlikely such research will be performed (and published) due to cost concerns and the lack of an immediate need for herbal therapy. That is not to say God has not granted us an herbal remedy somewhere within the plant kingdom. Chinese medicine has a long history of treating chronic illnesses with combinations of various plants. Personally I cannot make sense of the yin and yang and qi, but this does not negate the entire field of Chinese medicine. Since I have no experience in this field I can offer little advice. In his online article *Treatments for Thyroid Diseases with Chinese Herbal Medicine*, Subhuti Dharmananda, PhD discusses herbal remedies for hyper- and hypothyroidism in some detail, and lists 50 references and a dozen books.[25] Of note is that some of the Chinese treatments include thyroid replacement therapies with thyroxine or animal preparations, which are likely the effective ingredients.

Elsewhere the herb *Coleus forskohlii* has been shown to have a TSH-like effect in certain animals, but this has not yet been documented in humans. As

---

[25] *Treatments for Thyroid Diseases with Chinese Herbal Medicine*, Subhuti Dharmananda, PhD, online at: www.itmonline.org/arts/thyroid.htm

previously mentioned, nutraceutical desiccated bovine and porcine thyroid products are available over-the-counter without a prescription, though again I know of no physician nor patient who has used these.

If my own daughter suffered from hypothyroidism, I would first evaluate her disease with a series of blood tests to understand the extent of the problem. Additionally, I would stock up on levothyroxine while it is yet available, and investigate the nutraceutical sources of bovine and/or porcine thyroid products. Thirdly, I would learn how to harvest thyroid tissue from butchered pigs and/or cattle as a last resort. If all these resources are exhausted, I doubt that a ready supply of herbal therapies would be available either.

Prevention of hypothyroidism and iodine-deficiency goiter is another concern. With the addition of iodine to table salt, iodine-deficiency disease has essentially disappeared from America. Salt will be a valuable commodity if society collapses, and stocking up now on iodized salt is an inexpensive way to prepare. Those living near the ocean with access to shellfish, kelp, and other seafood are less likely to experience an iodine deficiency. According to the FDA Food and Nutrition Information Center, the recommended daily allowance is about 100 micrograms/day for children including infants, and 150 micrograms/day for adults. However, in 25+ years of medicine I've never encountered a person eating normal foods who needed to measure their intake. Iodine poisoning or overdose is also a potential concern, though I've never seen this either (except in patients taking amiodarone). Food alone does not contain sufficient iodine to exceed the upper limit of 1,000 micrograms daily (unless perhaps the entire diet is composed of kelp and seafood). Iodine poisoning may cause a brassy taste, stomach irritation, a rash, hyperthyroidism or hypothyroidism, with or without a goiter.

The current Morton Salt label indicates that 1/2 teaspoon of iodized salt would yield approximately 90% of the recommended daily allowance of iodine. This may seem like a lot of salt until you consider that a single can of Campbell's condensed soup contains twice that amount of sodium (without mention of iodine content). Sea salt, Kosher salt, and other forms of salt may not be iodized, so be sure to read the label. Pickling salt (for canning) does not contain iodine.

Thyroid disease – Hyperthyroidism (High thyroid)

Typical symptoms of hyperthyroidism are rapid heart rate, nervousness, hand tremors, insomnia, sweating, frequent bowel movements, feeling warm, fatigue or extra energy, and weight loss – basically the opposite of hypothyroidism. Some patients enjoy the symptoms of mild hyperthyroidism, especially the weight loss and energy boost they experience. But when the symptoms progress to palpitations, bulging eyes, shaking hands, sleeplessness, and diarrhea, people really start to worry that something serious is wrong. Rarely this leads to thyroid storm, a condition that includes high blood pressure, rapid heart rate, and possibly fever, confusion, delirium, shock, coma, and death.

Goiter, or swelling of the thyroid, may or may not be present. Sometimes the base of the neck just above the collarbone appears diffusely swollen, other times a goiter may be one-sided or feel lumpy (nodular). Occasionally the gland may be tender, but usually not. Most patients are unaware they even have an enlarged thyroid.

The most common cause of hyperthyroidism is Grave's disease, but other thyroid disorders may yield the same end result. Currently X-ray and ultrasound imaging in conjunction with blood testing (and occasionally biopsy) are used to delineate the exact problem. When these modalities are unavailable, the diagnosis will again be based on symptoms. Typical hyperthyroidism exhibits high T3 and T4 blood levels, and depressed TSH.

Most patients with hyperthyroidism are treated with inexpensive beta-blockers, the same medications that are used for high blood pressure. These drugs relieve symptoms of rapid heart rate, palpitations, high blood pressure, hand tremors, heat intolerance, and nervousness. Propranolol is most commonly used, at an initial dose of 10–20 mg every six hours, tapering up to a maximum of 80 mg every six hours if needed to control symptoms. Other options include metoprolol, atenolol, or any other beta-blocker. Asthmatics and certain other patients may be intolerant of beta-blockers. In this case, a calcium channel blocker such as diltiazem or verapamil may be used to decrease heart rate and blood pressure. However, the calcium channel blockers may not alleviate hand tremors, heat intolerance, or nervousness. Neither the beta-blockers nor calcium channel blockers correct the underlying condition of thyroid hyper-function. They merely control symptoms until the underlying inflammation burns itself out, which often results in hypothyroidism instead, usually years later, necessitating thyroid replacement therapy (see **Hypothyroidism**, above).

If beta-blockers are insufficient to control symptoms, antithyroid drugs are often prescribed for one to several years. Both methimazole (Tapazole) and propylthiouracil (PTU) suppress the organification of iodine and suppress thyroid hormone levels. Methimazole is usually prescribed in non-pregnant patients (at a dose of 15–30 mg a day), and may be used in conjunction with a beta-blocker. By a month or two the beta-blocker can usually be tapered, as long as symptoms don't recur. Propylthiouracil is preferred for pregnant hyperthyroid patients (100 mg up to three times daily) due to the rare incidence of birth defects with methimazole.

When blood tests are available, the dose of either medicine is titrated to maintain high-normal thyroid hormone levels. When blood tests are unavailable, again it's a matter of monitoring symptoms. This will eventually mean tapering the dose to see if symptoms recur. If they do, the medication can be reinstituted for several months before tapering again.

Unfortunately, either medication (methimazole or propylthiouracil) may cause agranulocytosis (low white blood cells, which fight infection), though this occurs less than 1% of the time, especially at low doses of medication. It is usually reversible upon stopping treatment. Detecting this condition is theoretically within the scope of a family doctor's training, if he or she still owns a functioning microscope and a few slides. Realistically, though, the routine blood testing that physicians perform now to monitor the disease is unlikely to be available after global catastrophe. Instead, monitoring for signs of infection is the more feasible approach, and patients should stop taking the drug if they develop a sudden fever, sore throat, aching joints, or other signs of infection.

If using the above medications is insufficient to control hyperthyroid symptoms, the current recommendation is to administer radioactive thyroid or to surgically excise the thyroid gland. At TEOTWAWKI radioactive iodine is unlikely to be a treatment option. Thyroidectomy requires a skilled surgeon willing to perform the surgery in possibly less than optimum conditions. Anyone considering either of these options at the current time, and who believes 2012 will bring Armageddon, should probably undergo definitive treatment while both radioactive iodine and thyroidectomy are still available. If you do so, you may want to ask your doctor if his or her goal is total ablation or removal of the thyroid or only partial. If the thyroid gland is entirely removed or rendered inactive, then lifelong thyroid replacement therapy will be necessary. If the gland is incompletely obliterated or removed, some residual functioning thyroid tissue may be adequate to supply sufficient hormones. Unfortunately, it's a guessing game as to exactly how much tissue to remove or precisely how much radioactive iodine is required to achieve this goal. After either treatment a patient could end up with just the right amount of functioning tissue, or too much, or too little. However, if the thyroid remains a bit overactive, the medications mentioned above are more likely to provide adequate symptom control. Most Grave's disease burns out with time, and hypothyroidism is usually the end result, though it may be several years down the road.

If you have hypothyroid disease now, consider:

Stocking up on several years' worth of levothyroxine or Armour thyroid

Having your doctor determine whether treatment is mandatory for you

Stocking nutraceutical desiccated thyroid (and having it analyzed)

Learning the exact cause and prognosis of your hypothyroidism

Ordering **Hypothyroidism – Answers for a Post-Apocalyptic World** at www.armageddonmedicine.net

If you have hyperthyroid disease now, consider:

Stocking up on several years worth of anti-thyroid medications

Definitive treatment with surgery or radioactive iodide

Everyone: stock iodized salt for your entire family and/or group

Thyroid protection from radiation

Are you worried about protecting your thyroid in the event of nuclear fall-out? You should be. I've devoted an entire chapter to this in **Section Nine** entitled **Special Topics**.

Vision

As one who relies on glasses for distance vision, assuring that I can see tops my list for disaster preparedness. Although some patients suffer glaucoma or cataracts, the majority of us have refractive errors correctable by eyeglasses or contacts. For anyone who's been putting off cataract surgery, now is the time to take action. Will there be an ophthalmologist to help you later?

For those who wear glasses or contacts, how many pairs are enough? Not just one. Will your vision – or that of your children – change over the next few years? Quite likely. For far-sighted people, those who use glasses only for reading, stocking up on a supply of inexpensive "cheaters" in several strengths is a great idea. The discount general stores offer reading glasses for a few bucks a pair – might as well get a dozen. For near-sighted folks, that is, those who use glasses for distance, unfortunately over-the-counter lenses are not available (though it seems to me that they should be). Save your old glasses when you get new ones – some correction is better than none. Also, check online for discount prescription lenses, available for under $10 with a prescription from your doctor (check out www.zennioptical.com). You don't have to buy your glasses the same place you have your eye exam. Your doctor is required to furnish you with a copy of your prescription upon request. For contact wearers, *un*opened contact lenses should remain sterile and viable for years beyond their printed expiration date. Though insurance will not pay for extra contacts or glasses, you can certainly secure an additional supply at your own expense.

Laser surgery is an additional option that affords long-term vision improvement. Even if bifocal correction is not available, if society collapses having good distance vision may be a higher priority for overall functioning, and again, stocking up on reading glasses will solve near-vision difficulties.

Chapter 24

Women's Health

Your mother discovers a lump in her breast. Your daughter's period is late. You're terrified you'll get pregnant once you run out of birth control pills. The men in charge think they have more important things to worry about. As in days of old, the sisterhood of women must stand together.

Women, this chapter is for you. Men, you can skip the following pages if you'd like.

Female health is centered around the breasts and reproductive organs. Breast problems are simpler and fewer, so let's begin there.

For menstruating women, breast problems fall into disorders of structure and those of function. Regarding structure, the breasts being composed of glandular tissue, are prone to cystic and glandular inflammation. Breasts that feel lumpy without a discrete mass are usually of little concern. **Fibrocystic breast** changes – generalized lumpiness and tenderness – are very common and often related to monthly hormonal changes. Avoiding caffeine often helps, as does application of heat or ice, or treatment with oral anti-inflammatory medicine such as ibuprofen. Rarely, a **breast cyst** will grow so large that draining it by puncturing it with a needle is helpful (but not mandatory). There really is no need for the layman to perform this procedure, although removing the fluid does relieve much of the discomfort. Unfortunately, the fluid often re-accumulates with time and the cyst may recur. Other potential problems with draining a cyst are accidental introduction of bacteria into the cyst, thus producing infection (although this is rare when using a sterile needle) and, in a thin woman, accidental puncture of the lung.

For women beyond the age of menopause, localized breast lumps are the biggest concern. Even then, most masses are not cancer, and if one is, it won't kill you overnight. In the days before MRI scans and chemotherapy, women were still treated successfully for **breast cancer** by surgery alone. Pathologic exam of breast tissue could still be performed by trained pathologists. However, if neither surgeon nor pathologist is available, the world will be a dangerous place, and not just for women with breast cancer. Odds of dying from trauma or infection will be much higher than the probability of dying from any sort of cancer. If life is stable enough that you don't have to worry about starvation, radiation, dehydration, pandemics, or marauders, then there will probably be doctors around to treat you.

Breast function is closely related to **lactation** (milk production). Any woman can nurse a baby. By any, I mean 99% of healthy women who've delivered a baby. Immediately after childbirth, a thin watery fluid is present (colostrum), until the mother's milk "comes in." In these first few days, any breast discomfort is likely related to **tender nipples**, often caused by excessive nursing. Don't allow your baby to turn you into a human pacifier. Even for a newborn, 10 minutes of nursing per breast every two to three hours is sufficient.

When, a few days later, the production of real milk does begin, the breasts become **engorged**, often painfully so. They may grow so tight you fear they may burst. It's a wonder breast tissue can build this much pressure without the milk simply running out. For a first-time mother, you won't understand the let-down reflex until it occurs. Usually let-down is triggered by a baby nursing, but it may also occur during orgasm, a hot shower, or even hearing your baby cry. The breasts may become tingly, or feel flushed, or perhaps relaxed, once the milk begins to flow on its own. At this point, the baby hardly needs to suck, and sometimes is barely able to keep up with the rapid flow of milk, which often drips spontaneously from the opposite breast.

However, until the let-down reflex is established, the breasts may become painfully engorged. The answer to engorged breasts is to empty them. This may be accomplished by the baby, or standing in a hot shower, or by using a mechanical pump, or learning to pump your own breasts manually, or even by a willing husband.

If for some reason you don't plan to nurse your baby (a curious choice in times of scarcity), empty your breasts only until the excess pressure is relieved. The milk supply will gradually lessen if the breasts aren't fully emptied, as occurs during natural weaning to solid food. On the other hand, for breast-feeding mothers, it is best to empty the breast completely to assure a continuous supply of milk.

If you have trouble getting the knack of nursing, don't allow someone who hasn't nursed a baby to talk you out of it. You CAN do it. A mid-wife or experienced mother is by far the best guide to encourage you in your efforts. Even women with **inverted nipples** are usually able to breast feed successfully.

When a lactating woman develops localized tenderness and redness of the breast, this is usually caused by **mastitis**, that is, inflammation and/or infection of the milk glands. This is NOT a reason to stop nursing. Emptying the breast completely helps relieve the problem. The baby will not get the infection by swallowing the mother's milk; stomach acid will kill any bacteria that are ingested. For a minor case, the combination of regular nursing and application of heat to the breast several times a day may be all that's needed. If symptoms don't improve within a day or two, or if they continue to worsen despite hot packs and nursing, antibiotics may be necessary. Don't wait until you're running a fever and the entire breast is red, hot, and swollen to begin antibiotics. The best antibiotics to use are usually amoxicillin-clavulanate or cephalexin, although ciprofloxacin, clindamycin, and trimethoprim-sulfamethoxazole may be used if necessary (TMP-SMX only for nursing mothers of infants over age 2 months). If you don't have antibiotics available, or start them too late, mastitis may lead to an **abscess** that may require lancing.

One note on the **male breast**: the most common problem is growth of breast tissue during puberty. It is not unusual for a young teenage boy to develop sufficient breast tissue to become self-conscious. Breast enlargement may be bilateral or one side only. The problem generally resolves when the individual reaches full sexual maturity (age 18–21). Reassurance is the answer and no treatment is necessary.

Moving to the **reproductive organs**, these are rarely a problem before puberty, but one issue bears addressing. The current recommendation for the HPV vaccine (**human papilloma virus** vaccine, **cervical cancer** vaccine, **genital warts** vaccine) is for all girls before periods begin, preferably about age 11–12. The administration of this vaccine to all prepubescent girls prior to any sexual intercourse should prevent most cases of cervical cancer, years down the road. Although I'm one to advise abstinence until marriage, this cannot be guaranteed. In a post-Armageddon situation where screening for and treatment of cervical dysplasia and cancer may be a thing of the past, immunization against this preventable cancer seems advisable. The Gardasil vaccine has also been approved for boys ages 9–26 to prevent genital warts. Hopefully as a by-product, the transmission of the virus to susceptible women will decrease as well.

Next, women often experience heavy periods, irregular bleeding, or excessive menstrual cramping. In most cases, these symptoms are aggravating but not actually dangerous. **Menstrual cramping** may decrease when women are more active physically. If not, NSAIDs may help alleviate the discomfort, as may a hot bath or hot compresses. Some women will simply have to slow down and rest a few days a month.

The problem with **irregular bleeding** is mainly one of difficulty becoming pregnant, or predicting one's cycle, or occasional heavy periods. Except for infertility or undiagnosed pregnancy, irregular periods are more aggravating than medically worrisome. Birth control pills help regulate the menstrual cycle, but don't actually correct the underlying hormonal imbalance. Women with irregular periods and/or a history of infertility should not assume they cannot become pregnant. Irregular bleeding is quite common as the cycle is becoming established (in teens) and as hormone levels are dropping (menopause).

Heavy periods are the greater concern, and can actually lead to anemia. Although birth control pills, ibuprofen, and naproxen often slow heavy menstrual bleeding, these medications may not be available. (For additional details on how high-dose hormones may be used to decrease excessive uterine bleeding, please consult a gynecology textbook.)

Anyone with heavy bleeding and symptoms of anemia (paleness, fatigue, short-windedness) should take supplemental iron, or make it a point to eat plenty of dark, green vegetables. Over the past few decades, I have seen only a few women bleed to the point of requiring blood transfusion. Although transfusions have been successfully performed for over a century, this is not a procedure you're likely to undergo in times of austerity. If, at the current time, you experience heavy periods, you might want to consider undergoing a surgical procedure to permanently curtail your bleeding problem. Again, in modern society women rarely curtail their activities during their menstrual periods, but for heavy bleeders, a few days of rest is often helpful.

Menstruating women are also likely to be concerned about **birth control**. If men cannot be counted on for consistent birth control now, it'll be no more likely in times of crisis. Take it on yourself to obtain a sufficient supply of condoms, pills, or other birth control for future needs. You may want to be fitted for a diaphragm, a device that could be used successfully for many years to come. Along the same line, ancient birth control methods included plugs of various materials that block the cervical opening to a greater or lesser degree, but not as efficiently as today's water-proof polymers. These plugs would sometimes be used in conjunction with olive oil or similar viscous fluid, to trap the motile spermatozoa. Post-coital douching has also been used since ancient times and is better than nothing, but not by much.

A woman closely attuned to her own body could employ the rhythm method successfully, avoiding the mid-cycle time of greatest fertility. Although the egg only lives two days or less, sperm can remain viable for a week after intercourse. For the woman with a regular, 28-day cycle this means avoiding sex beginning a day or two after bleeding has ceased, and continuing until at least 3 or 4 days after ovulation. For the woman with a longer or shorter cycle, ovulation occurs fairly consistently on the 14th day *before* a woman's next menstrual cycle begins, with a few days added or subtracted between the first day of menstruation and ovulation. The period of fertility begins a week before ovulation and lasts until about three days later. The safest bet is to only have sex the week before your period and the week of your period. (Safer yet, have no sex at all.) The chart below outlines the normal cycle. (If you desire pregnancy, having intercourse during the period of fertility increases the odds of success.)

NATURAL BIRTH CONTROL (the rhythm method)

Week 1	**Week 2**	**Week 3**	**Week 4**
Variable – usually 12–16 days		Consistently 14 days	
Bleeding		Ov.	
	Period of Fertility – Avoid Sex		

As for pregnancy, I'll only say a few words, and refer instead to the excellent books already written (see below). For most women this is a natural process, fret with occasional dire problems. A few things we've learned from modern medicine that bear on post-modern medicine are:

1. Drinking alcohol during pregnancy may cause fetal alcohol syndrome.
2. Although women over age 35 are at increased risk of having a baby with Down syndrome (1 in 400 at age 35, 1 in 35 at age 45), most babies born to older women are unaffected.

3. Smoking during pregnancy causes smaller babies and greater risk of complications (prematurity, placental problems).
4. Taking the vitamin folic acid around the period of conception and in the early months of pregnancy decreases the risk of certain birth defects (neural tube defects, spina bifida).
5. After a miscarriage, women usually do as well *without* a D & C as with one – good news for TEOTWAWKI.
6. Cerebral palsy is not caused by a difficult birth.
7. Avoiding transmission of bacteria from one laboring woman (or caregiver) to another greatly decreases the risk of maternal infection and death. Hand-washing or use of gloves may be life-saving.
8. Nursing a baby immediately after delivery releases a hormone that causes the uterus to contract, thus decreasing post-delivery bleeding.

For additional resources on pregnancy, childbirth, and nursing, please see the adjacent textbox for entire books devoted to these topics.

Menopause is a topic glossed over in medical training. As a woman in her fifties, I appreciate the trials and tribulations better than as a younger doctor.

The onset and course of menopause is quite variable. Although the average age of menopause (cessation of menstrual cycles) is about 50, age 37 is not considered premature. To date I have not encountered a woman still menstruating *naturally* beyond age 58, although this does occur in women taking hormones. For some women, regular cycles occur until menopause, then suddenly cease. More common is a pattern of tapering or irregular periods, often for years preceding true menopause. Although fertility decreases during this period, stopping birth control may result in an unexpected pregnancy.

Recommended Texts for Pregnancy, Labor, and Delivery

Childbirth Without Fear by Grantly Dick-Read

First published in 1933 as *Natural Childbirth*, this book forged the way to a better understanding of childbirth as a natural process. Every medical student, nurse, and midwife should read *Childbirth Without Fear* before stepping foot in the labor and delivery suite.

The Official Lamaze Guide by Judith Lothian and Charlotte DeVries

Written for the expectant mother, this excellent guide focuses on all aspects of pregnancy and delivery, not simply Lamaze breathing.

Pregnancy, Childbirth, and the Newborn by Simkin, Whalley, and Keppler

Another excellent complete guide intended for the pregnant mother. Everything a new mother would want to know.

Your Pregnancy and Childbirth – Month to Month (ACOG)

Compiled by the American College of Obstetricians and Gynecologists, this text offers additional technical information, and is geared toward understanding pregnancy and childbirth as experienced under the care of a modern obstetrician.

A Guide to Effective Care in Pregnancy and Childbirth (Oxford Univ. Press)

Written for the health professional, this text covers normal pregnancy as well as commonly encountered problems, including diabetes, hypertension, and multiple pregnancy. The tables included at the back of the book provide lists of interventions that have been proven beneficial and those now known to be harmful.

Essentials of Obstetrics and Gynecology by Hacker, Gambone, and Hobel

Written for medical students, this illustrated manual is a hands-on guide for those entering the field, also useful for any medical professional who may be dealing with women's health issues, including pregnancy, labor, and delivery.

Hot flashes, emotional swings, and worsening PMS may occur anytime as the hormones taper, even a decade before periods stop. Hot flashes usually only persist a few years beyond cessation of menses, but in some women they persist for decades. The herb Black cohosh is often effective at relieving hot flashes and sometimes hormone-related mood disturbances. Medical treatments for menopause include hormones (most effective), antidepressants (Paxil, Prozac, Effexor), clonidine, and gabapentin. Heavy periods are sometimes a problem in the pre-menopause years, and can usually be handled the same as in younger women (see above).

Osteoporosis occurs primarily in post-menopausal women. Adequate calcium intake and regular exercise help prevent the disease. Stockpiling calcium and vitamin D supplements for all women over the age of 35 is a consideration when dairy products are likely to be in limited supply. Dark green leafy vegetables are the most natural form of calcium for adults. If you have eggs available, don't throw the shells away. Eggshells may be ground to powder and ingested a little at a time, or used as fertilizer to increase the calcium content of vegetables.

If you already have osteoporosis and are taking a bisphosphonate (Fosamax, Actonel, or Boniva), consider requesting a long-term supply of alendronate (generic Fosamax), which is now quite inexpensive. These are all intended to be taken along with calcium and vitamin D.

Chapter 24 – Checklist

Items to include in your medical supplies:

- ☐ Antibiotics for treatment of mastitis (amoxicillin-clavulanate, cephalexin, ciprofloxacin, clindamycin, trimethoprim-sulfamethoxazole)
- ☐ NSAIDs to relieve menstrual cramping and to decrease heavy menstrual flow (ibuprofen, naproxen)
- ☐ Textbooks and books relating to pregnancy and childbirth, per text
- ☐ Birth control methods (diaphragm, pills, condoms, etc.)
- ☐ Black cohosh for menopause relief (or medications, per text)
- ☐ Folic acid containing vitamins for use before and during pregnancy
- ☐ Calcium with Vitamin D for women over age 35; possibly alendronate

Actions to take:

- ☐ Consider having your children vaccinated against human papilloma virus
- ☐ Consider definitive treatment for heavy periods (surgery)
- ☐ Quit smoking

SECTION EIGHT

Medication Concerns

Chapter 25

Simplifying Your Medication Regime

Substitute, consolidate, minimize

Are you a diabetic on metformin, glimepiride, lisinopril, and insulin? Are you hypertensive and taking a diuretic, a beta-blocker, an alpha-blocker, and a calcium channel blocker? As a heart patient, are you on Plavix, aspirin, nitroglycerin, Coreg, amiodarone, simvastatin, and Coumadin? For anyone with depression, asthma, arthritis, or other chronic disease, are you on a dozen different medicines you couldn't hope to sustain if the modern medical establishment collapses?

The trend in American medicine is more, more, more of everything. We treat patients based on statistical improvement within studied groups as opposed to (often un-measurable) individual improvement. *Will that fourth blood pressure medicine prolong your life? Does lowering your blood sugar another twenty points reduce the risk of blindness? Can you get by with only one inhaler instead of two or three?* These are all questions to consider now, before a crisis occurs and you find yourself suddenly adrift.

Generally speaking, within any therapeutic class of medication a patient may be taking, a single medicine affords the most improvement, with add-on drugs contributing less and less additional benefit (diminishing returns). High blood pressure is a perfect example of this: a single drug may lower your systolic blood pressure number by 20–30 points; the second decreases it another 10–15; the third another 5–7; the fourth possibly only 3–5. *At what point is additional medication just not worth it?*

In the current era of chart audits and treatment protocols, doctors expend much effort treating potential risks rather than current problems. Diabetics *should* have their eyes examined annually, their urine checked for protein, their blood sugar monitored, their feet inspected, their cholesterol recorded, their EKG analyzed. Yet little of this makes a person feel better. It's all to minimize the risk of future problems based on statistical likelihood of disease.

We practice medicine this way because we can. Doctors have hundreds of medications at our disposal. Insurance pays for expensive treatments we could not possibly afford on our own. Everyone deserves superlative treatment and no one should do without simply because they cannot afford the best in health care. Injections costing thousands of dollars apiece often provide little discernable benefit. Sometimes it seems the medical world has gone crazy. Although health care after an Armageddon event will provide its own challenges, it may come as a relief to physicians to be treating problems we can actually see, and patients may be happy to take only medications that make a discernable difference.

Preppers want to know which medications to stockpile and which not to bother with. The answers in this section are aimed at the general public. Your own situation may differ. If you're on a dozen medicines, you should have a doctor to whom you can address questions. The following is intended as a starting point only. Working with your own physician is essential.

Medications requiring drug monitoring may cause more harm than good when blood testing become unavailable. Coumadin (warfarin) comes to mind immediately. If you have atrial fibrillation or have had recurrent blood clots, you may be on this medication the rest of your life. Without monitoring, however, the question becomes: which is more dangerous, the risk of a blood clot or stroke, or the risk of excess bleeding? On the one hand, generic warfarin is cheap, effective, and therefore possibly appropriate for stockpiling. On the other hand, it can kill you fairly easily. Anyone choosing to continue warfarin had best also stockpile Vitamin K as an antidote. The alternative to warfarin is taking a single aspirin daily. Though it's not quite as effective at thinning the blood, it's considerably safer. As of late 2010 another new class of blood thinner has been released that does not require blood testing, but at $6 per pill (for Pradaxa), the cost may be prohibitive for stockpiling. Also, it has no antidote, and requires either transfusion or dialysis to reverse its blood-thinning properties, procedures which will be unavailable if hospitals are non-functional.

Other drugs requiring blood monitoring include many seizure drugs, lithium, digoxin, and theophylline. If your doctor requires periodic blood tests related to any drug you are taking, ask him would he prescribe the same medication if testing were unavailable. What alternatives would he consider? You'll want to find out now, while many choices exist, and when switching to alternate therapy can be accomplished under medical supervision.

Drugs with a high NNT (number needed to treat) are of questionable value to the individual patient. The NNT means the number of patients that must be treated in order to help one individual or to prevent one specific problem. For example, in a very high-risk individual, it may be worthwhile to continue Lipitor, a cholesterol-lowering drug. But would you do so if you knew it only decreased your risk of heart attack by 2%? Currently doctors figure it's reasonable to treat 10 people for the sake of 1. Though the great majority may not be helped, they suffer little harm. When a problem is prevented, and therefore does not occur, it's hard to know who would have experienced the problem to start with. This statistical method of thinking will change at the end of the world as we know it. For a list of interventions and their associated NNT, see the Table of NNTs at Bandolier (http://www.medicine.ox.ac.uk/bandolier/band50/b50-8.html). If you are taking any medication to prevent (as opposed to treat) a problem, ask your doctor what your odds are without it.

Polypharmacy, or the use of multiple medications, is an extremely common problem. I have patients who believe they can't live without their blood pressure pills, nerve pills, sleeping pills, pain pills, allergy pills, cholesterol pills, itching pills, arthritis pills, eye drops, nose sprays, hair tonics, inhalers, enemas, and skin creams, not to mention Viagra. In some cases, trying to eliminate any from the list is like pulling teeth. However, doctors are often to blame for piling one drug on top of another, especially when a patient has half a dozen physicians. Only rarely will one doctor discontinue another's therapy, not wanting to step on anyone's toes. If your goal is to simply your regimen, which I *am* recommending, this is a good time to confer with your family doctor. With so many drugs, patients often have no way of knowing which are providing the bulk of the benefit.

For example, how do you know which of your four blood pressure medicines are contributing the greatest benefit? Your doctor may be able to make an educated guess, but you may still have to taper off the others to find out.

If you are taking four diabetic medicines, could you discontinue one, two, or even three? Sometimes switching to insulin is the simplest alternative. If you're already on insulin, is it always necessary to take two kinds? Or could your doctor change you to one of the older insulins, available without a prescription, and therefore easier to stockpile?

Is an arthritic patient better off taking Celebrex, methotrexate, omeprazole, and tramadol, or could they do as well with prednisone plus Tylenol? There are pros and cons of every medical regimen, and what we view as undesirable today may become the treatment of choice tomorrow.

Multi-use drugs are great. *Wouldn't it be wonderful to treat both your migraines and high blood pressure with a single medication?* A beta-blocker or calcium channel blocker may work wonders for both conditions. *Or, wouldn't it be better to have a pain-killer you could use not only for your gout, but for any other pain as well?* Tramadol or ibuprofen would be preferable to colchicine in my estimation. Many blood pressure drugs benefit the heart and could work double-duty in a patient with angina.

Over-the-counter substitutes for prescription meds are both easier to stockpile and often less expensive. You may not even be aware that an OTC alternative exists. The chart on the following page lists several to consider.

If you're taking any medications on a chronic or regular basis, schedule a serious discussion with your doctor. Items to address include medication cost, long-term side-effects, medical monitoring, potential use for other conditions, relative contribution to your health or symptom control, risks of doing without, and risk of stopping abruptly, should you eventually run out of medicine.

This last is a real concern. Stopping a beta-blocker overnight may cause your heart to race dangerously. Discontinuing nerve pills or narcotics may lead to hallucinations or seizures. Lack of Synthroid may result in eventual coma. Now is the time to discuss potential consequences and how best to avoid them.

With the above suggestions in mind, talk to your doctor about simplifying your drug regimen, or that of your parents or children. It may take months to determine the ideal combination of medications, so don't wait until chaos strikes to begin.

Prescription Drug	Over-the-counter Alternative
Albuterol inhaler (for asthma or COPD) (Proventil, Ventolin, ProAir)	Primatene Mist (epinephrine inhaler) – BUT risk of increased HR or BP
Antivert (meclizine) (for dizziness/nausea)	Bonine, Dramamine, meclizine
Bactroban (antibiotic cream or ointment)	Bacitracin antibiotic cream or ointment
Celebrex (for arthritis or pain)	Ibuprofen, naproxen sodium, or aspirin, possibly along with OTC Prilosec or Prevacid
Clarinex (for allergies)	Claritin, Allegra, Benadryl, Zyrtec (generics)
Diflucan (fluconazole) (for yeast infection)	OTC Gyne-Lotrimin, Monistat, or generics
Flonase (fluticasone, Rhinocort, Veramyst) (for nasal allergies)	NasalCrom for chronic use; Afrin short-term
Lamisil pills (for toenail fungus)	Vicks VapoRub
Nexium, Aciphex, Protonix, Prilosec, omeprazole, Prevacid, lansoprazole (for heartburn and stomach acid)	Prilosec OTC, Prevacid 24, Pepcid, Zantac (generics)
Pataday, Patanol (for eye allergies)	Zaditor, Visine
Pyridium (for urinary burning)	Azo
Steroid skin cream (rashes)	Hydrocortisone 1% cream or ointment

Chapter 26

Use of Expired Medications

It's now a decade post-WWIII. Rummaging through the ruins of a burned-out pharmacy you discover a bounty of antibiotics and pain pills. According to the labels, the drugs expired five years ago. You stash them in your pockets anyway, but wonder, are they still safe? Will they be effective?

Use of expired medicines is a common concern among preppers, and with good reason. Once our current drug manufacturing capability and/or transportation system has been destroyed, it may take many years to reestablish.

The question of expiration brings to mind dates on canned food. *Does a can of tuna go bad overnight?* Logic would dictate this cannot be. My pastor told me only recently that he's been eating soup that expired in 2005. However, doctors advise against using medications beyond their expiration dates for many reasons, not the least of which is medical liability risk.

But is there any science to support the safety and efficacy of expired drugs? Can any generalizations be made? What special concerns exist with regard to specific formulations or drugs? How, exactly, does a medication "go bad?" Likewise, how are drug expiration dates actually determined?

Since 1979 the FDA has required all medications in their original packaging to be imprinted with an expiration date. This date does not indicate when a drug goes *bad*, but rather a date through which the drug is guaranteed to be *good*, similar to a "best if used by" date on a can of beans.

How are these dates determined? In two ways. The first is by real-time testing. Medications are stored under manufacturer-recommended conditions (which does not mean above the toilet in your hot, humid bathroom). At given intervals the medications are tested for appearance, drug content, and stability. Nowhere could I find that they are tested for safety specifically, but if the product does not appear to have degraded, the inference is that it is safe.

Secondly, drugs are tested under high-temperature stress conditions (accelerated degradation studies) to simulate longer time periods. Logically, if a medication has only been available for two years, five years of stability testing is unlikely to have been performed. However, if a medication remains stable for a specified time period under adverse conditions, one may presume it likely stable and therefore safe for much longer periods under optimum storage conditions.

Expiration dates are only found on the original packaging and apply to unopened meds that have been stored as directed. No guarantee is made for drugs exposed to extremes of temperature, humidity, or lighting.

This is in contrast to the date on your actual prescription bottle, a "do not use beyond" date. Pharmacists commonly purchase pills in bulk bottles of 1,000 then dispense them into smaller containers, generally with a shorter expiration date. The most liberal dating will be a year beyond which the original prescription was dispensed. Although the original bottle (which you may never see and that remains in the pharmacy, in the case of bulk meds) may have a date 2–3 years in the future, your own bottle will be dated for 1 year or less from purchase, due to uncertainty about actual storage conditions and patient use.

One tip on stocking up, then, is to request your prescription in the original packaging. Find out if your medication comes in bottles of 30, 60, 90 or 100, and request that it be dispensed in containers of that quantity. Your doctor will not necessarily know this information, but you can ask your pharmacist or look it up in a PDR (Physicians' Desk Reference). A used PDR can be purchased online for under $5. However, many generic drugs are not listed in the PDR, so you may have to ask your pharmacist regarding certain prescriptions. In the case of drugs re-packaged and dispensed in the typical dark plastic bottles, ask the pharmacy what the expiration date is on the original bulk drug bottle.

The primary source of information regarding the prolonged stability of medications comes from the Shelf Life Extension Program database. Rather than discard millions of dollars worth of expired drugs stockpiled for emergency use, the government tested representative lots of selected medications for extended stability. These stockpiled drugs are aimed at emergency use for injuries and infections (rather than chronic diseases such as diabetes, heart disease, and asthma). The most pertinent data for the layman are related to drugs to combat bacterial and viral infections.

In 2009 as a result of the H1N1 influenza scare, two antiviral (anti-influenza) drugs were granted an Emergency Use Authorization (which has since expired). At that time, tested lots of Relenza were granted approval for up to one year after the original expiration date, whereas Tamiflu products were approved for up to an additional 5 years. Tamiflu is easier to use, has fewer side-effects, and comes in sealed blister-packs of 10. (A full dose is one 75-mg tablet twice daily for 5 days, to be started within the first day or two of true influenza infection.)

Several antibiotics tested for extended use were found to be safe as well, for an additional one to several years. Of the lots tested, the following had their expiration date extended by the number of months indicated.

Medication name	Dosage form	Average extension in months (and range)
Amoxicillin sodium	Tablets	23 (22–23)
Ampicillin	Capsules	49 (22–64)
Cephalexin	Capsules	57 (28–135)
Ciprofloxacin	Tablets	55 (12–142)
Doxycycline Hyclate	Capsules	50 (37–66)
Erythromycin lactobionate	Powder	60 (38–83)
Sulfisoxazole	Tablets	56 (45–68)
Tetracycline HCl	Capsules	50 (17–133)
Silver sulfadiazine	Cream	57 (28–104)

A summary of the SLEP data is available in *The Journal of Pharmaceutical Sciences*, Vol. 95, No. 7, July 2006. Many of the tested medications were injectables for anesthetic, surgical, and hospital use.

The *Medical Letter*, a respected professional newsletter, addressed the topic of expired medications in both 1996 and 2002. Regarding safety, they advise:

"The only report of human toxicity that may have been caused by chemical or physical degradation of a pharmaceutical product is renal tubular damage that was associated with use of degraded tetracycline. . . Current tetracycline preparations have been reformulated with different fillers to minimize degradation and are unlikely to have this effect."[26]

Regarding safety, the same issue summarizes data from the FDA Shelf Life Extension Program: "84% of 1122 lots of 96 different drug products stored in military facilities in their unopened original containers would be expected to remain stable for an average of 57 months after their original expiration date."

Regarding selective drugs they report: captopril and TheoDur tablets remained chemically and physically stable for 1.5–9 years beyond their expiration dates; amantadine and rimantidine remained stable after storage for 25 years; another theophylline preparation retained 90% potency for about 30 years.

Liquid preparations may be much less stable, and degrade more quickly if frozen or heated. The *Medical Letter* advises that "Drugs in solution, particularly injectables, that have become cloudy or discolored or show signs of precipitation should not be used." For oral medications, color changes may be related to the dyes rather than the drugs, however. Epinephrine in EpiPens was noted to contain less than 90% potency at 10 months after the expiration date. The concern with eye drops is microbial contamination when the preservative becomes ineffective.

Overall then, the concern is not regarding safety, but rather effectiveness. "Many drugs stored under reasonable conditions retain 90% of their potency for

[26] *The Medical Letter*, Vol. 44, Issue 1142, October 28, 2002.

at least 5 years after the expiration date on the label, and sometimes much longer," per the *Medical Letter*.

Of the medications tested in the SLEP program, few if any were of the extended release variety. Because Americans like the convenience of once-daily dosing, many drugs have been developed with delayed-release technology. This includes any medicine with the following letters in the name: XR or XL (extended release), SR (sustained or slow release), CR (controlled release). The methods by which the medications are slowly released in the stomach or intestine have the potential to be effected by extremes of storage temperature or humidity. The release system may be via a semi-permeable membrane of the entire tablet, or on each individual granule within a capsule, or by a layered tablet designed to dissolve at different pH (acidity) levels. Under adverse conditions, the active drug may be released more quickly or more slowly than intended, yielding unpredictable clinical results. For example, an extended-release anti-hypertensive medication that enters the blood stream too quickly may lower your blood pressure too much or too rapidly. If released too slowly, it may not reduce your blood pressure adequately or at all.

Although I could find no specific data regarding stability of delayed-release medications, having your doctor change your medication now to an immediate-release preparation may be desirable. Of course, these rapid-release medications often must be taken more than once a day. Examples where switching from a delayed to an immediate release formulation is possible include Toprol XL, Wellbutrin SR and XL, Biaxin XL, Diltiazem SR, CR, and XL, Xanax XR, Effexor XR, and many others. If you are planning to stockpile extended-release medications, make sure you obtain them in the original factory-sealed packaging (that often includes a desiccant).

Another question is the stability of generic drugs versus name brand. Although I expect brand-name drugs would exhibit greater stability, cost is significantly more for most (but not all) preparations. Brand-name drugs must exhibit a bioavailability of 100% (+/- 5%) of the specified dose. Generic drugs have a 20% leeway. Therefore, from the outset, a generic drug may yield 80–125% of the specified dose. (I have no proof, but I would assume they err on the low side.) Some generic drugs are difficult to swallow, others crumble easily, or stick together, or become discolored. If possible, investigate the country of origin of your generic prescriptions. In this case, "Made in the USA" is a good sign.

Yet another concern lies with medications where blood levels are usually monitored. Of course, at TEOTWAWKI it's unlikely that blood testing will be performed. Drugs with "narrow therapeutic windows" pose a special concern. These drugs are ineffective at low dose but toxic at higher doses, with a small window between where the drug is therapeutic. Such drugs include digoxin, lithium, and theophylline. When serum drug levels or other biologic indices cannot be measured, dosing must be determined by clinical result and side-effects. Anti-seizure medications, thyroid preparations, and even insulin may fall in this category.

To sum it all up, the good news is that most tablets and capsules are very likely safe and quite likely effective for several years beyond the printed expiration date. Using expired medications may do for a decade beyond the end of the world as we know it.

(But then what?)

Chapter 27

Fish Antibiotics

By some fluke or loophole, fish antibiotics are available over-the-counter without a prescription, whereas canine, feline, and human antibiotics are not. For this reason preppers and survivalists question whether they can be safely substituted for human antibiotics. Some online pet supply sites list off-label dosing recommendations for pets such as cats and dogs, but are careful to state, "Not for use in humans."

Fish (aquarium) antibiotics include ampicillin, amoxicillin, penicillin, cephalexin, tetracycline, doxycycline, azithromycin, erythromycin, ciprofloxacin, clindamycin, metronidazole, and sulfamethoxazole-trimethoprim, as well as the antifungal drug ketoconazole. Generally speaking, the milligram amount of these tablets is of the same strength as that used in humans.

Given that these drugs are the same type and strength used by humans, why are they specifically labeled, "Not for use in humans?" The primary reason is that it is unlawful in the United States to dispense these drugs for human consumption without a physician's prescription. A person who purchases them and subsequently gives them to someone else would be considered practicing medicine without a license. Secondly, although even fish antibiotics are regulated by the FDA, safety for human consumption may be questionable, particularly with foreign manufacturers.

Here's an analogous question: would you eat dog food? Munching on a Milk-Bone might not seem objectionable, but would you chow down on a can of Alpo? (Though who knows . . . if it's a choice between Alpo and road-kill possum, I might go for the Alpo.)

However, it does appear that certain fish antibiotics are the same ones used for humans. Generic human antibiotics are USP grade, usually AB-rated. The United States Pharmacopeia (USP) sets standards for prescription and OTC drugs manufactured or sold in the USA. An AB rating indicates that the generic in question has been proven to meet bioequivalence to a reference standard (which is generally the brand name drug). To determine the rating of a fish antibiotic, find an online retailer whose advertising features an image of the medication in mind. Check the color and imprint against a pill identifier such as that at www.drugstore.com, then view additional details, searching for the manufacturer. Next find the manufacturer's Web site and search for products with the same imprint and appearance, to check if the drug is USP grade and AB-rated. Presumably these would be safe for human consumption.

However, as long as a supply of human medication is available, I cannot recommend the use of fish antibiotics. It isn't that doctors want to keep antibiotics all to themselves – there are reasons antibiotics are regulated. Safe and effective antibiotic use requires both knowledge and experience. True, a patient who's taken amoxicillin a dozen times for sinus infections would probably know how to handle a recurrence, but do you have the medical acumen to recognize and treat adverse antibiotic effects including allergy, rash, anaphylaxis, diarrhea, yeast infection, and drug-drug interactions? In this manual I have explained proper use of antibiotics in many scenarios, but that isn't to say that this volume contains all the medical knowledge that seven years of training and two decades of experience affords.

For human use, each of the antibiotics mentioned above is inexpensive and most are on the $4 list of prescription medications at discount pharmacies. For example, Wal-Mart offers 30 tablets of cephalexin 500 mg for $4, whereas online I find a price of $21 for the equivalent drug for fish. When my son took his dog to the veterinarian recently he was charged $42 for the same thing (which seems unethical). It really makes more sense to use human antibiotics on pets rather than the other way around.

If modern civilization were to end and my daughter was dying of pneumonia, would I treat her with fish antibiotics? Probably so. If she had a sinus infection today, would I send her to the pet store to save a visit to the doctor? No. For those looking to stock up on antibiotics or other drugs, I suggest reading the following chapter.

Chapter 28

How to Get Your Doctor to Help You Stockpile Medications

Picture this: Your doctor enters the room and asks, "How can I help you today?"

"I'd like enough medicine to survive the end of the world as we know it," you reply.

He narrows his eyes and responds, "Just how much Prozac would that require?"

Finding a physician to help you stockpile medications will be a challenge. Unless your doctor, too, believes Armageddon is nigh, he's not likely to grant your request.

Why not? Doctors are responsible for the medications we prescribe and the consequences, intended or unintended. Remember, every medication is a potential poison. You're probably glad your own physician has sufficient training to possess a valid medical license. Certain problems (and medications) require periodic monitoring regarding their effects on the human body. No doctor wants to be responsible for patients who won't comply with essential examination and testing. Would a car maker warranty your automobile engine if you refuse to change the oil?

Typically, doctors prescribe enough medication to cover a specific problem for an appropriate length of time. Antibiotics are usually dispensed for seven to ten days, blood pressure medicines for three to six months, diabetic medications for one to several months, and pain relievers until the underlying problem is expected to resolve.

Does your doctor prescribe you extra amoxicillin, just in case you get sick later this year? Not likely. When physicians prescribe more medication than is currently necessary, this often amounts to patients playing doctor with themselves or with others. Under our current system, this can be a felony. However, at TEOTWAWKI, many survivors will become their own doctor of necessity, and to do so, you will need a stockpile of medications.

Before I offer advice on how to get your doctor to help you with stockpiling, please realize that there are other obstacles to the acquisition of said drugs. Pharmacists have the right to refuse to fill a prescription that seems unreasonable or potentially harmful. Insurance companies usually limit payment for prescriptions to at most a 3-month supply at one time, and don't want to pay too far ahead in case either your disease state or your insurance changes. You'll have to pay out of your own pocket to get more medicine than this. Doctors cannot legally alter their prescriptions to say you are taking more medication than you actually are. Neither would it be ethical for you to lie about the situation.

So, how to get the medicine that you may need? One option is to convince your physician that the end of the world is near. That'll be tough. But think a moment, if your doctor really did think TEOTWAWKI is around the corner, he'd be doing his best to help you prepare.

Doctors do prescribe extra medication, along with directions for use, under special circumstances: antibiotics for potential traveler's diarrhea, anti-malarials for missionaries to Africa, six months of medications for someone wintering in Antarctica. Asking for medications for TEOTWAWKI is akin to doing the same for a trip around the world. After a national catastrophe, such a supply would be intended to span a gap of only a year or two. Although some medications probably do have a shelf-life of a decade beyond their expiration date, hopefully drug manufacturing and distribution will be re-established long before then.

Convincing your doctor to prescribe extra medication depends largely on the doctor-patient relationship. If your doctor trusts you, he or she is much more likely to assist you. Please realize that your doctor will think that he's doing you a fairly large favor. He may even question the legality of his own prescribing. Don't forget to be grateful. Also realize that even if a doctor writes more than a year's worth of refills, pharmacists cannot dispense them beyond a year of the original prescribing date. If you are convinced that you need more than a 12-month supply stockpiled, you'll need to discuss this openly with your doctor. Obviously a person could visit more than one doctor, which I don't recommend, especially if you don't tell each and every one of your physicians what you are doing. Dishonesty is a deal-breaker when it comes to trust.

In general, medications are prescribed for either acute problems or chronic problems. Acute problems include most infections and injuries. Chronic problems include asthma, diabetes, heart disease, hypothyroidism, mental illness, arthritis, and a host of others. Treatment of chronic conditions also includes modification of risk factors including high cholesterol and high blood pressure. Even antibiotics are sometimes prescribed long-term in certain situations, e.g. acne, rosacea, certain forms of colitis, and recurrent urinary infections.

Medications for acute problems include antibiotics, antivirals, anti-malarials, antifungals, anti-diarrheals, anti-emetics, migraine treatments, pain medications, heartburn relief, albuterol for asthma and COPD, nitroglycerin, corticosteroids, and anti-inflammatories, to name the most common.

Drugs for chronic problems and conditions include birth control pills, antidepressants, allergy medications, inhalers for asthma and COPD, anti-anginal drugs, acid-reducing drugs (proton pump inhibitors, histamine-2 blockers), anti-inflammatories, diabetic meds, thyroid replacement, and many others.

Without specifying which of these meds I'd advise for stockpiling, I'll tell you exactly how I'd like a patient to approach me to acquire an extra supply, an approach which I believe would work for other doctors as well.

First, begin establishing a trusting relationship with your doctor. If you don't think your physician even knows who you are, make an appointment for a physical or minor problem. *Don't* ask about stockpiling at this initial visit.

If your doctor asks you to follow-up for some reason, then do so. Follow directions. Be responsible. If he says no follow-up is needed, no doubt you can find another reason to come in within a month or so. Accompany another family member to their appointment to keep your face fresh in your doctor's memory. If there are multiple providers in your physician's office, try to see the same one each time to establish a relationship.

By the third time your doctor has seen you within a time frame of a few months, he's going to start knowing you, and more importantly, trusting you. You must act in a trustworthy manner by:

- Showing up for your appointments
- Not canceling appointments with insufficient warning
- Arriving on time (even if you must wait on the doctor)
- Taking your medications properly and knowing their correct names and dosing
- Trying to do your part in every way
- Being kind, pleasant, polite, and cheerful.

Of course, this is good advice even if TEOTWAWKI does not occur in our lifetime. (Doctors should follow the same advice.)

After doing the above, it's time to consider approaching the topic of stockpiling. Say that you have diabetes and want to be prepared. If you ask for a year's prescription, your doctor may figure you won't show up again, even though you've demonstrated responsibility to date. Ask for an extra three months instead and make 100% sure that you show up for your next scheduled visit. If you don't, your doctor will decide he cannot trust you. As in every relationship, once trust is broken, it takes much, much longer to re-establish.

Assuming you do keep your scheduled follow-up, remind the doctor that you have put back the extra medication, and that you'd like to have an additional three month's worth. Reassure him that you will again follow-up whenever he'd like you to return. (And especially for diabetics, do what your doctor suggests regarding blood sugar testing, weight loss, etc. – at the very least, try.) In this fashion, by establishing and confirming trust, you can build up an adequate stockpile. If your relationship is strong, he may trust you to get even a year's worth ahead of time. The same protocol would apply equally well to any of the chronic diseases mentioned above – and if you suffer from any of these, educating yourself is an excellent idea. Learn how to take care of yourself now so you'll be ready later.

For acute problems, such as bacterial infections, you'll want a supply of antibiotics on hand. Follow the above directions in establishing a trusting relationship. Then either when you are sick (or when you are not) ask for a supply of one appropriate antibiotic, perhaps a 30-day supply. Reassure your doctor that you will not use this medication as long as he is here to take care of you. If you get sick again, go back to your doctor and remind him of your plan. If he suggests antibiotics, request a new prescription, and perhaps another supply to stockpile. Trust, trust, trust. That's 99% of the equation.

With 2012 just around the corner, you should start now. None of us knows God's timeline, but waiting until the last minute is ill-advised.

From www.ArmageddonMedicine.net

Several readers of my blog have asked what dose of antibiotics to stockpile. As a general rule, I suggest that you *not* request multiple strengths of a single medicine, as few if any doctors would agree to this.

Here are my recommendations for the most appropriate doses of common antibiotics to stockpile and why, based on both cost and traditional dosing. If your doctor is willing to write antibiotics for stockpiling at all, these are the ones most likely to be prescribed.

1. **Amoxicillin** – Many pharmacies offer the 250 and 500 mg capsules at the same unit price. Amoxicillin *tablets* are also available, but may cost somewhat more than the capsules, depending on the pharmacy. Amoxicillin tablets may be split more easily (than the powder in the capsules can be divided) to provide a lower dose if needed for children or small adults. (Babies are usually administered a reconstituted powder, but few pediatricians would prescribe this for stockpiling.) The best single option is amoxicillin 500 mg tablets (or capsules).

2. **Cephalexin** – Again, cephalexin 250 and 500 mg capsules are priced the same, so the 500 mg capsule is the better deal. The powder could be divided to obtain a lower dose, or the medicine could be taken twice daily rather than three or four times daily (also true of amoxicillin, above) to yield a lower dose.

3. **Ciprofloxacin** – Because the 500 mg dose is used more commonly than the 250 mg dose, the higher dose is actually less expensive than the lower dose and may be split as needed. Except in dire emergencies, this drug is not used in children, so pediatric dosing does not apply.

4. **Doxycycline** – Available in either tablets or capsules at about the same cost, I suggest the 100 mg tablet, which may be split for lower dosing.

5. **Erythrocin** – Another case where the higher milligram dose may be cheaper than the lower dose, depending on the pharmacy. Check your local $4 list before asking your doctor for either the 250 or 500 mg tablet. In general, I would advise the higher dose.

6. **Metronidazole** – Another case of an adult medicine, though in this case, the higher dose is generally more expensive than the lower dose. Still, I'd recommend 500 mg tablets, which may be split if needed.

7. **SMZ-TMP DS** - The DS (double-strength) is used much more commonly than SMZ-TMP (single-strength), so again I recommend the higher dose, which also may be split for adult or pediatric use.

8. **Tetracycline** – The 250 mg and 500 mg capsules cost the same, so I'd go with the higher dose. Like doxycycline, tetracycline is not used in children whose teeth are still forming due to the potential for permanent staining.

Chapter 29

10 Essential OTC Drugs to Stockpile

The primary advantages of over-the-counter medications are their ready availability and relatively low cost. However, certain medications are actually less expensive by prescription, even though they are available OTC. Many conditions can be treated using these drugs, more than most people realize.

Anyone interested in stockpiling medications may want to think beyond his or her own personal use. Though family, friends, and future health needs come to mind first, the good of the immediate and greater community are an additional concern – consider all the people who have not prepared. They, too, may need medication. And though doctors and other medical personnel may begin with a large store of supplies, when these are exhausted, back-up supplies will become essential.

Medical supplies may become a valuable commodity for barter. If money is meaningless, people will trade one necessity for another. Musculoskeletal pain and stomach pain are probably the two most common conditions for which relief may bring a pretty penny. The following is a list of highly useful, affordable medications to stockpile not only for your personal use, but also for others in need whom you may encounter, and for possible bartering.

1. **Ibuprofen (Motrin, Advil, Nuprin)** – Among the OTC anti-inflammatory medications (NSAIDs), ibuprofen is probably the most versatile. Most commonly used for pain, it may be used to relieve headaches, earaches, sore throats, sinus pain, stiff neck, muscle strains, menstrual cramps, arthritis including gout, and back pain. It is also effective at reducing fever and is generally safe for use in children. It is usually not advisable for stomach-related pain, although may decrease the pain of kidney stones, kidney infections, and possibly bladder infections. The most common side-effect is stomach irritation or heartburn. When combined with acetaminophen, it is nearly as effective as codeine, tramadol, or hydrocodone in relieving more severe pain.

2. **Acetaminophen (Tylenol)** – Acetaminophen is the only OTC pain-reliever that is not an anti-inflammatory drug. It will not irritate the stomach like ibuprofen, aspirin, or naproxen may. It is useful for the same conditions as ibuprofen, though effectiveness varies according to patient. As mentioned above, it may be combined with ibuprofen in full doses for more severe pain. Side-effects are very few, though in high dose, especially when combined with alcohol, it can lead to liver failure. It is available in several pediatric dosages.

3. **Diphenhydramine (Benadryl)** – An inexpensive antihistamine, diphenhydramine is primarily used for respiratory infections and nasal allergies, in both adults and children. It is also useful for hives and itching, including itchy rashes such as poison ivy, and sometimes nausea. Although not all patients become drowsy when using diphenhydramine, many do so, making this medication effective for insomnia as well.

4. **Loperamide (Imodium)** – The most effective OTC medication for diarrhea is loperamide, which is available both as tablet form and liquid for children. It is often useful for relieving intestinal cramping as well.

5. **Pseudoephedrine (Sudafed)** – Pseudoephedrine is effective at relieving congestion of both the upper and lower respiratory tract due to most common causes including infection, allergy, chemical irritation, and mild asthma. It often has a stimulatory effect, like caffeine. The most common side-effects are those resembling a burst of adrenaline: rapid heart rate, palpitations, and increased blood pressure.

6. **Meclizine (Bonine, Dramamine)** – This anti-emetic drug is available both over the counter and by prescription. It relieves nausea, motion sickness, and vertigo-like dizziness. For some patients it causes drowsiness, and therefore may be used as a sleep aid. It is related to medications that are used for anxiety.

7. **Ranitidine (Zantac)** – Although several medications are available OTC for the treatment of heartburn and other acid-reducing conditions, ranitidine is among the best-tolerated and is also useful for relieving hives.

8. **Hydrocortisone cream** – The 1% version of hydrocortisone cream is the strongest steroid cream available over the counter. It is safe for use in both adults and children in treating inflamed and/or itchy rashes such as eczema, poison ivy, diaper rash, and other minor genital irritations.

9. **Bacitracin ointment** – This ointment is best used to prevent skin infections when the integrity of the skin has been breached, as by an abrasion, laceration, insect bite or sting. It also may be used to treat a superficial skin infection such as a mildly infected wound or impetigo. It is less likely to produce a topical skin allergy than other topical antibiotic preparations, such as those containing neomycin.

10. **Clotrimazole (Gyne-Lotrimin)** – The same antifungal medication clotrimazole is contained in both Lotrimin and Gyne-Lotrimin. Gyne-Lotrimin may be used to treat both female yeast infections and any other yeast or fungal infection that Lotrimin would treat, including athlete's foot, ringworm, diaper rashes, and skin fold irritations.

For under $50 a good supply of all of the above can be purchased. Several of these medications are also available at higher doses by prescription, and may actually be less expensive if obtained from a physician (ranitidine, meclizine, loperamide, and diphenhydramine), even paying full price.

Chapter 30

Herbal Medicine and Other Natural Remedies

Thinking outside the pill-box

Introduction

Allopathic doctors (M.D.s and some D.O.s) have little experience with herbal medication, yet we have the greatest likelihood of making some sense out of a thorny issue. Although I realize many people distrust the medical establishment, should you trust an herbalist more? What sort of training have the clerks at your local health food store undergone? Are they selling you a useful remedy or merely a bottle of hope? At least physicians are trying to get at the truth, which is often elusive and requires painstaking effort to ascertain. Biology is not a simple matter and neither is the treatment of disease.

Several other problems plague the practice of herbal medicine. All too often a morsel of legitimate data suggesting a *possible* beneficial effect is inflated by those with minimal scientific training, especially by those who stand to gain financially. Proving cinnamon lowers blood sugar slightly is not tantamount to a cure for diabetes. When a kernel of truth becomes a mountain of misinformation, significant damage may result. Anyone in the health care profession must remember: first, do no harm.

Secondly, anyone can sell herbs. The profit margin is large and expectations minimal. Have you ever noticed that nutraceuticals all carry the same warning, stating that the products have not been evaluated by the FDA and are not intended to treat any medical condition? Do you trust a teenager who directs you to the digestive aisle in the health food store more than you trust your own physician? Saying something is natural in no way makes it safe. Arsenic is natural. So are poison mushrooms. But patients buy these purported "natural cures" because they view them as harmless, and because they offer at least the illusion of control over one's own body.

Thirdly, large, high-quality, unbiased medical studies involving herbal products are very expensive to perform. Since no pharmaceutical company stands to gain from such research, it is unlikely to be undertaken, and smaller studies are rarely published in respected journals.

Fourth, the placebo effect is very strong. Doctors realize that a third of patients will have a therapeutic effect from almost any treatment at all. Although a patient may swear by a certain remedy, which indeed may appear effective for him or her, this does not prove the same treatment will help anyone else.

Fifth, herbs from foreign lands, though available currently, will not be easy to find at TEOTWAWKI, and even today most people do not recognize native plants. *Can you name the weeds in your yard other than dandelions? Can you recognize the difference between mandrake and ginseng? Do you know how to cultivate either?*

Sixth, even if a plant is beneficial, has a therapeutic dose been determined? *Are two leaves enough? Is six too many? Big leaves or small ones? Spring sprigs or autumn roots? Are there side-effects to be concerned about?* I often warn my patients that every medication is a potential poison, and the same can be said about every plant.

Despite all this, I do feel that herbal therapy is a vastly unexplored and underrated territory. There is no doubt that plant chemicals interact with those of the human body. Foxglove can help – or hinder – the heart. Caffeine can improve – or worsen – a headache. Opium can relieve pain, or cause addiction. Ma huang can decrease the appetite, or cause palpitations. The use of herbal preparations is even more complex than treatment with patent medications, which generally involve only a single chemical, whereas every plant contains hundreds of uniquely identifiable molecules.

Very gradually the body of evidence is mounting regarding the medicinal uses of various plants and herbs. My intention is to share what is scientifically known. Although Grandma may have some favorites of her own, and though she may indeed be proven correct, my aim is to share proven evidence. What science lacks, though, is Grandma's healing touch, and belief in a remedy is almost as important as the remedy itself.

Although I will address a few effective remedies below, since my experience with herbal remedies is limited, I refer you to the resources I would use myself to increase my knowledge base. These include:

The **American Family Physician**, available free online at:
http://www.aafp.org/online/en/home/publications/journals/afp.html

The **National Center for Complementary and Alternative Medicine**, free online at: http://nccam.nih.gov/

The **Alternative Medicine Foundation**, featuring hundreds of books and references, online at: http://www.amfoundation.org/herbinfo.htm

What follows is a discussion of the health benefits of certain plants and other natural remedies, and the scientific evidence in support of their use.

Cranberries

Cranberries and cranberry juice have long been touted as effective for treatment of urinary infections. *But are they?*

This is one of the many questions the Cochrane Collaboration has set out to answer. Though not involved in original research themselves, they pool data from research others have done, and try to give the best unbiased answer available.

Because cranberries are known to produce a substance that prevents certain bacteria from adhering to the bladder wall, theoretically eating cranberries could prevent or cure urinary infections. After reviewing 10 studies of 1049 participants the results are in: yes, the ingestion of cranberry juice or capsules can decrease the frequency of recurrent bladder infections in women. However, cranberries do not seem as effective in the elderly (male and female), nor in those who require a catheter.

Also, the Cochrane group concluded there were no good studies that assessed whether the ingestion of cranberries could treat an established urinary tract infection. They may help, they may not. In my clinical experience, I have seen simple bladder infections resolve with the combination of cranberry juice plus increased consumption of fluids. I have not, however, seen kidney infections or severe bladder infections resolve with this regimen. I have also seen women cure their own cystitis (bladder infection) with increased fluids alone. Drinking a gallon of water daily at the first hint of infection is sometimes sufficient to ward off a full-blown infection.

Today's standard of care for urinary tract infections is antibiotics. However, with bladder infections so common, when antibiotics are unavailable alternate therapies become vital, and the use of cranberries to prevent cystitis may be your best option.

Echinacea

The most common infection known to man is the common cold – and everyone knows there is no cure. But could an herb decrease the frequency of colds, or perhaps make them resolve a little sooner?

Echinacea has been studied for both the prevention and treatment of the common cold. Many different preparations using various species of *Echinacea* are already on the market, so should you invest in a stockpile?

The trials that studied whether *Echinacea* prevents colds showed no clear benefit. However, research regarding its effectiveness after the onset of cold symptoms suggests that preparations made from the herb of *Echinacea purpurea* may be effective in adults, whereas those made from the root do not seem to be. To date there is no clear evidence of benefit in children.

Every doctor has patients who seem to get over a cold in no time, and others in whom symptoms linger for weeks. If you are in the latter group, taking *Echinacea* (herb, not root) at the first sign of a cold may help shorten the duration and severity of symptoms. For those who seem to have superior immune systems, little benefit would be gained.

Honey

Does pouring honey on a burn sound like good medicine to you? Studies as recent as 2010 yield a surprising affirmative. The results should be enough to turn current medical burn treatment on its head (though I expect it won't.) Still, this is good news for those interested in caring for themselves when no doctor is available.

Honey has been used since antiquity in the care of skin wounds, which ought to count for something, but just because a remedy is well-established as folk medicine (such as the application of excrement to a baby's umbilical cord) does not mean it has documented proof of efficacy (and may, indeed, be harmful).

One recent study[27] compared today's gold standard of burn wound treatment (SSD, or silver sulfadiazine) with honey. Each patient had two or more similar burn wounds, one of which was treated with honey, the other with silver sulfadiazine. Amazingly, the honey-treated wounds not only healed more quickly, but also demonstrated *far* fewer harmful *Pseudomonas aeruginosa* bacteria within the healing wound. Another study[28] showed no bacterial resistance to medical-grade manuka honey among several bacteria that commonly develop antibiotic resistance, including MRSA (methicillin-resistant *S. aureus*). Whereas in the United States honey-impregnated dressings such as MEDIHONEY® are prescribed, elsewhere straight honey is employed. Readily-available clover honey has been used successfully on diabetic wounds in developing countries.

As I typed this section, I managed to burn my arm on a waffle iron. (Don't ask.) What an appropriate time to try a little of my own advice on my 1x3 inch mild second degree burn. Not having silver sulfadiazine at home, I hoped to compare generic bacitracin antibiotic ointment to KFC honey (yes, that's Kentucky Fried Chicken). After one day I could tell no difference and became too

---

[27] Honey compared with silver sulphadiazine in the treatment of superficial partial-thickness burns. *Int Wound J.* 2010 Oct;7(5):413–7.
[28] *Eur J Clin Microbiol Infect Dis.* 2010 Oct;29(10):1237–41.

busy to continue the experiment. The honey certainly caused no harm, and at least for that short a period, worked as well as bacitracin. (This is what scientists call anecdotal evidence – it doesn't prove a thing. Maybe peanut butter would have worked equally well. Best to go by the scientific studies referenced above.)

Another traditional use for honey is to soothe a cough. *But does it really work?* Again, yes, according to the Journal of Alternative and Complementary Medicine.[29] Children suffering from upper respiratory infections were assigned to four different treatment groups. The first received a half teaspoon of honey at bedtime, whereas the others were given either dextromethorphan, diphenhydramine, or no treatment. Those given the honey not only coughed less, but also slept better.

Is there any evidence that honey can be harmful? Certain honeys, such as wild honey obtained from the nectar of Rhododendron species in Nepal, may contain grayanotoxin, which, when ingested, may cause "mad honey poisoning." Symptoms include blurred or double vision, nausea, vomiting, and depressed heart function. A second concern is infants less than a year old, who may develop infant botulism upon ingesting honey, though this is rare.

In summary, honey has been proven effective for the treatment of certain wounds, including burns and some skin ulcers, and for soothing coughs in children with colds – and to do so more effectively than commonly used medications. Although medical-grade honey was used in most of the skin wound studies, standard commercial honey may work just as well. As with other wound dressings, I would suggest changing the dressing every 12 to 24 hours. To avoid contamination of the honey by the wound, it is better to apply the honey directly

---

[29] *J Altern Complement Med.* 2010 Jul;16(7):787–93.

to the dressing, (preferably a Telfa pad or other non-stick dressing), then apply the dressing to the wound.

Maggots

I count myself fortunate to have worked with a wonderful patient who benefitted from maggot therapy. Without her beloved maggots, she would have lost her feet.

This middle-aged woman with insulin-dependent diabetes mellitus had been in the hospital for a prolonged period, and developed pressure ulcers on her heels. These became infected clear down to the bone, with increasingly resistant bacteria. When nothing worked, including new-fangled antibiotic therapy (which caused the doctors to believe she had leukemia, though she didn't), they gave up and started talking amputation instead.

She, of course, was not fond of the idea and did some research on her own. She'd been told that, though maggot therapy had been shown to help chronic ulcers, her wounds were too deep for this to be effective. But, her feet being her own, she insisted the therapy be tried anyway. Medical maggots were obtained and applied to her ulcerated heels. Lo and behold, they cleared away the dead tissue and her feet began to improve. Months later, the wounds were closed, and the maggots had prevented the amputation her doctors had recommended (again illustrating that doctors don't know everything).

Maggots have long been used to perform rapid wound debridement, that is, to remove dead and dying tissue from soft tissue injuries. The use of maggots is also associated with the elimination of infection, decreased pain, and less odor. Wounds contaminated with resistant strains of *E. coli* and *staph* (including

MRSA) are sometimes curable with therapeutic myiasis (larval/maggot therapy) when antibiotic treatment has failed.

The benefits of maggot therapy were first noted in infected battlefield wounds. Soldiers who may have felt themselves doomed upon finding maggots feasting on their injured limbs actually did better than those whose wounds were spared the repulsive creatures. Anecdotal reports include using larval treatment for a variety of wounds including leg ulcers, bone infection, soft tissue infection, burns, pressure sores, and diabetic ulcers. The maggots not only consume necrotic tissue, thereby removing debris that may block the growth of healthy tissue, but also secrete chemicals that decrease or stop the growth of many types of bacteria.

Currently, larval therapy employs maggots raised specifically for the purpose. For cosmetic reasons, maggot therapists may cover the wound being treated with a containment bag that adheres to the adjacent normal skin. However, in a catastrophic scenario these will not be available, but you should be able to improvise a similar covering with little difficulty.

Medical maggots are the larvae of the common green bottle fly (*L. sericata*), the first insect to visit most corpses. Time of death may be estimated by their presence and life cycle (but that's another story). The fly is present worldwide, especially in warm, moist climates, and it is certainly possible to capture this insect during warm months and harvest its larvae for medical use.

Most conditions for which medical maggots would be employed are chronic conditions – open wounds that are not healing, such as injuries, burns, and pressure ulcers. Allowing a common green bottle fly to have access to such a wound and lay her eggs in it is one treatment option. Alternatively, the maggots may be harvested from a secondary source, for example, a piece of raw meat purposely exposed to green bottle flies. When the maggots hatch, from 8 to 72 hours later (depending on humidity and temperature), they may be transferred to the wound, where they may be left in place for about three days.

My patient who underwent maggot therapy advised keeping the wound sufficiently moist; otherwise the maggots die prematurely. A spray from a bottle of water or a drop of water periodically is sufficient. The wound does not necessarily need to be covered. After three days, the wound may be gently washed with clean water and the process repeated as needed. Necrotic tissue appears black or dark, and lacks the healthy pink of fresh and healing tissue. When the tissue is free of pus and appears a healthy pink, the job is done. Don't worry about the maggots turning into flies in the wound – the larval stage takes 4–8 days to complete, followed by a pupation period of 6–14 days before new flies emerge.

Other maggots may work equally well, but those of the common green bottle fly have been studied. If a wound becomes infested with maggots of an unknown type, it is probably fine to follow the treatment protocol above, at least for a few days. If the unknown maggots are achieving the desired goal, all is well. If you keep "spent" maggots in a ventilated jar and allow the pupae to reach adulthood, you can determine which sort of fly has been involved.

If standard medical care is unavailable, I would consider maggot therapy for the following conditions: burns skin deep or deeper, pressure ulcers (but remember treatment *must* include avoiding pressure to the ulcerated area), ragged wounds that have not been sutured (such as bites, gouges, deep scrapes), or any open wound that does not heal. One type of wound that will not permanently resolve with maggot therapy is an ulcerating skin cancer, which you probably won't be able to diagnose. That does not preclude maggot therapy, however. If you try this treatment and the wound improves but does not heal, a doctor may be able to excise the entire area, then close the new wound with sutures.

Fecal Transplant

What could be worse than maggot therapy? *How about eating feces?*

In recent years *C. diff*, or antibiotic-related colitis, has emerged as a major cause of recurrent diarrhea, especially in chronically ill patients who require frequent antibiotics. These patients have difficulty re-establishing the normal flora (normal bacteria) that live in the colon. One way to correct this problem is to transplant feces (poop) from one person to another. At least in the hands of a skilled operator, this procedure has a 90% cure rate.

How is this accomplished? Currently, the feces donor (preferably a spouse or close relative) is screened for HIV, hepatitis, and other potentially infectious diseases. The donor poo is collected, mixed in a blender with enough salt water to yield the desired consistency, then transferred to the donee either through an NG tube through the nose to the stomach, or via an enema. Administering the dose (several tablespoons) from above (via NG tube) usually provides a cure with a single dose. Enemas also work, but often require multiple repeat dosing.

If I were going to attempt this treatment without the benefits of modern medicine, I would first diagnose the condition as best I could. *C. diff* usually occurs during or shortly after a round of antibiotics, producing diarrhea with a particularly offensive odor. Hospital nurses are great at identifying the smell. Some patients have no symptoms beyond diarrhea, but many complain of abdominal pain, and some experience weakness and dehydration. Frail patients can certainly die from this infection. *C. diff* does not respond well to standard anti-diarrheal medication, which is *not* advisable with this infection. Another tip-off to the condition is diarrhea that at first seems like a typical intestinal virus, but then does not resolve within a few to several days, as would be expected of simple stomach flu.

Unless I had a patient demanding to undergo oral administration, I would pursue the enema route. (Of course, a nasogastric (NG) tube can be placed without any fancy equipment. If an NG tube is on hand, and a doctor or nurse familiar with insertion is available, then this is an option. Keep in mind, though, that the procedure may cause gagging, and you certainly don't want your patient to aspirate feces into his lungs, which is likely to produce a pneumonia worse than the *C. diff* infection you are hoping to cure.)

I would do my best to find the healthiest donor, preferably a spouse or other relative sharing the same home. The stool may be collected in a bowl, and stored in the refrigerator pending administration. Rather than contaminate your blender, consider smashing the feces with a fork or whisk while adding a little water to achieve a pudding-like consistency. A few lumps won't matter, as long as they are small enough to be administered with an enema bottle. If this is unavailable, any squirt-type bottle (such as a mustard bottle) may suffice. Squeeze a few ounces of the mix into the rectum, and have the patient try to retain the fluid as long as possible. Enemas often trigger a bowel movement or diarrhea, so be prepared. Repeat the procedure about every 2 days for up to several times. *Do not* force the liquid in under pressure – you don't want to puncture the colon or cause a perforation, which *will* kill your patient (unless you can perform abdominal surgery and administer I.V. antibiotics).

Neither I nor any doctor I know has actually used this treatment on a patient, but the concept is a simple one. Personally, I'd hope to have either metronidazole or vancomycin available. Still, the docs who advocate this treatment have used it on patients in whom these standard medications have been ineffective. A fecal transplant may sound like a last-ditch effort, but it may be the most viable option in a difficult future.

Probiotics

Diarrhea is rarely fatal in itself, but the dehydration that accompanies it may be lethal, especially in infants and children. Because acute diarrhea may be caused by many types of infection, most of which are viral, antibiotic therapy is not usually effective.

As part of the diarrheal syndrome, healthy/helpful bacteria may be eliminated from the gut. *Does reintroducing these normal, helpful bacteria shorten the length of diarrhea?* The Cochrane Collaboration reviewed 63 trials including 8014 people and found:

1. No bad side-effects of probiotics
2. Shorter duration of diarrhea in those who took probiotics (about 25 hours less)
3. Reduced number of bowel movements in those on probiotics (one less BM per day)

Probiotics are sold in health food stores, drug stores, even supermarkets, in a variety of formulations. *Which is best?* Doctors don't yet have the answer, and there is no standardization as to what these remedies must contain. Probiotic treatment is not life-saving, but feeling better a day sooner may be worth it for you or your children. Trying them out now while they are readily available over-the-counter may help you decide whether it's worth purchasing a supply for future use.

Special Populations

The majority of this book deals with adult care, from the late teenage years through an age of about seventy. Much of the information applies to people of all ages, but certain populations deserve special attention regarding medication concerns, in particular children, pregnant women, and the elderly.

Children are not little adults. Their metabolism is accelerated, their growth or maturing organs may be altered by drugs, they may not recognize worrisome side-effects, they often respond to medicines quite differently than adults, and they have less leeway for dosing errors, especially infants. Although scaled-down dosages can often be approximated based on age, this rule does not apply for all drugs, and dosage based on weight is preferable. For the most part I have not indicated pediatric dosing, and refer the reader to readily available pediatric dosing recommendations in product inserts, the Physicians' Desk Reference® (PDR®), or pediatric textbooks.

Approximate pediatric dosing for many medications

Ages 12 years and above	Full adult dose
Ages 6–11 years	One-half adult dose
Ages 2–5 years	One-fourth adult dose
Under age 2 years	One-eighth adult dose

Best to consult a pediatric text for correct dosing of infants, per weight.

Likewise, when treating a pregnant (or potentially pregnant) woman, remember that any drug or other treatment you advise may have an effect on the unborn infant. Some drugs can cause birth defects (for example, the ACE-inhibitors, used for high blood pressure), or permanently stain developing teeth (the tetracycline drugs), or cause miscarriage or induce labor (misoprostol). Again, when administering a drug to a pregnant female it is always best to first check a pharmacology reference such as the PDR® or *Drugs in Pregnancy and Lactation: A Reference Guide to Fetal and Neonatal Risk* by Briggs, Freeman, and Yaffe. Of the over-the-counter preparations, those that are generally recognized as safe include: acetaminophen, chlorpheniramine, pseudoephedrine, Kaopectate, Maalox, Tums, Mylanta, Tagamet, Pepcid, and Zantac. An abundance of free, reliable information is available on the subject at the American Family Physician Web site at www.aafp.org.

The elderly present additional challenges regarding medication dosing. Metabolism slows as we age, and as liver and kidney function decline, the rate at which drugs are eliminated from the body slows. Even half the normal adult dose of a medication may produce drowsiness, disorientation, change in blood pressure or heart rate, urinary retention, constipation, or a myriad of other symptoms. Additionally, the elderly are often taking multiple other drugs which may react badly with any new medication. The rule for treating the elderly is to start low and go slow. If a low dose is tolerated, the amount can always be increased if needed.

I often tell my patients that every medicine is a potential poison. Although doctors must base treatment on how the majority of humans respond to a specific medication, we all remain individuals, and treatment must be individualized. This is where the art of medicine meets science, and a careful observer can spell the difference between success and disaster.

Listen to what patients say – they often lead you to the correct answer. Ignoring their input will greatly limit your potential as a healer.

SECTION NINE

Special Topics

Chapter 31

Chernobyl, Nuclear Fallout, and You

Beyond government advice

You've taken precautions, retreated to your underground bunker, complete with a supply of potassium iodide and enough food and water for a year. In yesterday's terrorist attack the targets were not high-rise and government buildings – 9/11 was only a practice run. This time nuclear power plants across the country were struck, resulting in a dozen simultaneous disasters. News service is spotty at best, and you're pretty sure it's been censored. Do you dose your children with potassium iodide now, or wait for health officials to give the word?

With the 2011 nuclear disaster in Japan, U.S. awareness of potential exposure to radioactive fallout has skyrocketed. Suppliers ran out of potassium iodide (KI) tablets within days. People who had little clue as to its actual benefit bought it anyway, assuming the miracle pills would protect them from all harm.

Doctors across America visited the CDC Web site to update their knowledge base, as worried patients sought reassurance. If you've read the official recommendations yourself, you may have noticed that they assume a controlled disaster, one in which the government is there for us, with communication intact and doctors readily available to advise patients. But what if you're simply on your own?

Before moving to the next level, let's review the problem and current advice.

As part of a nuclear event, radioactive iodide (I-131) is likely to contaminate the atmosphere, first locally, then distributed by prevailing winds. Humans (and animals) will be at risk for inhaling or ingesting the radioactive iodide. Although very high dosage may threaten the body as a whole, the primary concern with typical exposure is the thyroid. About a third of the radioactive iodide that enters the entire body will accumulate in the thyroid, where iodide is needed to manufacture thyroid hormone. With so much radioactivity concentrated in an area smaller than a chicken egg, the exposure in the thyroid gland may be hundreds to thousands of times higher than elsewhere in the body. The end result may be thyroid cancer, between 3 and 10 years down the line, especially in young children.

Flooding the thyroid *pre-exposure* with normal iodide slows the gland's subsequent absorption and resultant concentration of both normal and radioactive iodide for at least a day, meaning even if you are exposed, the amount of radioactivity localized within the gland will not increase to potentially dangerous levels. However, even potassium iodide cannot protect your body from radiation sickness due to a massive radiation dose, nor can it prevent radioactive iodide from entering your body in the first place. Nor does it protect against any other radioactive isotope. Post-exposure, potassium iodide administration is futile. It will not "dilute" the radioactive iodide already concentrated in the thyroid nor will it reverse any damage that has already occurred.

With this in mind, the CDC recommends taking potassium iodide only on the advice of public health officials or your doctor. They seem to assume these resources will always be available. However, that assumption seems a bit naïve. If communication is disrupted, how will you get word? The online radiation counter monitoring radiation levels in your locale may not be there to assist you (see www.radiationnetwork.com).

If you're concerned about radiation exposure, it makes sense to purchase a home Geiger counter *now* (available online for $200–1200). Don't plan on waiting until the next nuclear threat. Within a week of Japan's March 2011 tsunami and nuclear plant breaches, both potassium iodide and Geiger counters had disappeared from both retail suppliers *and* wholesalers as well!

There are only three U.S. manufactures of potassium iodide, all of whom sell to the public. Any of the products may be used for any age. The pills may be split to achieve a lower dose. The accompanying chart shows the available products and Web sites.

Company	Product	Web site
Anbex, Inc., Williamsburg, Virginia	Iosat Tablets (130 mg)	http://www.anbex.com
Recipharm AB, Jordbro, Sweden	ThyroSafe Tablets (65 mg)	http://www.thyrosafe.com
Fleming & Company Pharmaceuticals, Fenton, Mo.	ThyroShield Solution (65 mg/mL)	http://www.thyroshield.com

Our current recommendations for potassium iodide administration are based on the post-Chernobyl cases of thyroid cancer in radiation-exposed children. The incidence of thyroid cancer increased between 30- and 100-fold in children under the age of 4 years, in a dose-dependent fashion.

The following chart outlines FDA-recommended dosing for potassium iodide (KI) according to age and group, if the product is administered.

Group	Predicted Thyroid Exposure (cGy)	Dose
Adults over age 40 years	Only treat if over 500	130 mg
Adults over 18 through 40 years	≥10	130 mg
Pregnant or lactating women	≥5	130 mg
Adolescents, adult-size (>150 lb)	≥5	130 mg
Adolescents over 12 through 18 years (<150 lb)	≥5	65 mg
Children over 3 years through 12 years	≥5	65 mg
Children over 1 month through 3 years	≥5	32 mg
Birth through 1 month	≥5	16 mg

Notice that the chart says *predicted* thyroid exposure. As long as public health officials are available to supply this information, all's fine and dandy. But lacking that, how will you decide and what should you do? Once started, how long should you take the medication and how will you know when it's safe to stop? What if you already have thyroid disease? This is where you must weigh the potential benefits versus the potential hazards.

What are the drawbacks of taking potassium iodide anyway? Again, the Chernobyl experience provides valuable information. According to the FDA's

Guidance report (see **Resources**, at end of chapter) over 10.5 million Polish children (under age 16) and 7 million Polish adults received at least one dose of potassium iodide. That's a larger cohort than any pharmaceutical company is ever going to study. Side-effects were considered generally mild and not clinically significant. Up to 2% of children experienced some gastrointestinal distress, which was thought to be due to the bad taste of SSKI (saturated solution of potassium iodide). About 1% of both adults and children experienced a rash, and only two individuals were noted to have an allergic reaction, both in adults known to have iodine sensitivity. A minimal risk of transiently depressed thyroid function is also possible, but no clinically relevant harm was noted.

In summary, the risk of a single dose of KI is quite small. Pregnant women, nursing mothers, and those with underlying thyroid disease are recommended to take a single initial dose, with subsequent dosing determined in conjunction with a physician (if possible). Others are advised to continue the recommended daily dose until the risk is passed.

Again we're back to the question, how does one decide for oneself if/when the government is not there to advise? The only answer is to have a way of measuring radiation exposure yourself, using personal dosimeters, rate meters, and possibly a Geiger counter (all available for purchase online). Any increase above background levels may indicate an impending exposure. Since even very low levels of radiation may lead to cancer in children, you cannot wait until levels skyrocket to initiate treatment. A doubling of background levels today may predate a 100-fold increase tomorrow. When the risk is high, it is better to be safe than sorry. Since a single dose of potassium iodide offers very little likelihood of harm, and since *not* taking it may lead to childhood thyroid cancer,

I would err on the side of administering the first dose to children and pregnant women, reassessing the need for additional doses on a daily basis.

Remember that radioactive iodide may be both inhaled and ingested. Contaminated plants (and animals who eat them) should not be used for food for at least 2–3 months after radiation levels have dropped. (See the resources below for specifics.)

Regarding continued administration of potassium iodide, are there any risks? If exposure to radioactive iodide continues for days, or weeks, or months, should you continue giving KI to your children or take it yourself? To date, there is little data regarding this question. Nuclear accidents and explosions have been isolated events, with a rapid decline in radiation levels. For on-going exposure, the dose of KI will need to be repeated every day or two.

The short answer is, yes, there are risks. Gastrointestinal disturbances would likely increase in number, as would the incidence of minor rashes. Some individuals may experience inflammation of the salivary glands.

The biggest concern is transient hypothyroidism, which is reversible and of little concern in older children and adults. However, in neonates even short-term lack of sufficient thyroid hormone (a few to several weeks) may result in permanent intellectual impairment. The current recommendation is to monitor KI-treated infants closely for the development of hypothyroidism, instituting thyroid replacement therapy if the TSH level increases. (Refer to entry on **Thyroid Disease** for a more detailed explanation. In brief, serum thyroid stimulating hormone (TSH) increases with low thyroid and decreases with high thyroid conditions.) If society collapses, there is little likelihood you'll be able to determine your child's TSH level. Therefore, treating infants who take KI beyond several days presumptively with levothyroxine is a consideration, which would normally be accomplished with close monitoring of serum TSH and thyroid hormone levels, under the care of a pediatric endocrinologist. Hypothyroid children are treated with the approximate dosing in the table below, using divided and crushed levothyroxine tablets. Times will have to be desperate indeed for parents to undertake this on behalf of their child.

Synthroid (levothyroxine) dose for pediatric hypothyroidism

Age	Daily Dose in mcg/kg/day
0–3 months	10–15
3–6 months	8–10
6–12 months	6–8
1–5 years	5–6
6–12 years	4–5
Over 12 years but still growing	2–3
Over 12 years, growth completed	1.7

(The above information is summarized from the Synthroid product insert available at: http://www.rxabbott.com/pdf/Synthroid.pdf. Note dosing is in micrograms, not milligrams.)

This brings up the question regarding alternatives to prolonged KI therapy. I have not seen the topic addressed in the medical literature, but theoretically, taking full-dose thyroid replacement therapy (approximately 100–200 micrograms, or 0.1–0.2 milligrams, daily, for adults) should turn off the thyroid's production of hormone and possibly decrease the absorption of iodide. Levothyroxine has been used successfully in patients *without* thyroid disease as an adjunct in the treatment of depression. In these patients, doctors monitor for suppression of TSH to avoid iatrogenic *hyper*thyroidism. These patients with normal thyroid functioning who take levothyroxine (for depression) seem to do quite well at replacement-level doses, and thyroid function returns to normal levels when medication is discontinued. (The usual concerns regarding initiating thyroid replacement therapy in the elderly and special populations would apply, and are beyond the scope of this book. In brief, elderly patients are started at approximately one-quarter the total daily dose, and gradually increased to full dose over 2–3 months.) Determining whether treating babies (exposed to prolonged radioactive iodide) with levothyroxine is effective in preventing thyroid cancer is a study that will never be done (unless widespread nuclear catastrophe strikes).

A second possible alternative is kelp. It is known that ingestion of a high-iodide diet can induce reversible hypothyroidism, and so it is theoretically possible to prevent absorption of radioactive I-131 by ingesting kelp (harvested before a nuclear event). Correct dosing is difficult to advise, but if it's the only option available, it is a consideration.

As for patients who already suffer thyroid dysfunction, little if any problem is expected to occur with a single dose of KI, although repeat doses beyond a few consecutive days may cause thyroid function to decrease (or possibly increase, especially in hyperthyroid patients). Normally, under current conditions, any thyroid patient taking potassium iodide beyond a few days should have their TSH (thyroid stimulating hormone) monitored, but again, this will not be possible in a truly widespread catastrophe. For a prolonged situation, thyroid patients may want to dose themselves once or twice a week instead of daily. One thing to keep in mind is that most people, especially adults, exposed to I-131 do *not* develop thyroid cancer.

Potential thyroid cancer may be the least of our concerns if our food supply, water supply, and national security are threatened. Having potassium iodide available is really only a small part of medical prepping. People die quickly of dehydration, pneumonia, influenza, tetanus, rabies, cholera, diphtheria, smallpox, polio, trauma, hypothermia – these don't take years to develop. Do get a supply of potassium iodide, just in case. But in your medical prepping, focus on the long list of potentially lethal, common, preventable, and curable conditions.

A full treatise on radioactive iodide exposure is beyond the scope of this book, but many free references are available online, as listed below.

ADDITIONAL FREE RESOURCES

Potassium Iodide (KI) Key Facts

http://emergency.cdc.gov/radiation/ki.asp

Guidance: Potassium Iodide as a Thyroid Blocking Agent in Radiation Emergencies

http://www.fda.gov/downloads/Drugs/GuidanceComplianceRegulatoryInformation/Guidances/ucm080542.pdf

Frequently Asked Questions about a Radiation Emergency

http://emergency.cdc.gov/radiation/pdf/emergencyfaq.pdf

Nuclear War Survival Skills – free online book

http://www.oism.org/nwss/s73p904.htm

Chapter 32

Bioterrorism

If you visit American city,

You will find it very pretty.

Just two things of which you must beware:

Don't drink the water and don't breathe the air.

- Tom Lehrer, lyrics to "Pollution"

The CDC Web site lists over two dozen potential biological agents on its bioterrorism Web site, along with national and local plans to ensure the safety of U.S. citizens, should an attack occur.[30] Naturally these plans assume a functioning federal government, coordinated health care system, and nationwide communication.

The real question is: *what can you do yourself to prepare for when the government is crippled and chaos descends?*

Personally, I doubt that biological assault will play a large role in post-Armageddon medicine. An epidemic or biologic poison may wreak havoc in the short-term, but in weeks or months (or perhaps years) things will settle down, and the usual maladies will be the norm. Neither plague nor smallpox will last

---

[30] CDC, Bioterrorism Agents, at: http://emergency.cdc.gov/agent/agentlist-category.asp

forever. Better to know how to treat hundreds of common conditions than worry about a few unlikely diseases.

Still, if you're reading this book, you're looking to prepare for both Armageddon and beyond, and no doubt want to protect your family to the best of your ability from every possible threat. Asking your personal physician for advice is not likely to yield much useful information, so let's dig in with a logical approach to what you may encounter.

Bioterrorism is not a single entity. It includes the purposeful dissemination of highly contagious diseases (such as smallpox and hemorrhagic fevers), weaponization of microbes which ordinarily cause little disease in humans (anthrax), distribution of biologic poisons (such as ricin or botulinum toxins), food safety threats (*E. coli*, *Salmonella*, and *Shigella*), and waterborne illnesses (cholera and *Cryptosporidium*). The causative organisms are invisible to the naked eye and therefore undetectable without special equipment. Most of these conditions will not be recognized until someone has succumbed.

The CDC categorizes these threats further according to priority, with the most dangerous and easily disseminated agents listed as Category A (anthrax, botulism, plague, smallpox, tularemia, viral hemorrhagic fevers), lesser threats as Category B (food and water threats, brucellosis, psittacosis, Q fever, ricin and epsilon toxins, glanders, melioidosis), and potential future threats as Category C (emerging infectious diseases). Of these deadly diseases, most people are only aware of the bioweapon potential of anthrax, plague, and smallpox, and most physicians have not treated even a single case of any of them.

Bioterrorist agents do not come with labels attached. Diarrhea from intentional food poisoning from *Salmonella* will look very much like diarrhea from accidental exposure. *How are you going to tell the difference? How would your local health department distinguish the two?*

As with outbreaks of any disease, the answer lies in **patterns of illness**. A single case of botulism is an oddity. Two *may* be coincidence; three is an epidemic – or bioterrorism – until proven otherwise. Your local health department would search for unusual clusters of illness related by time, location, age group, or symptoms. If society falls apart, this job may fall to you.

Before moving on to specific symptoms and diseases, the role of prevention should be reiterated. Review **Chapter Six**, which covers medical quarantine and isolation. These measures should help guard against highly contagious microbes such as smallpox, plague, and viral hemorrhagic fevers. Second, safeguard your food and water supplies. Make sure both are protected from human fecal contamination. Cook meats, vegetables, seafood, and eggs thoroughly. Boil or sterilize drinking water unless it is clearly safe. Know the source of your water supply and evaluate its vulnerability to airborne contamination. Stockpile bottled water for emergency use.

Bioterrorism – Free Download

Diagnosis and Management of Foodborne Illnesses,

A Primer for Physicians and Other Health Care Professionals

http://www.cdc.gov/mmwr/preview/mmwrhtml/rr5304a1.htm

Also, bioterrorists are likeliest to strike areas of dense population, or target individuals in positions of authority or national defense. Joe Smith in the boondocks is unlikely to be on the radar. Do what you can to live similarly, and keep quiet about your location and preparations.

Next, educate yourself regarding specific entities. For purposes of this discussion, we will look to possible real-life scenarios.

An outbreak of a blistering rash

> *Three young men and one older gentleman in your group have fallen ill with what initially looked like the flu – fever, headache, body aches, and fatigue. You isolated them according to protocol, and so far, no one else has fallen ill. On the third day, one patient notices red spots in his mouth, which the others develop a day or two later. Over the next few days, they all develop a rash, starting as spots on the face, then moving to the arms and legs. Their fevers drop and each feels a little better as the red spots become red bumps, then fluid-filled blisters.*
>
> *It's only chicken pox! – one mother cries with relief. Or is it? Is there anything suspicious about this situation?*

It would be very odd for four adults to fall ill with a common childhood disease. Most adults should be immune to chicken pox. Could each have somehow missed the disease years ago? Since the children have all been vaccinated against chicken pox, will they be spared? Is there anything else all four have in common?

This is where you'll have to do some detective work. They all appear to have the same infection, but when and where did it originate? Had they travelled anywhere in the days – or weeks – prior to their illness?

Contagious diseases, especially viral illnesses, have an incubation period during which the causative organism multiplies before producing symptoms. If you find no commonality in the last several days, looking back 3–4 weeks should identify most opportunities for simultaneous exposure.

While you're pondering these questions, a fifth person became ill, the young wife of the man who first showed flu-like symptoms. The only other wife, that of the older gentleman, has shown no sign of illness, even though she has insisted on bringing him food on several occasions.

Now the first four are sicker than ever. They're all burning up with fever, and the blisters have turned to hard, pus-filled knots, like BBs under the skin. One young man has started to cough and is having trouble breathing. His chest aches and he's no longer able to eat. One week later he dies. Will the others succumb? Will your entire group?

Anyone who's seen chicken pox will recognize these symptoms as atypical. With chicken pox, hard BB-like bumps do not form, and the pox are concentrated more on the torso than on the arms and legs. Only rarely will anyone die of chicken pox. These symptoms are characteristic of smallpox, which carries a 30% fatality rate.

You maintain strict isolation and are relieved when no one else becomes ill. Over the next two weeks the pustules become covered with scabs, which eventually fall off. Are you out of the woods yet?

You still must discover the origin of the disease. How is smallpox spread? How is it weaponized? How long is it contagious? Is anyone immune? Is there anything you can do to protect your community?

Smallpox is caused by the variola virus, not the varicella virus of chicken pox (pox means spotted). It is a potential bioterrorism agent because there is no effective treatment except vaccination. The aggressive worldwide immunization campaign wiped out smallpox in our country as of 1949, with the last case anywhere occurring in Somalia in 1977. Those of us middle-aged and older still sport the scar of vaccination, a practice discontinued once the disease was successfully eradicated. To the best of medical knowledge, no smallpox virus exists in "the wild" – though laboratory stockpiles remain in the U.S., Russia, and perhaps elsewhere (in the hands of terrorists?)

Normally transmission requires close contact with an infected person during the period of contagion (see chart, next page). It can also be transmitted through fomites, such as bedding or clothing contaminated with viral particles.

Unfortunately, the virus can also be spread through the air within enclosed spaces. Buildings, airplanes, subways, trains, and buses are all potential routes of purposeful exposure. Since the virus is sensitive to sunlight and heat, with at least 90% of the virus dying outdoors within 24 hours, smallpox is unlikely to be an effective outdoor bioweapon. In the hands of a terrorist, aerosolized smallpox would likely be released in a crowded, indoor facility for maximum effect. Should an outbreak occur while the government is yet intact, the CDC plans an organized vaccination program for all potentially exposed persons, with enough vaccine stockpiled for every person within U.S. borders. Details about the vaccine are available at the CDC Web site.[31]

---

[31] Frequently Asked Questions About Smallpox Vaccine, at: http://www.bt.cdc.gov/agent/smallpox/vaccination/faq.asp

Smallpox Symptoms and Contagion

Period	Days	Comments
Incubation period	7–17 days post-exposure	No symptoms and not contagious CDC uses 18-day isolation period for potentially infected individuals
Prodrome	2–4 days	Flu-like illness, sometimes contagious Fever, body aches, headache, fatigue
Initial rash	About 4 days	Most contagious period. Red spots begin in mouth, then head, moving quickly to arms and legs. Spots turn to red bumps, then fluid-filled blisters with a central depression. Unlike chicken pox, which may come in crops over several days, all smallpox lesions develop within a few days.
Pustular rash	About 5 days	Still contagious Pus-filled bumps that feel like a BB under the skin
Scabs and pustules	About 6 days	Still contagious. Scabs starting to form
Resolving scabs	About 6 days	Still contagious. Scabs start to fall off
All scabs gone		No longer contagious. Pitted scars.

With or without the CDC, should a single case be identified in your locale, there are measures you can take to protect yourself. Avoid public gatherings, especially indoors. Avoid public transportation. Quarantine anyone with potential exposure for 18 days before declaring them healthy. Isolate anyone with a fever or flu-like symptoms for a week, observing for development of the typical rash. Do not assume that individuals with a history of vaccination are immune. The vaccine is known to offer effective protection for only 3–5 years, with dwindling immunity thereafter.

In reviewing the history of those ill in your group, you realize that the four initial cases occurred among those who had ventured a trip to the city for supplies. While there, they had come across a lethargic, abandoned child, whom they had carried to a local church.

What will you do when an act of kindness may endanger your entire family? Leaving the ethics of that question for you to decide, the good news is that the four who recovered from smallpox should now be immune. If additional cases are encountered despite your best efforts, these are the most logical care-givers. The older woman who did not succumb despite repeat exposure may have residual or perhaps natural immunity to the disease. In our scenario, she should have been isolated for 18 days to make sure. Anyone pretending to be well who isn't (such as a well-intentioned spouse or parent) could endanger the entire community. Fortunately, your pre-planning and prompt isolation of the infected individuals prevented the spread of smallpox throughout your entire group, and spared the 3 in 10 who would have died a miserable death.

Epidemic regional paralysis

It's a beautiful autumn in NYC. The streets are full of residents and tourists enjoying the brisk fall air and tasty Oktoberfest street fare. With Ground Zero construction progress well underway, the memory of the 2001 terrorist attacks is beginning to fade.

Scanning the local news, you read a blurb about three students admitted to the hospital with what is thought to be Guillain-Barré syndrome. Is this mere coincidence? Each complained of blurred vision and difficulty speaking, followed by trouble breathing. Fortunately, each is in stable, though critical condition on ventilator support.

Over the course of a week the hospitals are flooded with thousands of patients suffering similar complaints. ICUs are running out of respirators. People are beginning to die. It's now headline news and panic is setting in. The CDC has determined this isn't Guillain-Barré syndrome. It's epidemic-level botulism, source unknown, although home-canned and commercially-canned foods have been ruled out.

With new cases occurring every day, people are leaving the city in droves. Though it's not contagious, the common factor has not yet been identified. Should you and your family get out of Dodge?

Have you ever wondered what happened to the 19,000 liters of liquid botulinum toxin the United Nations claims were produced under Saddam Hussein's reign in Iraq? Did you know he got his nasty *Clostridium botulinum* culture for weaponization from the United States?[32] Most everyone has heard about botulism from contaminated canned goods (see **Chapter 23**), but what about the toxin used as a bioweapon?

Botulinum toxin is one of the deadliest in nature and it's not that hard to produce. Simply *don't* follow the rules for proper canning techniques and in a short time you'll have a homemade bioweapon yourself. Ratchet this up a few notches to produce purified toxin (as in Botox) and you're on your way to bioterrorism. The toxin is known to be effective in tainted food and thought to be active as an inhaled aerosol as well.

---

[32] History of Bioterrorism: Botulism, at: http://www2c.cdc.gov/podcasts/player.asp?f=8#transcript.

With sufficient supportive care (including weeks to months on a ventilator) the paralysis of botulism can be overcome. However, a widespread terrorist attack could easily overwhelm current medical resources.

What is the goal of terrorism anyway? Surely terrorists know they cannot stand against the U.S. military. But they are capable of inciting widespread panic and causing our government to divert enormous amounts of money, time, and effort chasing a moving target. How much did it cost to develop and maintain a stockpile of hundreds of thousands of doses of smallpox vaccine for a potential threat that has never been realized?

If there were an outbreak in New York City, health officials would look for a pattern of illness. Homes would be searched for tainted canned goods. Patients would be evaluated for location of residence and employment. Workplaces would be searched. How many personnel would this tie up? How much money would be spent? How many would die in the meantime?

Back to our case history:

> *The epidemic cannot be well-isolated, but seems centered on the island of Manhattan. With numerous but sporadic cases occurring throughout the city, inhaled toxin seems unlikely. No particular neighborhood nor workplace has been implicated.*
>
> *The one thing patients have had in common is purchasing food from various street vendors. With Oktoberfest comes sausage, the original source of botulism. The city shuts down all street vendors selling meat products but still the outbreak continues.*

If one had access to the preformed toxin, how easy would it be to inject a little into bottles or packages of condiments and distribute them randomly throughout the city? Leave a few packets of tainted mustard at every vendor or cafeteria. An evil-minded terrorist could not wipe out the population this way, but he could bring the city to its knees.

In a future without access to intensive medical care, there will be no effective treatment for botulism. Prevention is the only answer. If a foodborne outbreak occurs, avoid public eating places, rely on your personal stockpiles if possible, and make sure to thoroughly heat *all* other food you purchase and consume (as outlined in **Chapter 23**).

Botulism – Free Download

Free 42-page downloadable CDC handbook

Botulism in the United States, 1899 –1996,

Handbook for Epidemiologists, Clinicians, and Laboratory Workers

http://www.cdc.gov/ncidod/dbmd/diseaseinfo/files/botulism.pdf

Epidemic flu syndrome

It's the 4th of July and your family is looking forward to the evening concert, with fireworks to follow. Your wife is afraid of hot ashes falling on the children, but you laugh and insist on being in the midst of the action. It's true, smoke and powdery ashes do fall on the crowd, but that's all part of the fun. Your kids have a great time and your wife breathes a sigh of relief that no one's hair caught fire.

Life returns to normal, however 3–4 days later your kids come down with sore throats, and you feel a little feverish and achy yourself. A summer cold, you suppose, probably caught from the crowd. You take some ibuprofen and go to work anyway. Give it a few days and all will be well.

But it isn't. Over the next few days everyone in the family develops a cough, and your youngest, who has a touch of asthma, says her chest hurts. Your wife takes her to the pediatrician, who diagnoses viral bronchitis. "It's going around," he says. "I've seen dozens of cases just this week." Reassured, your wife picks up a bottle of cough medicine on the way home.

The next day your own chest starts to hurt and you feel a little short of breath as you head for the office. Several co-workers are absent, and word is they have a similar illness. By afternoon you're coughing so hard you decide to leave. Arriving home you find the kids sharing your king-size bed with your wife, all feverish, coughing, and miserable. You carve out a spot for yourself and join them. If things aren't better by morning, you'll go to the doctor.

Things aren't better, in fact they're worse. Your family doctor is home sick herself, so you drag the entire troop to the Urgent Care Center. The parking lot is full, but you decide to wait it out, sheltering your family in a corner of the waiting room where half the occupants are coughing as well.

"It looks like a virus, but I'll give you amoxicillin, just in case," the doctor says after a quick look at everyone. You don't wonder that he's wearing a mask.

"That stuff never works," your wife chimes. "How about a Z-Pak?" The doctor shakes his head, but complies.

Everyone takes their medicine and heads back to bed. You're too achy to sleep and turn on the news. The community-wide illness is the headline story: thirty dead already and hospitals over capacity. The CDC has been called in. Are you safe?

Unless a bioterrorist announces his deeds, this is how things would go. Don't expect your doctor to diagnose infection due to a bioweapon, at least not immediately. Many different organisms can cause the same set of symptoms. How will you know if you have a common flu – or anthrax? What better place to disperse an inhaled bioweapon than in a crowd where powdery debris and clouds of smoke are expected?

Is this anthrax? You won't know without a culture, sophisticated equipment, and someone to use it appropriately. Could it be plague? Or how about tularemia? Can your doctor tell the difference without laboratory testing? (Yes, yes, and doubtful.)

Before microbiology, diagnosis was made based on clinical syndrome. Plague was recognized and feared long before its cause was known. Inhalation anthrax, known as woolsorter's disease, was recognized in the 1800s in mill workers exposed to products from infected animals. Again, pattern of illness is most often the clue to a specific diagnosis.

In the realm of bioterrorism there are three possible basic scenarios: 1) the health care system is sufficiently intact to identify the problem and distribute appropriate vaccination and/or treatment; 2) the system is intact but overwhelmed, leaving many without access to professional care; or 3) the system is broken and you're on your own. If communication breaks down, it doesn't matter if Johns Hopkins has the answer, when you don't yourself.

Discussing every possible bioterrorist scenario would require hundreds of pages. This information is freely available on the CDC bioterrorism Web site,[33] where agent-specific fact sheets on anthrax, botulism, brucellosis, plague, smallpox, tularemia, and viral hemorrhagic fevers are offered for downloading and printing.

Again, quarantine, isolation, safeguarding of food and water supplies, and crowd avoidance are the mainstays of protecting yourself. Beyond that, the table below summarizes treatments for various bioweapons. In cases where antibiotics are effective, treatment is usually started with intravenous therapy, but assuming this option is not available, oral therapy may be effective. Appropriate dosages for children are outlined in detail at the CDC Web site and discussed briefly below.

From the chart (next page) you can see that ciprofloxacin and doxycycline are relied on most heavily, with up to 60 days (120 tabs) of either required per person per incident. For a large family this could approach 1,000 doses of medicine for a single exposure. Even doctors rarely keep this much medication on hand. If you are truly concerned, you'll need to do some serious stockpiling. Fortunately, 60 tablets of either cost as little as $10 at discount pharmacies (if your doctor is willing to prescribe them for you.)

Under ordinary circumstances, neither of these drugs is commonly used in children. Doxycycline can cause permanent discoloration of forming teeth (graying or yellowing), and so is avoided in children less than 8 years old.

[33] Bioterrorism, at: http://emergency.cdc.gov/bioterrorism/

Bioweapon	Preferred adult treatment	Comments
Inhalation anthrax	Ciprofloxacin 500 mg or doxycycline 100 mg twice daily for 60 days (Begin with I.V. therapy, if available)	Oral penicillin, ampicillin, clarithromycin, and clindamycin may be effective as well, but penicillin and ampicillin may induce resistance and should not be used alone.
Botulism	Antitoxin plus intensive medical support including ventilation for weeks to months	Antibiotics ineffective
Brucellosis	Doxycycline 100 mg twice daily plus rifampin 600 mg once daily for 60 days	Treatment for post-exposure prophylaxis is 21 days. Normally only 100–200 cases in USA per year, but higher elsewhere. Avoid eating unpasteurized cheeses, which may transmit infection
Pneumonic plague	Give antibiotics within first 24 hours or death is likely. I.V. streptomycin, gentamicin, doxycycline, ciprofloxacin, or chloramphenicol, if available. Oral meds: ciprofloxacin 500 mg or doxycycline 100 mg twice daily; or chloramphenicol 25 mg per kg, four times daily (10–21 days total) No vaccine yet available	Post-exposure prophylaxis: Oral meds: 7 days of either ciprofloxacin 500 mg or doxycycline 100 mg twice daily; or chloramphenicol 25 mg per kg, four times daily Levaquin, Avelox, tetracyclines are likely effective, and probably TMP-SMX as well
Smallpox	Vaccination	Antibiotics are NOT effective
Tularemia	Preferred: Streptomycin, 1g IM twice daily or gentamicin, 5 mg/kg I.M. or I.V. once daily Doxycycline, 100 mg I.V. or ciprofloxacin 400 mg I.V. twice daily; or chloramphenicol, 15 mg/kg I.V. 4 times daily Oral meds: ciprofloxacin 500 mg or doxycycline 100 mg twice daily; or chloramphenicol 25 mg per kg, four times daily	Post-exposure prophylaxis: Oral meds: 14 days of either ciprofloxacin 500 mg or doxycycline 100 mg twice daily; or chloramphenicol 25 mg per kg, four times daily Levaquin, Avelox, tetracyclines are likely effective, and probably TMP-SMX as well

	Treatment duration Ciprofloxacin – 10 days Doxycycline – 21 days	
Viral hemorrhagic fevers	No cure or treatment Infection causes damage to the vascular system with death due to multi-organ system failure	Usually endemic to a particular area, with infection due to contact with infected animal; however, human-to-human transmission can occur

Ciprofloxacin is rarely used in children under 18 years old due to concern about joint or cartilage damage, though the drug is officially indicated for pediatric use in anthrax post-exposure prophylaxis. In the case of serious illness or exposure, where the expected benefits outweigh the potential risks, pediatric dosing for these medications is as follows:

Doxycycline 2.2 mg/kg (maximum 100 mg) orally twice daily

Ciprofloxacin 15 mg/kg (maximum 500 mg) orally twice daily

What about other methods for reducing transmission? Face masks are effective – IF they are used consistently, meaning *always* when in the presence of any potentially infective individual (and do you necessarily know who is and isn't infective?) Gloves or hand washing (or hand sanitizer) is effective IF done consistently, before touching your nose, mouth, or eyes. Droplet-borne infection may enter through any of these orifices. The eye must be considered part of the respiratory system as well, since the tear ducts drain into the back of the nose. For the third time I'll reiterate that quarantine, isolation, safeguarding of food and water supplies, and crowd avoidance are the mainstays of protecting yourself. Avoiding mosquitoes, fleas, ticks, and animals which may carry these pests will also help avoid vector-borne illnesses.

Lastly, what about the family we left heading for bed after taking azithromycin? Will they live? Not if it's plague, maybe if it's anthrax, possibly if it's tularemia.

Although the "Z-Pak" is usually effective for ordinary infections, azithromycin does not make the preferred list for any bioweapon. Having doxycycline or ciprofloxacin on hand may save your life if the medication is started at the first sign of symptoms during a documented epidemic or immediately upon possible exposure to a susceptible infection. This opposes the usual medical advice to wait a few days to see if your body heals itself. These bioweapons are so deadly that waiting can be the end of you.

With all this said, I'll repeat that I doubt bioterrorism will play a large role in Armageddon medicine. If one does believe in true Armageddon, perhaps one should prepare a defense against prophesied woes of Biblical proportion, or better yet, seek a saving relationship with our Creator.

And the fifth angel sounded, and I saw a star fall from heaven unto the earth: and to him was given the key of the bottomless pit. And he opened the bottomless pit; and there arose a smoke out of the pit, as the smoke of a great furnace; and the sun and the air were darkened by reason of the smoke of the pit. And there came out of the smoke locusts upon the earth: and unto them was given power, as the scorpions of the earth have power. And it was commanded them that they should not hurt the grass of the earth, neither any green thing, neither any tree; but only those men which have not the seal of God in their foreheads. And to them it was given that they should not kill them, but that they should be tormented five months: and their torment was as the torment of a scorpion, when he striketh a man. And in those days shall men seek death, and shall not find it; and shall desire to die, and death shall flee from them.

Revelation 9:1-6 (King James Version)

Additional free resources to download

Bioterrorism Readiness Plan: A Template for Healthcare Facilities at:

http://www.cdc.gov/ncidod/dhqp/pdf/bt/13apr99apic-cdcbioterrorism.pdf

Botulism in the United States, 1899 –1996, Handbook for Epidemiologists, Clinicians, and Laboratory Workers

http://www.cdc.gov/ncidod/dbmd/diseaseinfo/files/botulism.pdf.

General Fact Sheets on Specific Bioterrorism Agents

http://emergency.cdc.gov/bioterrorism/factsheets.asp

SECTION TEN

Toward Becoming a Healer

Chapter 33

How to Take a Medical History

Though you've had no formal training, you've become the de facto medical expert. Birthing and raising four children has given you more practical knowledge than anyone else in your group. People are always coming to you and asking, "What do you think this rash is?" or "What should I do about my headache?" You wish you knew more. A real doctor could do a real physical exam. You feel like you're just guessing at it. You wish someone could teach you how to do a better job.

Every doctor once stood in your shoes – not knowing where to begin. Fortunately, you don't have to be a medical student to learn how to perform a thorough history and physical that will yield useful information for correct diagnosis and treatment.

When faced with a medical problem, the answer is always the same: start with the patient history. Even Dr. House would agree. A student whose headache disappears on the weekends does not have a brain tumor. A drooling lumberjack who's been attacked by a raccoon does not have a stroke, he has rabies.

Doctors are trained to begin with a patient's current complaint and proceed from there, organizing the medical history into manageable sections with a specified order, so nothing is forgotten or omitted.

The **chief complaint (CC)** is the single most important reason a patient is seeing you, in the patient's own words. Appendicitis is a diagnosis, not a complaint. Typical chief complaints include "sore throat," "dog bite," or "chest pain." Of course, patients often complain of multiple problems or injuries. When they stem from a single cause, this is usually listed as the chief complaint, for example, a motor vehicle accident causing multiple lacerations or fractures. Often a patient with an acute problem tries to "tack on" additional concerns they've had for months (a practice you'll soon grow to dislike, if you practice medicine for any length of time). Stay focused on the problem before you, unless the secondary problem is truly urgent or highly relevant. A months-old problem is rarely an emergency and can be addressed at a later time. However, beware that an acute problem may be the impetus driving a patient to seek care for a chronic problem (such as rectal bleeding) that they've been trying to ignore, but which may be more serious in the long run.

Next comes the **HPI**, or **history of present illness**. *When did the problem start? Did it come on all at once or begin gradually? Has the patient had similar symptoms before?* A 10-year history of migraines is less worrisome than the recent onset of incapacitating headaches. *Are the symptoms getting better, worse, or unchanging?* Nearly any problem that is worsening is of more immediate concern. *Does anything relieve the symptoms or make them increase?* Patients with appendicitis usually prefer to remain still, whereas kidney stone patients are often restless. Aspirin may decrease the pain of a broken rib, but will likely worsen a stomach ulcer. Ask about other associated symptoms – a person who can't breathe may not mention a swollen leg, the potential source of a blood clot.

Additional **current medical history** is also relevant. *Is the patient taking any **medications**, and if so, what and why?* This should include both prescription and OTC drugs, including herbal preparations. *Does the patient have any **other known conditions,*** including diabetes, asthma, heart disease, allergies, etc.?

Don't forget to inquire about past medications and reactions. *Does the patient have any **drug allergies** or **intolerances**?* You cannot cure your cousin's pneumonia with amoxicillin if she's highly allergic to it. Oral corticosteroids will not alleviate your nephew's asthma if they always make him vomit. Don't forget to ask about other allergies, in particular those to stinging insects, which may cause life-threatening anaphylaxis.

The **past medical history** (PMH) may seem irrelevant in a patient with a straightforward complaint, but what if you learned that the spelunker scratched by a rabid bat had already undergone pre-exposure vaccination? You'll be happier to reassure him that he's immune than hand him a death sentence. A patient with emphysema may simply be in his normal state of health if he huffs and puffs climbing the stairs, whereas in a recent trauma victim this may signal a blood clot or collapsed lung. Much of the time doctors can determine the diagnosis and likely course of treatment even *before* examining the patient, especially when they ask the right questions.

The past medical history should include several sub-sections. **Travel history** is vital. Even as I write, travelers from Japan are being screened for radioactivity. Adopting a child from Haiti will require pre-testing for TB, typhoid, worms, hepatitis, malaria, and syphilis. *Could your recently arrived patient be unknowingly harboring cholera that may threaten your entire community?* Although heartburn is usually caused by acid reflux, a patient's **occupational history** may lead to a different diagnosis in a sword swallower.

Always inquire about prior **surgery**. A carpenter may fail to mention his childhood appendectomy, but it certainly matters when he's doubled over with abdominal pain. A grandmother on the brink of coma may revive with a little levothyroxine, once you've uncovered her thyroidectomy of 20 years ago. A pregnant mother with three prior Cesarean sections may be at risk for uterine rupture if she goes into labor. It is easy to miss a scar on physical exam if it's hidden in a skin fold or covered by hair.

Hospitalizations for problems other than surgery are also relevant. An asthmatic who's been hospitalized a dozen times is in a different ballpark from someone who wheezes a little when holding a cat. A depressed patient with a history of electroconvulsive shock therapy is at much greater risk of suicide than someone who's never missed a day of work.

Recreational drug use includes tobacco, alcohol, caffeine, marijuana, cocaine, crack, LSD, methamphetamine, and certain prescription/street drugs. An alcoholic or drug-dependent patient may become unexpectedly violent if protracted vomiting precludes imbibing, thus triggering withdrawal symptoms.

An **immunization history** is vital for the safety of both the patient and his or her caregivers. In 2010, anyone presenting with a cough, fever, body aches, and chills was diagnosed with H1N1 influenza – unless they'd already been immunized against it, in which case bronchitis or pneumonia would be more likely. If you accidentally stick yourself with a blood-contaminated needle, you'll find your interest in your patient's immune status skyrockets.

Family history often helps determine a patient's risk status. If four generations of relatives have all died at age 40 of a heart attack, your 38-year-old patient has significant cause for concern. The medical status of non-blood relatives is also important. I wouldn't have suspected AIDs in my patient with thrush had I not been informed her ex-husband was HIV positive.

If a patient is unknown to you, his or her **social history** may well be relevant. Are they living alone? Is there anyone to help out? Will they die of exposure while you're focusing on ulcer symptoms? Patients do not exist in isolation. We are all dependent on our family, friends, and environment for food, shelter, and emotional support.

In a straightforward case, acquiring the needed medical history may take only a few moments. In a complicated situation, or one where communication is compromised, it could take half an hour or longer, and need to be re-visited several times throughout the course of an illness. Always keep an open mind; you may not have every piece to the puzzle.

Chapter 34

How to Perform a Physical Exam

You've labored over the patient's history, documenting every burp, hiccup, and BM. After an hour of questioning, you still have no idea why this patient's stomach is hurting so badly. Maybe a real doctor could decipher the problem, but you admit you have no clue. Your patient is sick of your inquiries and begs for relief. Should you give a shot of morphine and hope for the best? (Not that you have any morphine, anyway.) Will your first real patient die before your very eyes? Are you a total failure as a healer?

Although a physician can often make the correct diagnosis based on history alone, this is not always possible. Of the remaining cases, the majority can be determined by performing a careful **physical examination**. More often than not, medical testing is simply to confirm what the doctor already suspects, not to make the specific diagnosis. At least half the time labs and X-rays make little difference in a patient's outcome (and my suspicion is the number is closer to 90%).

Most non-professionals would be surprised to hear a doctor claim that a layman can learn to perform a satisfactory physical examination. But please realize, you're not starting from ignorance: you already know what normal is, at least in a general sense. *The* most important aspect of performing a physical examination is differentiating the abnormal from normal. When encountering a medical problem, doing a physical exam should be the *second step* in determining the best course of action or therapy. The first step is *always* to obtain the best history that time permits, as outlined above. The third step is putting it all together to establish a working diagnosis, with the final step being arriving at a plan of action.

When patients come to see their physician for the "annual physical," they seem to think this is something magical. Somehow the doctor will discover a problem of which they're unaware, or that isn't apparent when looking in a mirror. Occasionally this proves true. More often, however, if the patient isn't experiencing symptoms suggestive of a particular problem, the physician will not discover (nor look for) an unsuspected condition.

In current times, a physical examination is often viewed as a health maintenance visit, i.e., a medical encounter aimed at optimizing your current health and preventing future problems (like changing your oil and rotating your tires). Screening tests (such as blood work to assay your cholesterol level, or a PPD test to assess your TB status) might be administered, and advice rendered regarding ideal weight goals or tobacco cessation, along with recommendations regarding updating immunizations and other age-related concerns.

A health maintenance examination would be quite different at the end of the world as we know it. It's too late to get vaccines, cigarettes are hard to come by, and everyone's losing weight on the apocalyptic diet. Rather than advise my patients to avoid red meat and exercise more, I'd be telling them to dress properly, to make sure they had well-fitting shoes, to try to consume enough calories, protein, and vitamins, and to become a fanatic about skin care, the first line of defense against serious infection.

In hard times, physical examinations will be symptom-driven, that is, focused on the affected body part. In a patient with a hacking cough, for example, the condition of the feet might seem irrelevant, but forgetting about them altogether may be a fatal mistake. A 60-year-old woman who complains of a persistent cough may fail to mention that her legs are hugely swollen. Both her cough and swollen legs may be due to congestive heart failure. If time and circumstance allow, it is always best to perform a complete physical examination unless the diagnosis is readily apparent. When my own son was in a motor vehicle accident, he complained of left shin pain, unaware that his opposite femur (thigh bone) was shattered. Paramedics realize that accident victims frequently suffer injuries which patients cannot immediately perceive, and therefore these professionals take extreme care to protect susceptible body parts (such as the neck) until later examination and testing confirm no harm has been sustained.

The first job for a potential healer is to learn to distinguish the normal from the abnormal. The best way to begin is by examining patients who are currently well. Make yourself familiar with the wide range of what is normal in people of various sizes and ages. If you are to be the health care giver in a group, you may think it is a waste of time to examine patients before they become ill, but I can assure you, it is not. Recognizing a patient's current normal anatomy and physiology is a huge advantage when it comes to detecting future abnormalities. Even sick patients usually have most body parts functioning normally, and documenting the normal helps rule out a multitude of conditions. Although the eventual goal of performing a physical examination is to make the proper diagnosis, the immediate goal is first to uncover what is and is not normal, and in what way. After the examination is completed, the pieces of the puzzle can be assembled into a working diagnosis.

Doctors are always learning from their patients. Do swollen legs hurt? You won't find the answer to this in most textbooks. (Sometimes they do, sometimes they don't. It's quite a complex question.) Only exposure to patient after patient will build your knowledge base. Not that book-learning can't help – but hands-on experience builds a deeper level of understanding than books alone can provide.

In making a diagnosis, doctors look for patterns. An older woman with a cough and swollen legs reveals a pattern consistent with congestive heart failure, though numerous other causes exist. A single swollen leg with a cough suggests a blood clot to the lung. In a teenager thrown from a motorcycle, a hugely swollen thigh suggests a fractured femur. A particular finding on examination may alert you to seek another abnormality consistent with a typical pattern of illness or injury, but beware of tunnel vision that may lead you astray or blind you to an alternate diagnosis or additional potential problems. For all these reasons it is best to perform a complete physical examination whenever possible.

Medical students are taught from the beginning to always follow the same routine when performing a physical examination, usually starting at the top and working their way down. This way nothing is omitted or overlooked. Even a cursory exam is better than no exam at all. Reminding yourself to scan the whole patient will shield you from many an error. With these general recommendations as introduction, let us begin.

A **general description** of the patient is always helpful. Whether you are keeping medical records or not, this is a good place to start. *Does the patient look* *generally sick or well? Are they thin or heavy? Are they young or old? Male or female? Active or lethargic? Alert? Thinking clearly? Cooperative?* If you had to identify the person you're describing from a lineup, could you do so from your description?

Doctors use a variety of abbreviations as a shortcut. A few of the more common ones include:

WDWN	well developed, well nourished
WF, WM	white female, white male
BF, BM	black female, black male
AOC	alert, oriented, cooperative
NAD	no acute distress

For example, I would be described as a WDWN WF in NAD – AOC. Be careful to use only standard abbreviations that others can easily understand. (The first time I saw the abbreviation SOB in a medical record, I was appalled, unaware that this stood for "short of breath.")

It may not be so important to keep records if you're only taking care of those in your immediate group, or if you are moving from location to location. But if you'll be remaining in one place and will serve as a resource person for a large population (and if you have the supplies necessary to maintain records), it would be a good idea to write at least a short note to reference in case the patient returns. This not only helps the patient, but also the health care provider, especially when a problem has not resolved with the initial treatment. Often you'll wish you had a better record of what happened before.

Next, will you be doing **vital signs**? If you have a stethoscope and blood pressure cuff you can perform a heart rate, respiratory rate, and blood pressure. Of these, heart rate and respiratory rate are most important and certainly can be measured without any medical equipment, though a watch with a second hand would be nice. If you can feel a good pulse at the wrist or side of the neck, then the pulse rate should equal the heart rate. If you cannot feel the pulse adequately, listening to the heart directly is preferred. This does not require a stethoscope – just put your ear against the patient's chest. If you don't like this idea, buy yourself a couple of inexpensive stethoscopes now.

A normal **heart rate** is about 60 to 100 beats per minute (higher in babies, however – per chart below). If you're going to be the on-going health resource for a group of people, you might want to document a baseline physical exam on everyone before they get sick. A heart rate of 100 may indicate a problem in a person who normally runs only 50; likewise, a pulse of 50 is dangerously low in a newborn whose heart rate should be twice that or more.

Approximate Normal Resting Heart Rate

Age	**Heart rate** (in beats per minute)
Newborns, up to one month	70–190 (usually mid-range)
Infants, one month to one year	80–120
Children, 1–10 years	70–130 (generally decreases with age)
Children age 11 and up; and adults	60–100
Adult well-trained athletes	40–60

Respiratory rate can normally be measured simply by observing a patient breathe. About 10 to 14 breaths per minute is normal in a healthy adult at rest, but will be higher in infants as well as patients with fever, anxiety, heart trouble, breathing difficulties, or a multitude of other problems. Again, establishing a baseline would be ideal.

hypertensive patient. These are ideals, where statistically the least amount of end-organ damage is done (to the heart, kidneys, brain, and circulation). A fair number of older adults need their blood pressure a little higher to prevent dizziness or weakness. If dietary practices change, the population's average blood pressure will drop, due to decreased salt and food intake, increased exercise, and associated weight loss. Treatment goals will need to be modified, with anti-hypertensive medicine possibly reserved for those with extremely high readings. Again, monitoring blood pressure may be more relevant for the patient at risk for low blood pressure, or more specifically, the need for additional fluid intake.

Measuring **height** and **weight** is also often useful, especially for comparison purposes across time. How will you know if your patient has lost weight if it hasn't been recorded? You can't necessarily go by the fit of a person's clothing. In children, height and weight are recorded to assess proper growth and nutrition, especially when appropriate interventions are readily available. If there's no food to be had, however, monitoring a child's slow starvation makes little sense. Tracking height and weight measurements over months and years will probably be a luxury after an Armageddon event. What does make sense, though, is having a scale to assess acute changes. For example, infectious diarrhea may be epidemic, and a change in weight is one of the easiest ways to assess for dehydration. An older-type spring scale or balance scale is preferable to the newer electronic varieties, unless you have an unlimited stock of batteries.

Lastly, get a supply of traditional, mercury thermometers, both oral and rectal. **Temperature** is an exceedingly useful vital sign, and may suggest infection, inflammation, hyperthermia, hypothermia, hyperthyroidism, hypothyroidism, drug reaction, or even good health. The skill of reading a mercury thermometer seems to be a fading art in this digital age. Become an expert before the need arises. If the thermometer is cold, you may not be able to see the mercury on the scale, since it will be condensed into the bulb end. If you cannot determine the temperature, make sure the thermometer is at body temperature before trying to read the result. You may need to tilt the thermometer back and forth in the light a little, until it shimmers into view.

Two other measurements are sometimes included as vital signs: **BMI** and **LMP**. BMI, or body mass index, is currently measured to detect overweight conditions associated with increased body fat, which increase the risk of cardiovascular, neoplastic, and metabolic diseases. In an austere environment, underweight conditions are more likely to be the rule. If the possibility exists for a long-term relationship with a patient, or conditions exists where some useful decision can be determined based on this information, then go ahead and calculate the BMI. Otherwise, it is senseless. To obtain a person's BMI, divide the patient's mass (in kg) by the square of his or her height (in meters). Using pounds and inches, the formula is BMI = [mass (lb) x 703] divided by [height $(in)]^2$. Approximate BMI standards are given in the chart below:

Body Mass Index – BMI	Weight classification
Less than 15	Emaciated
15–18	Underweight
18–24	Normal
25–29	Overweight
30–39	Obese
Greater than 40	Morbidly obese

Generally speaking, it should be obvious if a person is emaciated, so the above adds little useful information. However, if the opportunity exists to both aid and monitor long-term nutritional status, the measurement may be of some value.

Lastly, **LMP** is short for last menstrual period, which is definitely valuable information. If the date is over a month prior, the patient may be pregnant, which might suggest certain diagnoses or raise a caution when using particular medications. If a patient appears pregnant and is encountering a problem, say abdominal pain, the LMP will help guide you to consider relevant conditions, for example labor pains versus intestinal cramping.

Once the general appearance and vital signs have been noted, start at the top and continue downward with your examination.

Head: Examine the shape of the head, the scalp, the hair, and the bones. This is particularly important in trauma victims. *Is the head shaped normally? Is there any deformity or bleeding, any tenderness, bruising, or swelling?* Hematomas ("goose eggs" or blood collections under the skin) are common from blunt trauma, but generally resolve without intervention unless underlying fracture is present. A bone that has any "give" to it is a bad sign (except in an infant with an open fontanel), and probably indicates a skull fracture, with the possibility of current or future brain swelling, which may lead to stroke-like symptoms or even death. Anyone with a skull fracture should be referred to a hospital if at all possible. If a fracture is suspected, pay careful attention to the neurologic exam (see below). For practical purposes, the facial bones should be included as part of the head examination. Tapping over the cheek bones or forehead may reveal tenderness in a patient with sinusitis (inflammation or infection in the sinus cavities).

Although the scalp and hair may be considered part of the skin exam, these findings are often noted under head examination. *Is the hair normal or perhaps thinning, broken off near the scalp (as in scalp fungus), or infested with lice or nits? Is the skin normal, or flaky (as in psoriasis, eczema, or seborrhea), or red, or bumpy (as in sunburn, bug bites, chemical dermatitis, or hives)? Are there any open wounds?* Scalp lacerations are exceedingly common and even small ones bleed like crazy. You won't be able to assess the depth if bleeding is profuse. Apply firm enough pressure to stop the oozing, and continue to do so for 10–15 minutes, or even longer if necessary. When the bleeding has stopped, gently blot the blood away and re-examine the scalp using as little trauma as possible.

EENT: eyes, ears, nose, throat (and mouth). The most sensible approach is to assess these structures for conditions you can actually treat, or that may indicate an emergency. Unless you have an ophthalmologist available, there is little reason to use an ophthalmoscope to detect retinal damage or cataracts, and skill with this instrument is difficult to acquire. A simple flashlight (or even sunlight) will suffice for most eye examinations. *Have the whites of the eyes turned red (conjunctivitis, pinkeye) or yellow (jaundice, icterus)? Are there any bumps or pimples (styes), or any rash or swelling (as in allergies)? Are the pupils approximately evenly sized? Do the eyeballs move together, at the same time? Is the vision normal or at least the patient's usual?* Abnormalities of the last three may indicate a neurologic (brain) problem.

Neurologic conditions involving the ears may cause loss of hearing, balance difficulties, tinnitus (ringing in the ears), or bleeding from the ear (with a skull fracture or other trauma). Also look for bumps (nodules) in the ear lobe, which may point to a cyst or abscess. Use a flashlight (or otoscope, if available) and exam the ear canal for swelling, redness, odor, or discharge, which usually indicate an ear canal infection. You will not be able to see the ear drum without an otoscope. If you have one, you should also be able to detect excess earwax that may be blocking the ear canal. A normal ear drum is grayish to slightly silvery. A little pink may be normal (or indicate mild infection). A bright red ear drum, especially if it appears to be bubbling outward, usually indicates a middle ear infection (otitis media).

Does the external nose look normal, or possibly askew, swollen, or bruised, consistent with trauma? Can the person breathe adequately or are the airways swollen? Is there any bleeding? Is the mucus (snot) clear or white, or thick yellow and gooey? A penlight is a handy device for nasal examination, but sunlight works as well. You will not be able to see very far up the nose without a lighted scope or nasal retractor. In children who may have inserted an object into the nose, be sure to look for toys, beads, and other foreign bodies.

The examination of the mouth and throat begins with the lips. *Any cold sores (think herpes virus), cracking (sun exposure, eczema, dehydration, malnutrition), paleness (consider anemia), or bleeding (laceration, trauma, bleeding disorder)?* Assess the inside of the cheeks and gums for ulcers, lacerations, redness, swelling, or growths. White spots on the cheeks and/or tongue often indicate thrush (yeast infection). White spots or pus on the tonsils or back of the throat usually indicate throat infection (tonsillitis, strep). With respiratory infections, drainage of mucus is often visible down the back of the throat (posterior pharynx). Also assess for oral signs of dehydration – *is there any saliva, or is the tongue cracked and dry* (also common with certain medicines)? A foul odor may indicate merely bad breath and poor dental hygiene, but is sometimes a sign of infection.

Neck: Moving downward, first take a step back and observe the neck. *Is any abnormality or asymmetry visible? Is the hollow at the base of the neck anteriorly (in front) identifiable or possibly obscured (by fat or a goiter)? Can you see swollen glands?* Ask the patient to move the neck forward and backward, to lean it side to side, and to rotate (twist) it in all directions. *Does it move easily, without discomfort?* Next, feel for any swelling around the glands on the sides and back of the neck. Palpate the front of the neck, noting any swelling or tenderness at the base (goiter). Check the carotid pulses on both sides by palpating just below the angle of the jaw. The carotid artery pulse is one of the easiest to find. A weak or rapid pulse may indicate anemia, dehydration, general illness, or a host of other conditions.

Chest: The chest exam (other than the heart and lungs) is sometimes overlooked but shouldn't be. Trauma victims often experience fractured ribs or clavicles (collar bones). As always, simply look at the chest – front, back, and sides – to begin. *Any bruising, bleeding, or lacerations?* Palpate each rib individually for tenderness if trauma has occurred. Tenderness is also common on a non-traumatic basis where the ribs join the sternum or where the bony part of the ribs attaches to the cartilage (costochondritis). *Next, is there any rash?* Scattered welts may be hives or bug bites. Pale or light brown splotches on the upper back may be a minor fungus. A band of red sores or blisters that goes half-way around the chest is likely shingles.

Breast: checking the breasts for cancer may be unnecessary if no treatment for cancer exists, but other conditions are not uncommon. An enlarging mass in a younger woman (under age 40) is likely a cyst or localized infection. Sometimes simply aspirating the fluid into a syringe will eliminate a cystic mass. In an older woman, cancer is more likely. The undersides of the breast may be reddened (from friction or a yeast infection) or develop abscesses (boils). In a nursing mother, localized breast tenderness (and sometimes redness and swelling) usually indicates mastitis (infection of the milk glands). Tenderness of both breasts is more likely to be from hormone stimulation or engorgement. New mothers (with neither medical personnel nor experienced mothers to advise them) may encounter difficulties if they have to decipher breast-feeding on their own. Inverted nipples may make it difficult for an infant to latch on. Sore, cracked nipples may hurt too much to permit nursing.

Lungs: lung sounds can be detected with a stethoscope or simply by applying one's ear to the chest. Either way, it is easier to distinguish breath sounds in a thin patient than in a heaver one. Breast tissue often obscures breath or heart sounds in a woman and occasionally in men as well. Again, begin with observation: *does the breathing appear normal, rapid, shallow, or labored? Does the chest seem to move as it should, that is, expand symmetrically on inhalation and contract on exhalation? Does the right side move the same as the left?* Any asymmetry suggests injury (collapsed or perforated lung, paralysis). *Does the air seem to pass in and out without obstruction?*

When examining the lungs, doctors listen specifically for certain sounds. **Rhonchi** are course rattles, heard more often on expiration, but sometimes on inspiration, associated with bronchitis, COPD, and sometimes pneumonia. They result from mucus rattling in the bronchial tubes as air passes through. **Rales** are a much softer sound heard in areas of partial lung collapse or congestion. This faint crackle, like the sound of rubbing a lock of hair between your fingers, is that of moist alveoli (air sacs in the lung) popping open on inspiration. An examiner with high frequency hearing loss may be unable to discern rales. Patients with heart failure or swelling in their legs may exhibit rales at the base of the lungs posteriorly, usually bilaterally. (Gravity causes fluids to accumulate more at the base of the lungs than toward the top.) Patients with pneumonia may have rales isolated to a single lung or part of a lung. Fairly often, even in patients with pneumonia, no abnormal sounds may be detected. Sometimes this is due to lack of air flow – similar to having too little air to blow a whistle. If air flow later increases, both normal and abnormal breath sounds may become louder. This is also true of **wheezing**, a raspy sound usually heard more so on expiration than on inspiration. Wheezing may not be apparent with normal breathing at rest. Asking a patient to inhale more deeply and exhale a little more rapidly may bring out the presence of a wheeze. YouTube offers several videos demonstrating all these lung sounds.

When you ask patients to breathe deeply, don't be surprised if they take a deep breath and hold it, thinking this will assist you. In reality, nothing can be heard when the breath is held, that is, when no air is moving. What you're aiming at is rapid enough airflow to rattle any mucus or bring out a wheeze. If a patient cannot understand your instructions, simply demonstrate the depth and rate of breathing you desire.

In a patient with obvious respiratory difficulties, you should begin your exam with the heart and lungs, returning later to complete the remainder of the history and physical. Don't spend time inspecting and documenting a minor scalp wound if the patient cannot breathe. Also, don't forget about inhaled foreign bodies (teeth, dentures, food, vomit), which may be blocking the airway or causing a wheeze or rattle.

Heart: Both now and at the end of civilization as we know it, the most useful cardiac exam consists of listening for the heart rate and the heart rhythm. Although heart murmurs and heart enlargement are potential concerns, they are difficult for the layman to assess and little treatment could be offered in an Armageddon scenario.

The heart rate should be fairly steady, and is generally 60–100 beats per minute in otherwise healthy adults (see vital signs above). In a younger adult or a child, the heart rate often increases a little on inhalation and decreases a little on expiration, possibly as much as 10–20 beats per minute. This is considered normal, and may or may not be noticeable.

The heart rhythm is a second consideration: *does the heart beat regularly like the bass drum in a marching band, or skip helter-skelter? Is it sometimes irregular and sometimes regular? Is there an occasional skip or extra beat?* In younger adults, the heart rate is almost always regular. Before middle age, an irregular heart beat is more suggestive of an acute problem than intrinsic heart disease (think drug or medication use, poisoning, or hyperthyroidism). Beyond age about 60, skipped or early beats become quite common, and often go unnoticed by the patient, usually requiring no treatment. Atrial fibrillation is a frequent cause of a highly variable heart rhythm in adults. The acute onset of atrial fibrillation is very likely to cause symptoms of shortness of breath or fatigue. It may be difficult to count the pulse, which may vary significantly over the course of several beats, and the rate determined by listening directly to the heart may appear higher than that obtained by measuring the pulse elsewhere.

Probably the most useful consideration is whether a patient's heart rate and rhythm are normal for himself or herself. It's one thing to have had atrial fibrillation for twenty years and another to develop it overnight. Many adults are aware they experience some irregular heartbeats and suffer no ill consequences, but in a patient recently started on a pharmaceutical or herbal product, the meaning may be entirely different, possibly indicating toxicity or intolerance.

Abdomen: Generally speaking, the abdominal exam includes the portion of the torso between the lower ribs and the pelvic bones. It should also include the flanks, or sides of the abdomen where kidney pain often occurs. The extreme lower abdomen overlaps the pelvic organs, and symptoms here may indicate a problem of the reproductive or urinary systems.

Again, begin with **inspection** of the abdomen. *Is it lean, emaciated, protuberant, or discolored? Are there any bulges consistent with a hernia? If protuberant, is the size of the abdomen consistent with fat deposition elsewhere in the body or is the protuberance in contrast to emaciated limbs, an indicator of protein malnutrition? Are there any bruises or other discolorations, or perhaps small bruises or puncture marks consistent with insulin or blood thinner injections?*

Next, **listen** to the abdomen for bowel sounds, especially in a patient who reports a digestive disturbance. Everyone knows what a stomach rumble sounds like, and everyone should be exhibiting them at least periodically. When auscultating with a stethoscope (or simply your ear), you should hear something "moving" within a minute or less. If you don't, then listen for another minute. Total absence of bowel sounds may indicate a serious problem. Occasionally you'll hear an abundance of rumbling, whooshing, or squishing. This is usually normal and simply indicates active digestion. Occasionally it is abnormal, and may indicate overly active bowels, consistent with the rapid passage of food through the intestines (with or without discomfort), or sometimes obstruction of the passage of food (which usually is quite painful).

Thirdly, **palpate** the abdomen for tenderness. This is one of the easier exams to perform, as patients are usually able to say, yes, it hurts here and not there. For the most part, tenderness will overlie the affected part. Upper abdominal pain is commonly related to the stomach, but rarely reflects a urinary infection – and there are exceptions to every rule. You may want to have a human anatomy book on hand to help you understand the layout of the internal organs. A very simple diagram is represented in the table below. The abdominal exam is usually performed with the examiner standing on the patient's right side, with the patient's head toward the physician's left.

	AFFECTED ORGANS TO CONSIDER BASED ON SYMPTOM LOCATION		
	Patient's right	**Middle**	**Patient's left**
Upper	Gallbladder Liver Kidney (toward side) Ascending colon Small intestines	Stomach Duodenum Gallbladder Small intestines Transverse colon	Stomach Kidney (toward side) Colon Pancreas – spleen Small intestines
Mid	Small intestines Ureter to kidney Ascending colon Gallbladder	Small intestines Stomach Transverse colon	Descending colon Ureter to kidney Small intestines Pancreas – spleen
Lower	Ascending colon with appendix Ureter to kidney Ovary Small intestines	Bladder Uterus Sigmoid colon Small intestines	Descending colon Ureter to kidney Ovary Small intestines

Knowing which organs are where will help you decipher what is going on. The ordered lists above indicate the approximate relative likelihood of a certain organ causing a problem in a particular area. About 80% of the time, pain or tenderness will be in the expected location. An acid stomach will hurt in the upper abdomen, not the lower. Another 15% of cases will exhibit symptoms in the next adjacent zone, and perhaps 5% will simply be in the "wrong" place. Appendicitis symptoms usually occur in the patient's right lower quadrant, and if not, then one zone "next-door" – but they could occur anywhere or nowhere specifically. With the abdominal exam you must keep an open mind as to which organ is involved, but in general, upper abdominal pain is usually stomach-related, lower abdominal pain is usually digestive, pelvic, or urinary, and mid-abdominal pain is usually intestinal. Don't forget the flanks, where the ureters or kidneys may exhibit tenderness or pain.

Palpating the abdomen is also helpful in discovering enlarged organs or growths, particularly the liver or uterus (think pregnancy). Acute liver enlargement nearly always causes tenderness, whereas with chronic liver enlargement this is uncommon. Liver enlargement is always a sign of something wrong. Normally an examiner cannot actually feel the liver edge, but if you find it protruding below the lower ribcage, it is probably enlarged. Sometimes during deep inspiration the liver will be pushed down to where the lower border can be palpated, which may not be abnormal. However, if the lower edge of the liver can be felt when the lungs are deflated, this is an abnormal finding.

Another useful test, if you have a keen ear, is **percussion**. This consists of tapping over the abdomen (which contains abundant gas and should, therefore, sound hollow), in contrast to tapping over a solid organ such as the liver (which has less echo and therefore sounds more solid). Because the abdomen is a soft surface, it is ineffective to tap directly on the patient's body. Rather, apply your left middle finger flat against the patient's abdomen, and use your right middle finger to tap on your left middle finger between the two finger (interphalangeal) joints. *Is a patient's right upper quadrant tenderness due to an enlarged liver or perhaps gallbladder inflammation?* Palpating and percussing this area may help you distinguish the two.

In a postmenopausal female or male of the same age, a palpable abdominal mass is considered a tumor until proven otherwise. One exception to this is when the stool can be palpated along the left lower abdomen, usually only possible in a slender, constipated individual. This is most commonly observed in women, adolescents, and children.

In a middle-aged or older male, what looks suspiciously like an early pregnancy is probably a distended bladder caused by urinary obstruction due to an enlarged prostate. In extreme cases, a distended bladder may hold as much as a gallon of urine.

In a female of menstruating age, an enlarged uterus should be considered a pregnancy until proven otherwise. If you can detect a separate, rapid heartbeat using a stethoscope or simply your ear, the pregnancy is at least a good 5–6 months along. The uterus reaches the height of the belly button by about 5 months. If you can actually observe the baby moving, the pregnancy is likely at least 7 months completed.

Genitourinary: As mentioned above, there is significant overlap in symptoms due to disorders of the pelvic and abdominal organs, even though in males the genital organs are not contained within the abdominal-pelvic cavity. Lower abdominal symptoms may be caused by digestive, urinary, or reproductive organ malfunction or disease.

The examination of the male is easier to perform for a layman than a female exam. Visual inspection is, as usual, the place to begin your exam. *Is the penis straight, curved, retracted, or normal length? Is the patient circumcised, or does the foreskin cover the head (glans) of the penis? If not circumcised, does the foreskin retract easily? Is there any redness or odor? Are there any bumps, ulcers, or lesions along the shaft of the penis?* Bumps or warty lesions often indicate human papilloma virus (venereal warts, HPV). Small blisters or clusters of blisters are typical of herpes virus infections, whereas larger ulcers may indicate syphilis or chancroid. (By now you're considering stocking up on gloves.)

Next, is there any visible discharge or pus from the opening of the penis (the urethral meatus)? Gonorrhea usually produces a visible discharge, but chlamydia may do so as well (and many patients with one infection have the other.) Trichomonas usually causes burning on urination without a discharge.

Moving downward, is the scrotum tender or swollen? Can the testicles be palpated within the scrotal sac? Are they about the same size? Testes (testicles) are always a little tender, but extreme tenderness indicates a problem, usually infection, but occasionally signals a dangerous twisting (or torsion). If the scrotal sac is quite enlarged, there may be a hernia, hydrocele, or varicocele (which feels like a bag of worms). Tenderness of the testicles may indicate infection (such as with mumps), but may be difficult to differentiate from tenderness of the epididymis, lying just behind the testicles (as in epididymitis). Gradual testicular enlargement over weeks to months, accompanied by little if any tenderness, may indicate a tumor.

The female exam begins with visually inspecting the external genitalia. *Is there any swelling of the outer genitalia, any redness, blisters, bumps, or cystic areas?* Common problems include the erythema (redness and irritation) associated with a yeast infection, the bumps or warty growths consistent with HPV, small blisters consistent with herpes, and swollen, tender abscesses consistent with skin infections, or infected cysts or glands.

The internal exam will be limited without appropriate lighting and a vaginal speculum to hold the tissues apart. Nevertheless, you may be able to determine visually if a discharge or blood is present. Palpating the cervix may be performed using the index and/or middle finger. Often the cervix is quite deeply situated and may be difficult to reach for an examiner with small hands. In a non-pregnant woman, cervical tenderness is probably the most important consideration, looking for signs of infection. Pap tests will be irrelevant unless a cytologist can interpret the slides and a surgeon can do something about the result.

In a pregnant female, note the presence of blood or leaking fluid. In a laboring patient the degree to which the cervix has dilated can be determined by feel with practice. The normal cervical opening is only about an eighth- to a quarter-inch. A fully dilated cervix has an opening of approximately10 cm. Determining the degree of dilation is a skill best learned from a physician or midwife using a hands-on approach. The first several times you perform this exam you'll likely have no idea what you're feeling.

Rectal: Although the rectum is part of the digestive system, it is commonly examined along with the genitalia due to location. Note any swelling or tenderness at the anal opening (consistent with hemorrhoids) or in the gluteal fold (the "butt-crack," consistent with a peri-rectal abscess, a fairly common infection). Observe for redness or rash, as this is a common area for a yeast infection, especially in infants, but also in adults taking antibiotics. Use a single finger to check internally, feeling for any masses or tenderness, and examine the color of any stool, particularly if blood is present.

Back: the older I get, the less worried I am about back pain. By middle age who hasn't had it? But back pain is not a single entity, and may actually be of more concern in a younger patient than in an older one.

Probably the most important consideration is determining whether back pain is internal or external, that is, relating to the "guts" and internal organs, as opposed to the muscles and bones (musculoskeletal system). Sometimes patients can tell the difference, sometimes they can't. Pain on movement is commonly musculoskeletal, whereas tenderness to palpation is usually internal, but there is a great deal of overlap between the two.

Of the internal organs, the kidneys are most commonly implicated as the cause of back pain, especially when the discomfort is one-sided and situated just below the ribs posteriorly. Tapping (gently pounding) over an inflamed or swollen kidney will frequently cause more discomfort than palpation (pressing) alone elicits. Other organs that may cause back pain include the stomach, large intestine, gallbladder, pancreas, bladder, uterus, prostate, heart, and aorta . . . pretty much any internal organ. Back pain caused by an internal organ other than the kidney may be difficult to pinpoint, especially if additional, more typical, symptoms are lacking. (Even as a physician, it once took me a few weeks to decide that my left-sided back pain was stomach-related and due to some ibuprofen I'd been taking. It simply did not have the quality of pain I'd been expecting.) As with abdominal symptoms, it is wise to keep an open mind when diagnosing the cause of back pain.

Even with back pain it is important to begin with a visual inspection. *Is there any sign of trauma, any abrasion, bruising, or swelling?* A cluster or band of red splotches or blisters may indicate a shingles outbreak, which both you and the patient may miss if you don't lift or remove the patient's shirt.

Note whether the back is twisted or symmetric. The curvature of scoliosis often becomes more prominent and thus more easily detected when the patient bends forward from the waist, revealing the asymmetry. Elderly patients commonly have chronic compression fractures of the thoracic (chest) and cervical (neck) spine, causing them to exhibit a hunched-over appearance (kyphosis). An abnormally straight back may indicate a spinal problem or muscle spasm.

As part of the visual inspection, examine the patient's ability to move. *Can he touch his fingertips to the floor? Lean side to side? Twist freely (rotate)? Lean backward? Do any of these movements trigger other symptoms, such as leg pain or numbness, indicative of a pinched nerve?* For the most part, probably 9 out of 10 times, pain on movement accompanied by decreased range of motion (ability to bend and twist) indicates a mechanical (musculoskeletal) problem such as a back strain or disc injury. However, a bad kidney infection will sometimes hurt worse with movement as well.

Examination of the back should be performed with the patient in the standing and/or sitting position. Additionally, as the patient lies on his back for the abdominal exam (which should not be omitted in the patient with back pain), have him lift one leg at a time, straight up, without bending the knee. When this movement is significantly reduced on one side only, it often indicates a slipped disk that is pinching a nerve. Many patients with back pain cannot lie comfortably flat on their back, which causes the abdominal muscles to tense. To get a good abdominal exam, have them bend their knees up a little, which will relax the abdominal muscles.

Extremities: Moving downward and outward now brings us to examination of the extremities (arms and legs). The focus of this exam is somewhat age-dependent. In younger patients acute injury is the main concern, whereas chronic and degenerative conditions plague the older generation.

For the younger or injured patient, look first for visible abnormalities: bruising, swelling, deformity, bones sticking through the skin. *Does the patient prefer a certain position due to pain or inability to move?* When he broke his femur, my son kept his injured limb in a frog leg position, one I've never seen him assume otherwise. When a patient maintains what appears to be an awkward position, this often indicates an underlying injury to the bone, joint, or sometimes muscle.

After documenting the obvious, don't forget to examine other areas. The pain of a fractured femur may trump that of a broken neck. The brain sometimes has trouble processing pain signals from multiple areas, distracting the patient from secondary injuries. When the mechanism of injury, say a car wreck, suggests the likelihood of additional injuries, it is always best to protect susceptible parts (especially the head, neck, and back) until it is clear no injury has occurred. Having a patient wear a cervical collar a few days may cause discomfort, but it won't lead to the permanent injury *not* doing so may allow. This is a reminder that physical examination is not a one-time exercise. As a patient's condition progresses, the examination of relevant parts should be repeated. Some areas may improve while others seem to worsen. Swelling and bruising in particular tend to worsen in the days following an injury.

Injuries to the extremities typically occur either *at* or *between* the joints. In general, injuries of the joints are more difficult to treat, take longer to resolve, and are more likely to result in permanent deformity or pain. Early immobilization of a weight-bearing joint may prevent worse damage from continued use. A damaged joint is usually swollen, occasionally reddened, often "squishy" (with fluid), usually tender, and almost always quite painful, causing the patient to resist movement. When a joint swells within minutes, this is a sign of bleeding within the joint capsule, whereas fluid that accumulates over several hours or days is usually synovial (joint) fluid, the body's reaction to joint injury. Pay special attention to lacerations or deep abrasions overlying an injured joint, as this places the joint at greater risk of infection.

Injuries in between joints (for example, midway between the elbow and wrist, or between the ankle and knee) are either soft tissue injuries (crush injury, bruise, laceration) or bony injuries (breaks, fractures). Though you might expect that a force severe enough to break a bone would also cause overlying soft tissue injury, this is often not the case. Bones are more brittle than skin, fat, and muscle, and will snap when sudden bending or twisting force is applied. My own son's femur was snapped into three pieces, with not a scratch on his leg. However, when soft tissue injury is present, always consider the possibility of an underlying fracture. With soft tissue injuries alone, a person can often walk or move the affected limb fairly normally, which is usually not the case with a fracture.

In an older patient, say over about 50 years old, I always check for edema (swelling). Minimal swelling is more common in women than men, especially in those who've had children (which often causes minor, permanent damage to the leg veins) or in anyone who carries a great deal of weight in his or her abdomen. Swelling is also more common in hotter weather, and when people have been on their feet a long time. Because swelling is gravity dependent, it will usually accumulate first in the feet or ankles, sometimes making it difficult to see the ankle bones. As additional fluid accumulates, it "moves up" the legs. Firmly pressing over the shin bone will reveal a dent afterwards, as the extracellular fluid is temporarily displaced. The higher along the shin that you can make a dent, the more fluid has accumulated. By the time enough fluid has accrued to detect in this fashion, it will cause an increase in weight of at least a pound or two, and sometimes as much as twenty. Thick ankles that won't indent may simply be fat or naturally thick. Visible swelling that does not indent, and in which the overlying skin has the texture of an orange peel, is nearly always chronic and usually indicates lymphatic obstruction.

Any time significant swelling is present, reconsider the heart and lung exam. There is no shame in checking again for a closer listen. In a person about sixty or older, new or worsening edema may reflect poor heart function, caused by either heart damage or heart rhythm abnormalities. Patients often deny or fail to mention shortness of breath or chest pain, and may not notice a rapid heart rate. I've had older patients (and sometimes younger) visit my office, oblivious to the fact their heart was racing at over 150 beats per minute. One reason for this is that such a rapid heart rate may result in insufficient blood flow to the brain, which may cloud the thinking. This is especially common with the recent onset of atrial fibrillation.

Difficulty breathing often accompanies leg swelling when inadequate heart function is the cause, but you may not notice this when the patient is at rest. If in doubt, take the patient for a short walk, and observe whether the breathing seems appropriate. I once had a patient who required crutches, but I was unsure if she could handle them. Though she'd given no history of breathing problems, a 10-second trial of crutch-walking threw her into heart failure. A week later, she underwent heart valve replacement! She'd attributed her shortness of breath to aging and obesity, and never thought to mention it.

Skin: always, always, always give the skin at least a quick once-over. At a minimum, take note of the condition of the visible skin – the face, hands, arms, maybe legs. *Is the face ghost-white?* This may be your first clue to anemia or blood loss. *Are the hands covered with tiny scratches*? Infection from a pet kitten may be the cause of the patient's tender armpits. *Is the patient constantly scratching?* Lifting the shirt may reveal a case of hives or bug bites – and you'll certainly want to know if you need to delouse a patient before everyone becomes infested.

In trauma patients, check for scratches, bruises, and lacerations. In sick patients, look for generalized rashes of which they may be unaware. In patients with a skin complaint in one location, be sure to check elsewhere for the same problem.

Most patients will not spontaneously remove their shoes and socks for a medical exam. Even if you think this is unnecessary, at least consider the question in every patient. Anyone exposed to the elements for prolonged periods may have a foot fungus, frostbite, or blisters. Foot pain may well be due to an infection that has spread from the skin. Gout may show up as swelling and redness overlying the big toe joint.

For more specifics regarding examination of the skin, please refer to **Chapter 13**.

Neurologic: for the layman, this part of the exam may be frightening. *What mystery lies behind the knee-jerk exam? How can you tell if someone's had a stroke? Does numbness indicate a brain problem or could it be something else? How can you tell a blood clot from a pinched nerved?*

Although the neurologic exam can be daunting, taking a practical approach will dissolve much of the mystery. For the purpose of this discussion, I will focus only on common findings that are likely to be clinically useful.

The first part of the neurologic exam is the **mental status exam**. *Is the person awake, alert, and aware of his or her surroundings? Can you entertain a normal conversation or are the patient's responses off the wall?* The biggest question, whatever their current status, is: *is this the patient's normal state?* An 80-year-old may be quite forgetful, but a teenager shouldn't be. Anyone whose brain doesn't seem to be working normally has something going on. Usually this boils down to one of two conditions: a *localized* brain problem or a *systemic* (whole body) condition, such as infection or metabolic disorder.

Next, the **special senses** should be considered: hearing, vision, taste, and smell. On a practical note, the last two are rarely assessed, though patients often mention loss of taste or smell in conjunction with upper respiratory infections. Hearing or vision loss is much more significant. Without special equipment, measuring vision or hearing will require the cooperation of an alert patient.

Hearing can be quickly assessed by the patient's response to quiet speech or whispering. Most **hearing loss** is high-frequency loss, in which patients have difficulty distinguishing consonants, especially when background noise is present or if they are unable to see the speaker's face. If I suspect hearing loss, I perform two quick tests.

For the first, I demonstrate what I'd like the patient to listen for by rubbing my fingers together in front of his or her face. Most patients can detect this high-pitched sound when it is right in front of them. For the test itself, I spread my arms wide apart, and while the patient listens with eyes closed, I rub my fingers together (which you should be able to hear at arm's length), slowly edging my hand closer to the patient's ear. The patient is asked to say "yes" when they are able to detect the sound. Practice now, while you're reading this, and again later with your friends and relatives. You'll find young people can detect the sound immediately, whereas many older folks cannot do so until your hand is an inch from their ear. Often one side is worse than the other.

Next, I have the patient repeat consonants after me as I hold a piece of paper in front of my mouth, blocking their visual cues. Even young children should be able to respond with a high degree of accuracy. Patients with high-frequency hearing loss have difficulty distinguishing the following groups of consonants: t/p/k, s/sh/f, d/t, and g/k. "Pick" may sound like "tip," "seat" may be confused with "feet." Imagine how confusing a conversion can be if key words are constantly mistaken. For an excellent example of how a person with hearing loss perceives conversation and other sounds, visit:
http://appl.phonak.com/hearinglossdemo.htm.

The above tests do not specify the cause of hearing loss, but may guide or confirm your exam otherwise. In the elderly, hearing loss is usually neurologic, age-related presbycusis. In the young, hearing loss is usually related to infection, wax build-up, blocked sinuses or eustachian tubes, trauma, or foreign body in the ear canal.

To determine **vision**, you may want to invest in an inexpensive eye chart, but otherwise it is fine to simply ask the patient to read printed material (for near vision) or identify a book title (or equivalent item) from across the room. Use your own (hopefully good) vision to judge by. Examine the patient's vision using each eye individually and both together.

But what good is an eye exam, you may ask, if you can't do anything about a visual problem? While it's true you probably can't cure glaucoma or cataracts, an eye exam may help you determine if something serious is present. Many a time a patient has said, "I can't see," when what they really mean is it's just a little blurry, and on vision testing, they have little or no discernible loss. This can be very reassuring for both doctor and patient.

Examining **facial expression** and facial muscle movement is the next question to consider. *Is the lady sitting before you having a stroke?* What if one side of her face seems a little droopy, and spittle is collecting at the corner of her mouth? Her one eye doesn't seem to close or open all the way, and her speech seems a little slurred.

In a case like this, if you have the opportunity, get the patient to a hospital right away. She may, indeed, be having a **stroke**, and time is of the essence. But assuming hospital care is not an option, then what?

Again, the patient history is important. *How old is the patient? Has she had a prior stroke? Did the symptoms come on gradually or within minutes? Are the arm and leg weak on the affected side? Is the speech normal or not?* There will be little you can do about a stroke (other than giving an aspirin), but not everything that looks like a stroke is a stroke. In the diabetic patient, a hypoglycemic (low blood sugar) spell may resemble a stroke, but is reversible upon raising the blood sugar. A hemiplegic migraine may cause temporary one-sided weakness, paralysis, or numbness, which resolves as the migraine headache improves. More common is **Bell's palsy**, which resembles a stroke, but has a slower onset (over hours to days), and usually occurs in middle-aged or younger people. When the onset occurs during sleep, the patient may awaken with one side of the face paralyzed. Bell's palsy does not cause dizziness, loss of vision, or any symptoms in the arms or legs. A stroke is a problem inside the brain, whereas Bell's palsy is a temporary paralysis of a group of nerves in the face. A Bell's palsy patient usually *cannot* lift the eyebrow on the affected side, whereas a stroke victim usually *can*. Your patients will love and adore you if you can reassure them they are not having a stroke.

Next, what about the **reflexes**? In my opinion, there is little reason for a layman to learn to check the knee reflex or similar reflexes of the ankle and arm. The evaluation of reflexes rarely adds anything that isn't apparent through the history or other components of the physical examination. The reflex response is highly dependent on the patient's ability to relax and on operator error as well. It is much more important whether a patient can simply move the arms and legs on their own.

Much more common than strokes or Bell's palsy are **pinched nerves**. Even with a pinched nerve, the examination isn't nearly as helpful as the history. A patient may complain of terrible pain or numbness, whereas your exam seems to reveal no apparent abnormality. At least 9 out of 10 patients who say their hands or feet are numb can still detect the sharpness of a pin. The other 10% may not be able to tell the difference between the prick of needle and the touch of a cotton swab. Either way, if a patient says they feel numb, they probably are, to a degree.

Whenever a patient complains of **numbness**, or the sensation of the arm or hand falling asleep, obtaining an accurate pattern of symptoms is essential. This may be possible through history-taking alone, but the physical exam can be quite helpful. For example, nearly every patient I've seen with carpal tunnel syndrome has said the entire hand is numb; however, on careful testing, the little finger and outer half of the ring finger are actually normal.

Specific patterns of localized pain, numbness, weakness, or tingling are the rule for pinched nerves, and can usually explain the level where the nerve is being pinched. Symptoms travelling down one or both arms are commonly from a problem in the neck. When the thumb and adjacent 2-½ fingers are affected, this is a pinched median nerve in the wrist (carpal tunnel syndrome). When the little finger and perhaps the ring finger are half asleep, this is usually an ulnar nerve irritation stemming from the back of the elbow. Pain running down the posterior (back) or side of the leg is usually from a pinched nerve at the level of the lumbar spine.

Again, when patients experience numbness, they often question whether they're experiencing a stroke, a blood clot, or other circulation problem. Pinched nerves are far more common than any of these, especially in patients about 60 years of age and younger. We have not covered assessing arterial circulation in the legs because (despite television commercials) peripheral arterial disease is relatively rare and there won't be much you can do about it. Taking an aspirin a day (as for heart disease) will be the primary intervention.

If you've read and studied this chapter, you will have more medical understanding than 90% of the general population, and definitely more than a fledgling medical student. *Do you know how doctors begin to act like physicians?* They put on a white coat and are taught to call themselves Doctor (or at least, Student Doctor). If you want to be a healer, start thinking of yourself as one. Don't be surprised if other people look to you as the local expert before you believe you're qualified. Recognize your limitations, and do what you can to help others without causing harm, seeking outside help (if available) whenever you are unsure (books count). Don't blame yourself when you find you are only human – every doctor, every healer, has limitations – except for the Great Physician.

Conclusion

In completing this text I acknowledge that it is only a beginning. Though I've tried to address most problems encountered in family medicine, had time allowed I could have added thousands of pages on additional topics – post-Armageddon pediatrics, childbirth, geriatrics, orthopedics, dentistry, and much more. Thankfully, others have written excellent resources which can supplement your medical library, many of which are listed in Appendix A.

I've entitled this book *Armageddon Medicine* for three reasons: the words flow well and are easily remembered; the title conveys the idea of end-of-life-as-we-know-it concerns; and despite America's current blessings, I believe this era of abundance may come to an end in my lifetime, possibly quite soon. Pray that I am wrong and that you'll never need this book.

* * *

"Heaven and earth shall pass away: but my words shall not pass away.

But of that day and that hour knoweth no man,

no, not the angels which are in heaven, neither the Son, but the Father.

Take ye heed, watch and pray: for ye know not when the time is."

– Mark 13:31-33 (King James Version)

Appendix A

Resources

Medical Books and Textbooks

The medical references and textbooks listed below are excellent for both outpatient and (uncomplicated) inpatient medical care. They address real problems in real patients. Most of the books I have used myself as a family physician. I have purposely chosen certain older books (circa 1990s) for several reasons: 1) they were state of the art several years ago; 2) they rely less on today's complex technology; 3) the basics of diagnosis and many diseases have not changed much otherwise; and 4) with cost a consideration, an excellent library may be compiled inexpensively. If you are especially interested in a particular field, you may want to procure both a current and an older version of the same title.

Wilderness Medicine Books and Textbooks

This manual has not attempted to duplicate information found in already-existing wilderness medicine resources. Three books are suggested below for readers possessing various degrees of medical knowledge, from beginner to professional.

Free Downloads

Free downloadable online resources referenced throughout the text are compiled here for easy access.

Medical Textbook Title	Author/Editor
101 Ways to Save Money on Health Care	Cynthia J. Koelker, MD
(The) 5-Minute Pediatric Consult	M. William Schwartz, Louis M. Bell, Peter M. Bingham, and Esther K. Chung
(The) 5-Minute Clinical Consult	Frank J. Domino
Bedside Diagnostic Examination	Elmer L. DeGowin and Richard L. DeGowin
Clinical Dermatology	Thomas P. Habif
Clinical Sports Medicine	Peter Brukner and Karim Khan
Common Skin Disorders	Ernst Epstein
Conn's Current Therapy	Robert E. Rakel MD, Rick D. Kellerman, and Edward T. Bope MD
Dr. Spock's Baby and Child Care	Benjamin Spock, MD
Emergency Orthopedics	Robert Simon and Scott Sherman
French's Index of Differential Diagnosis	Mark Kinirons and Harold Ellis
Goodman and Gilman's Pharmacological Basis of Therapeutics Digital Edition	Laurence Brunton, Keith Parker, John Lazo, Iain Buxton, et al.
Grant's Atlas of Anatomy	Anne M.R. Agur and Arthur F. Dalley
Handbook of Fractures	Clayton R. Perry, John A. Elstrom and Arsen M. Pankovich
(The) Harriet Lane Handbook: A Manual for Pediatric House Officers	Johns Hopkins Hospital
Hypothyroidism – Answers for a Post-Apocalyptic World	Cynthia J. Koelker, M.D.
Manual of Obstetrics: Diagnosis and Therapy (A Little, Brown Spiral Manual)	Kenneth R. Niswander, M.D.
Manual of Pediatric Therapeutics (A Little, Brown Spiral Manual)	John w. Graef
Manual of Surgical Therapeutics (Little, Brown Spiral Manual)	Lloyd M. Nyhus and Robert E. Condon

(The) Merck Manual of Diagnosis and Therapy	Mark H. Beers, Robert S. Porter, and Thomas V. Jones
(The) Merck Manual of Medical Information, Home Edition	Mark H. Beers
Physicians' Desk Reference	PDR Staff
Principles of Ambulatory Medicine	Randol Barker, et al.
Rapid Interpretation of EKGs	Dale Dubin
Sanford Guide to Antimicrobial Therapy	David N. Gilbert
Textbook of Family Practice	Robert E. Rakel
Textbook of Physical Diagnosis (with DVD)	Mark H. Swartz
Vander's Human Physiology	Eric Widmaier
(The) Washington Manual of Medical Therapeutics	Washington University School of Medicine
(The) Washington Manual of Outpatient Internal Medicine	Washington University School of Medicine
Where There is No Dentist	David Werner, Jane Maxwell, Carol Thuman (Hesperian Foundation)
Where There is No Doctor	Murray Dickson (Hesperian Foundation)

Wilderness Medicine Books

Wilderness First Responder – How to Recognize, Treat, and Prevent Emergencies in the Backcountry *(appropriate for the layman)*	Buck Tilton, MS, WEMT
Wilderness Medicine – Beyond First Aid *(appropriate for those with some mid-level knowledge or interest)*	William W. Forgey, M.D.
Field Guide to Wilderness Medicine *(appropriate for physicians and trained medical providers)*	Paul S. Auerbach, Howard J. Donner, Eric A. Weiss

Free Downloads

Botanicals in Dermatology: An Evidence-based Review

http://www.medscape.com/viewarticle/723144

Botulism in the United States, 1899–1996, Handbook for Epidemiologists, Clinicians, and Laboratory Workers

http://www.cdc.gov/ncidod/dbmd/diseaseinfo/files/botulism.pdf

Diagnosis and Management of Foodborne Illnesses, A Primer for Physicians and Other Health Care Professionals

http://www.cdc.gov/mmwr/preview/mmwrhtml/rr5304a1.htm

Haiti Cholera Training Manual: A Full Course for Healthcare Providers

http://www.cdc.gov/haiticholera/pdf/haiticholera_trainingmanual_en.pdf

Nuclear War Survival Skills

http://www.oism.org/nwss/s73p904.htm

Sexually Transmitted Diseases Treatment Guidelines, 2010

http://www.cdc.gov/std/treatment/2010/STD-Treatment-2010-RR5912.pdf

(The) Ship Captain's Medical Guide

http://www.dft.gov.uk/mca/mcga07-home/workingatsea/mcga-medicalcertandadvice/mcga-dqs_st_shs_ships_capt_medical_guide.htm

USDA Complete Guide to Home Canning 2009 Revision

http://www.uga.edu/nchfp/publications/publications_usda.html

Where There is No Dentist

http://www.hesperian.org/publications_download.php

Where There is No Doctor

http://www.hesperian.org/publications_download.php

Appendix B

Medical Kit

The following chart details medical kits/supplies for individuals, families, community groups, and professional services. Quantities listed assume standard rates of injury and illness in a general population over the course of 1–3 years. If you are expecting mass chaos, you may want to procure a greater stockpile of injury and infection related supplies. Anyone providing medical services for even a small community will need the equivalent of a well-stocked physician's office with pharmacy.

Medical supplies are often less costly when purchased from a medical supply house (such as Henry Schein or Moore Medical), some of which will sell directly to the public. Certain items may actually cost less from your local pharmacy, especially heavy or liquid items such as hydrogen peroxide that are expensive to ship.

Before purchasing, consider whether you are able to use the supplies yourself or are hoping to encounter a professional to use them in the future. Choice of products will naturally vary according to the age and gender of family and/or group members.

Persons currently experiencing specific health issues should also prepare accordingly. What follows are general guidelines only for conditions common in a mixed population.

	Basic	Intermediate	Advanced
INTENDED USE	Family or Personal	Small group	Professional
WOUND CARE			
Skin prep/cleansers			
Hydrogen peroxide	1 bottle	5 bottles	20 bottles
Alcohol, isopropyl	1 bottle	5 bottles	20 bottles
Alcohol, isopropyl, 200 pads/box	1 box	5 boxes	20 boxes
Iodine prep pads, 100/box	-	1 box	5 boxes
Hibiclens, 16-oz bottle	1 bottle	2 bottles	5 bottles
Razors, pack of 10	1 pack	2 packs	5 packs
Sterile saline, bottles	2 bottles	5 bottles	20 bottles
Baby brush for scrubbing	1	2	5
Gloves, nitrile, 100/box	1 box	5 boxes	20 boxes
Gloves, sterile, 50 pair/box	-	1 box	5 boxes
Wound closure			
Steri-Strip Wound Closures			
1/4 x 4″ (over-the-counter)	1 Box of 30 strips	-	-
1/8 x 3″ – 50 packets/box	-	-	1 box
1/4 x 3″ – 50 packets/box	-	1 box	2 boxes
1/2 x 4″ – 50 packets/box	-	1 box	1 box

	Basic	Intermediate	Advanced
Duct tape	1 roll	1 roll	3 rolls
Stapler, skin, disposable	1	5	25
Staple remover, disposable	1	5	25
Laceration tray, single use (with instruments, no suture)	2	10	50
Suture material (with needle)			
4-0 absorbable, 12/box	-	-	1box
3-0 non-absorbable, 12/box	-	1 box	2 boxes
4-0 non-absorbable, 12/box	1 box	2 boxes	5 boxes
5-0 non-absorbable, 12/box	-	1 box	2 boxes
Suture removal kit	2	20	100
Local anesthesia			
Lidocaine, 1 or 2%, plain, 50 cc	1 bottle	2 bottles	10 bottles
Lidocaine, 2% with epinephrine	-	2 bottles	10 bottles
Diphenhydramine Inj. 50 mg/ml, 1 cc	-	1 vial	5 vials
Syringe with needle 3cc, 25 gauge	5 syringes	1 box of 100	3 boxes of 100
Dressings			
Band-Aids, standard, 100/box	1–3 boxes	5–10 boxes	20–100 boxes
Band-Aids, 2x4″ 50/box	1 box	5 boxes	10–20 boxes
Bacitracin Ointment, 1 oz. tube	2 tubes	5 tubes	10–100 tubes
Bacitracin 0.9 gm foil packs, 144/box	-	1 box	1 case (12x144)
Telfa, non-stick dressing, 3x4″	20 pads	100 pads	500 pads

	Basic	Intermediate	Advanced
Feminine napkins (for large wounds)	1 box	5 boxes	25 boxes
Honey (for burns)	1 bottle	2 bottles	5 bottles
Gauze			
Gauze rolls, non-sterile, 2″	1 box of 5	1 box of 96	1 box of 96
Gauze rolls, non-sterile, 4″	1 box of 5	1 box of 96	1 box of 96
Gauze rolls, non-sterile, 3″	-	-	2 boxes of 96
Gauze, sterile, 2x2″	-	1 box of 100	5 boxes of 100
Gauze, sterile, 3x3″	1 box of 25	1 box of 100	5 boxes of 100
Gauze, sterile, 4x4″	1 box of 25	1 box of 100	5 boxes of 100
Coban, Self-Adherent Wrap			
1″ and 4″ – box of 12 rolls	-	-	1 box each
2″ and 3″ – box of 12 rolls	-	-	3 boxes each
Coban, OTC, 3″	1 box of 5	2 boxes of 5	-
Medical tape, assorted sizes	5 rolls	25 rolls	100 rolls
Bandage scissors	1	2	10

INJURY TREATMENT

	Basic	Intermediate	Advanced
Elastic compression wrap (Ace)			
2″	1 roll	2 rolls	5 rolls
3″	1 roll	1 box of 10	5 boxes of 10
4″	1 roll	1 box of 10	5 boxes of 10
6″	-	3 rolls	1 box of 10
Cervical collar	-	1	5
Sling	1	5	20

	Basic	Intermediate	Advanced
Splints and braces			
Finger	-	-	2 dozen assorted
Wrist, pair of right and left	1 pair	2 pair	10 pair
Figure-of-eight	-	-	2
Knee	1	2	5
Ankle	1	2	10
Lumbar	-	-	2
Post-op Shoe	-	2	5
Crutches			
Adult, adjustable	1 pair	2 pair	4 pair
Child, adjustable	1 pair	1 pair	2 pair
Walker	-	1	2
Wheelchair	-	1	2
Plaster casting, 2″, 3″, 4″ 12/box	-	-	1 box each
Cast-cutter	-	-	1–2
Eye tray			
Fluoresceine strips, 100/box	-	-	1 box
Penlight, Fluoro-Dot	-	-	2 lights
Proparacaine Ophth. Sol, 15 ml	-	-	2 bottles
Erythromycin Ophthalmic Ointment 3.5 gm	-	-	2 tubes
Saline eye rinse	-	-	Optional
Ophthalmoscope + power source	-	-	1

	Basic	Intermediate	Advanced
MINOR SURGERY and OTHER TREATMENT			
Scalpels, disposable, #10, 11, 15	-	-	5 boxes each
OTC Wart-freezing canisters	-	1	5
Hyfercator and tips (box 100)	-	-	1
Instruments			
Suture scissors	1	1	3
Splinter forceps	1	1	3
Smooth pick-ups	-	1	3
Toothed pick-ups	-	1	3
Needle holder, various sizes	-	-	3
Curved forceps	-	-	3
Smooth forceps	-	1	3
Toenail clippers	1	1	3
Instrument holder	-	1	2
Disinfectant (Cidex), quarts	-	Use alcohol	12+ quarts
Local anesthetic (see Wound Care)			
Suture material (see Wound Care)			
Ear-irrigation syringe	-	1	5
PHYSICAL EXAMINATION			
Stethoscope	1	2	5
Watch/clock with second hand	1	2	3
Scale, non-electronic	1	1	2

	Basic	Intermediate	Advanced
BP machine (mercury preferred)	1	1	2
BP cuff	1 large	1 large	1 each S, M, L, XL
Otoscope with tips, light, power	1	1	2
Ophthalmoscope with light, power	-	-	1
Reflex hammer	-	-	2
Peak flow meter	-	1	2
EKG machine (and paper)	-	-	1
Q-tips, box of 500	OTC Q-tips	OTC Q-tips	2 boxes of 500
Sterile tongue depressors, 100/box	1 box	5 boxes	10 boxes
Non-sterile depressors, 500/box	-	1 box	5 boxes
Charts or notebook	Optional	Yes	Yes
Ball-point pen	Several	Several	Dozens

LABORATORY

Microscope with light source	-	-	1
Microscope slides and cover slips	-	-	200/500
Immersion oil	-	-	2 bottles
Bunsen burner or equivalent	-	-	1
Gram stain kit	-	-	1
Centrifuge	-	-	1
Test tubes, box of 100	-	-	1 box
Transfer pipettes, 500/box	-	-	1 box
Hemacytometer	-	-	1 kit

	Basic	Intermediate	Advanced
Urinalysis Multistix 10 SG, 100/bt	1 bottle	1 bottle	10 bottles
Blood glucose tester	-	1	2
Blood glucose test strips	-	100	500
Rapid Strep Kit	-	-	2
Pregnancy Test Kit, 25 tests	-	OTC kits	2
KOH solution	-	-	2 bottles

OTC MEDICATIONS – SEE APPENDIX C

PRESCRIPTION MEDICATIONS

Allergies/colds/flu

Benzonatate 100 mg cap	100	300	1,000
Diphenhydramine 50 mg cap	100	300	1,000
Pseudoephedrine 30 mg	100	300	1,000

Antibiotics, oral

Amoxicillin 500 mg tabs	100	500	5,000
Amoxicillin-clavulanate 500 mg	100	500	5,000
Cephalexin 500 mg caps	100	500	5,000
Ciprofloxacin 500 mg tabs	100	500	5,000
Doxycycline 100 mg caps	100	500	5,000
Erythromycin 400 or 500 mg	100	500	5,000
Metronidazole 500 mg	100	500	5,000
Penicillin 500 mg	100	500	5,000

	Basic	Intermediate	Advanced
Tetracycline 500 mg caps	100	500	5,000
Trimethoprim-Sulfa DS	100	500	5,000

Antibiotics, topical and ophthalmic

Bactroban 30 gm tube	1	5	50
Erythromycin ophth ointment	1	5	10
Gentamicin 0.1% ointment	-	-	5
Gentamicin 0.3% ophth soln	-	-	2
Sulfacet Sodium 10% ophth soln	1	5	10
Tobramycin 0.3% ophth soln	-	-	2

Antifungals

Nystatin/Triamcinolone Cr 30 gm	1 tube	5 tubes	30 tubes
Nystatin Cream 30 gm	1 tube	5 tubes	30 tubes
Fluconazole 100 mg tabs	5	30	300
Terbinafine 250 mg tabs	-	-	300

Arthritis

Allopurinol 300 mg tab	-	100	1,000
Dexamethasone 4 mg tab	-	100	2,000
Diclofenac DR 75 mg tab	-	100	1,000
Indomethacin 25 mg cap	-	100	1,000
Meloxicam 15 mg tab	-	100	1,000
Naproxen 500 mg tab	Use OTC	300	3,000

	Basic	Intermediate	Advanced
Asthma			
Albuterol HFA Inhaler	1	3	30
Albuterol 4 mg tabs	-	100	1,000
Albuterol 0.083% soln 3 ml	-	25 vials	500 vials
Ipratropium 0.02% soln 2.5 ml	-	-	100 vials
Prednisone 20 mg tabs	100	300	5,000
Blood pressure and heart			
Atenolol 100 mg tab	100	500	2,000
Clonidine 0.2 mg tab	-	-	1,000
Digoxin 0.25 mg tab	100	300	1,000
Diltiazem 120 mg tab	-	-	1,000
Doxazosin 8 mg tab	-	-	1,000
Furosemide 20 mg tab	-	100	1,000
Hydrochlorothiazide 50 mg tab	-	-	1,000
Isosorbide Mononitr. ER 30mg	-	-	500
Lisinopril 20 mg tab	-	100	1,000
Triam.-HCTZ 75/50 mg tab	100	300	2,000
Verapamil 120 mg tab	-	100	1,000
Warfarin 5 mg tab	-	-	1,000
Diabetes			
Glimepiride 4 mg tabs	100	300	5,000
Glipizide 10 mg tabs	-	300	5,000

	Basic	Intermediate	Advanced
Glyburide 5 mg tabs	-	300	5,000
Metformin 500 mg tabs	100	300	5,000
Insulin 70/30	If diabetic	5 vials	100 vials
Insulin Lantus or NPH	If diabetic	5 vials	30 vials
Blood glucose monitor	If diabetic	1	5
Blood glucose test strips	If diabetic	200	1,000

Gastrointestinal

Belladonna Alkaloid/PB tab	-	100	1,000
Dicyclomine 20 mg tab	30	100	1,000
Famotidine 20 mg tab	100	500	3,000
Lansoprazole 30 mg	30	100	1,000
Meclizine 25 mg	30	100	500
Metoclopramide 10 mg tab	-	-	500
Omeprazole 20 mg	30	100	1,000
Promethazine 25 mg tab	30	100	500
Ranitidine 300 mg tab	100	500	3,000

Mental health

Alprazolam 0.5 mg	-	30	1,000
Amitriptyline 50 mg tab	-	-	500
Buspirone 10 mg tab	100	300	2,000
Citalopram 40 mg	100	300	2,000
Doxepin HCL 50 mg	-	-	500
Fluoxetine 20 mg cap	100	300	2,000

	Basic	Intermediate	Advanced
Haloperidol 5 mg tab	-	-	200
Lorazepam 1 mg	30	100	1,000
Lithium Carbonate 300 mg cap	-	-	1,000
Nortriptyline 25 mg cap	-	-	500
Paroxetine 20 mg tab	100	300	2,000
Prochlorperazine 10 mg tab	-	-	500
Temazepam 30 mg	-	-	1,000
Thioridazine 50 mg tab	-	-	500
Trazodone 50 mg tab	-	-	1,000
Zolpidem 10 mg tab	30	200	2,000

Pain medications (also see Arthritis)

	Basic	Intermediate	Advanced
Acetaminophen with codeine #3	30	200	5,000
Baclofen 10 mg tab	-	-	1,000
Cyclobenzaprine 10 mg tab	-	100	1,000
Ibuprofen 800 mg tab	Use OTC	Use OTC	5,000
Tramadol 50 mg	100	500	5,000
Vicodin 5/325 mg	30	200	5,000

Skin Conditions (also see Antifungals and Antibiotics)

	Basic	Intermediate	Advanced
Fluocinonide 0.05% cream 30 gm	-	-	50
Hydrocortisone 2.5% cr. 30 gm	1	5	50
Silver Sulfadiazine 1% cream 50 gm	1	5	50
Triamcinolone 0.1% cream 80 gm	1	5	50

	Basic	Intermediate	Advanced
MISCELLANEOUS			
Condoms	100	300	1,000
Female diaphragms	-	-	10, assorted
Birth control pills	As needed	As needed	12 packs, min.
Oxygen concentrator & tubing	As needed	1	2–3
Goggles and/or face shield	-	1	2
I.V. tubing and supplies	-	-	100
Nebulizer	As needed	1	3
Charting supplies	Optional	Optional	300 charts

Appendix C

Useful OTC Medications

MENTAL CONDITIONS

(Drugs in this category are primarily used for problems other than mental illness)

Common name	Other names	Primary use	Other possible uses
Benadryl	Diphenhydramine	Allergies, colds	Anxiety, insomnia
Bonine	Meclizine Dramamine	Nausea, vomiting, motion sickness	Anxiety, insomnia
Caffeine	Caffeine	Mental alertness	Headaches, to increase a slow heart rate
Nyquil	Nighttime cold medicine	Colds and flu	Anxiety, insomnia
Sudafed	Pseudoephedrine	Sinus congestion	To increase mental alertness
Zyrtec	Cetirizine	Allergies	Anxiety, insomnia

SKIN CONDITIONS and INFECTIONS

Benadryl	Diphenhydramine	Hives, itching	See respiratory and mental health
Clearasil	Benzoyl peroxide	Acne	
Cetirizine	Zyrtec	Hives, itching	See respiratory and mental illness

Cortaid 10	1% hydrocortisone	Itchy rashes	Poison ivy, eczema, atopic dermatitis, metal allergy
Lamisil cream	Terbinafine	Fungal rashes	Athlete's foot, jock itch, yeast diaper rash, ringworm
Lotrimin	Clotrimazole	Fungal/yeast rashes and infections	Athlete's foot, jock itch, yeast diaper rash, ringworm
Nix	Permethrin	Head lice	Crabs, body lice
Nizoral Shampoo	Ketoconazole	Dandruff	Yeast infections, seborrhea, jock itch, diaper rash
Pepcid	Famotidine	Heartburn	Hives
Rid	Piperonyl butoxide, Pyrethrum Extract	Head lice	Crabs, body lice
Selsun	Selenium sulfide	Dandruff	Seborrhea
Tinactin	Tolnaftate	Fungal infections	Athlete's foot, jock itch, yeast diaper rash, ringworm
Zantac	Ranitidine	Heartburn	Hives

PAIN and INFLAMMATION

Aleve	Naproxen sodium	Pain, arthritis	Fever, inflammation, painful periods, heavy periods, gout, backache, strains, sprains, headaches
Aspercreme	Aspirin cream	Local pain, arthritis	
Aspirin	Acetylsalicylic acid	Pain, arthritis	Fever, inflammation, painful periods, heavy periods, gout, backache, strains, sprains, headaches Blood thinner
Capsaicin C		Local pain, arthritis	

Motrin	Ibuprofen, Advil, Nuprin	Pain, arthritis	Fever, inflammation, painful periods, heavy periods, gout, backache, strains, sprains, headache
Tylenol	Acetaminophen	Pain	Fever, headache

EARS, EYES, NOSE, MOUTH, THROAT

Afrin spray	Oxymetazoline	Nasal congestion	Allergies, colds, sinus headache
Allegra	Fexofenadine	Allergies	Hives, itching, runny nose, sinus headache
Benadryl	Diphenhydramine	Runny nose	Allergies, colds, post-nasal drainage, hives, itching, insomnia, anxiety
Claritin	Loratadine	Allergies	Hives, itching, runny nose, sinus headache
Fluoride		Prevent tooth decay	
MiraLAX	Polyethylene Glycol	Laxative	Constipation prevention and relief
Mucinex	Guaifenesin	Expectorant	Thin nasal mucus, decrease cough, decrease sensation of post-nasal drainage
NasalCrom	Cromolyn sodium	Nasal allergies	Asthma, allergic conjunctivitis
Robitussin DM	Guaifenesin dextromethorphan	Cough relief	
Sudafed	Pseudoephedrine	Nasal decongestant	Chest decongestant, mental alertness, energy boost
Visine	Tetrahydrozoline	Relieves red eyes	Eye allergies, minor eye irritation
Zaditor	Ketotifen	Allergic eyes	

BRONCHIAL TUBES and LUNGS			
Caffeine	Caffeine	Mental alertness	Bronchodilator, opens lungs
NasalCrom	Cromolyn sodium	Nasal allergies	Controller medication for asthma, when inhaled deeply
Primatene Mist	Epinephrine	Bronchodilator, for immediate relief	Bee sting allergy, anaphylaxis
Primatene Tablets	Ephedrine, guaifenesin	Bronchodilator, for temporary relief of mild asthma	Decongestant for bronchitis

HEART and CIRCULATION			
Aqua-Ban	Panabrom	PMS	Diuretic
Aspirin	Acetylsalicylic acid	Pain, fever	Blood thinner
Caffeine		Stimulant	To raise slow heart rate (questionably effective)
L-Arginine		Increases exercise tolerance in patients with *stable* angina	
Sudafed	Pseudoephedrine	Decongestant	To raise slow heart rate (questionably effective)

STOMACH, DIGESTION, and INTESTINES			
Alli	Orlistat	Fat malabsorption to promote weight loss	Constipation
Beano	Alpha-galacto-sidase enzyme	Prevents gas symptoms from beans	May also help prevent gas from broccoli, onions, other foods

Bonine	Meclizine, Dramamine	Nausea, vomiting	Motion sickness, anxiety, insomnia, dizziness, vertigo
Colace	Docusate, Surfak	Stool softener laxative	
Gas-Ex	Simethicone	Gas relief	Burping, belching, flatus, bloating, abdominal pressure
Gentian Violet	Purple dye	Antifungal	Thrush, yeast, vaginal yeast
Imodium	Loperamide	Diarrhea	Intestinal cramps, irritable bowel syndrome
Maalox, or Mylanta, or Rolaids	Aluminum and magnesium hydroxide (or calcium)	Heartburn	Abdominal discomfort, acid stomach Calcium formulation good for osteoporosis treatment or prevention
Milk of Magnesia	Magnesium hydroxide	Constipation	
Pepcid	Famotidine	Heartburn	Acid stomach, gastric or duodenal ulcer, hives
Pepto-Bismol Kaopectate	Bismuth subsalicylate	Upset stomach, indigestion, heartburn, diarrhea, nausea	Traveler's diarrhea
Prevacid	Lansoprazole	Heartburn	Acid stomach, duodenal ulcer, gastric ulcer, GERD
Prilosec	Omeprazole	Heartburn	Acid stomach, duodenal ulcer, gastric ulcer, GERD
Tagamet	Cimetidine	Heartburn	Acid stomach, gastric or duodenal ulcer, GERD, hives
Tums	Calcium carbonate	Heartburn	Calcium supplement to prevent or treat osteoporosis
Zantac	Ranitidine	Heartburn	Acid stomach, gastric or duodenal ulcer, GERD, hives

URINARY			
Azo Standard	Phenazopyridine	Short-term urinary pain relief	Bladder pain, passing kidney stones
Saw palmetto	Saw palmetto	Prevent further prostatic growth	

GENITAL and REPRODUCTIVE			
Aqua-Ban	Panabrom	PMS symptoms, bloating	Diuretic, swelling
Black cohosh		Menopausal symptoms	
Condoms		Contraception	STD prevention
Gynelotrimin	Clotrimazole	Yeast infection	Athlete's foot, ringworm, yeast diaper rash, jock itch
Midol		PMS symptoms	
Monistat	Miconazole	Yeast infection	Athlete's foot, ringworm, yeast diaper rash, jock itch
Saw palmetto		Prevent further prostatic growth	

ENDOCRINE and ELECTROLYTES			
Iodized salt		Goiter prevention Hypothyroidism prevention	
Desiccated thyroid		Treatment of hypothyroidism	

Potassium chloride		Potassium replacement	Substitute for prescription potassium supplements
Potassium iodide		Prevention of thyroid cancer after I-131 exposure	

OTHER

Condoms		Contraception	STD prevention
Urine HCG	Pregnancy test	Diagnose pregnancy	
Ovulation kit	LH	Predict ovulation	
MultiStix 10 SG	Urine test strips	Identify infection	Check for ketones and diabetes

INDEX

1

2

A

B

C

D

E

F

G

H

I

J

K

L

M

N

O

P

Q

R

S

T

U

V

W

X

Y

Z

www.ingramcontent.com/pod-product-compliance
Lightning Source LLC
LaVergne TN
LVHW082013200926
848481LV00010B/2855
* 9 7 8 0 9 8 2 5 0 8 1 2 1 *